ADVANCES IN
PHARMACOLOGY AND THERAPEUTICS II

Volume 5

TOXICOLOGY AND EXPERIMENTAL MODELS

ADVANCES IN PHARMACOLOGY AND THERAPEUTICS II

Proceedings of the 8th International Congress of Pharmacology, Tokyo, 1981

Editors: H.YOSHIDA, Y. HAGIHARA, S. EBASHI, Japan

Volume 1   CNS PHARMACOLOGY - NEUROPEPTIDES
Volume 2   NEUROTRANSMITTERS - RECEPTORS
Volume 3   CARDIO-RENAL & CELL PHARMACOLOGY
Volume 4   BIOCHEMICAL-IMMUNOLOGICAL PHARMACOLOGY
Volume 5   TOXICOLOGY & EXPERIMENTAL MODELS
Volume 6   CLINICAL PHARMACOLOGY - TEACHING IN PHARMACOLOGY

(Each Volume is available separately)

SATELLITE SYMPOSIA OF THE 8TH INTERNATIONAL CONGRESS OF PHARMACOLOGY PUBLISHED BY PERGAMON PRESS:

DHAWAN: Current Status of Centrally Acting Peptides

FUJII, CHANNING & MARTINI: Non-steroidal Regulators in Reproductive Biology & Medicine

IZUMI & OKA: Synthesis, Storage & Secretion of Adrenal Catecholamines: Dynamic Integration of Functions

KOHSAKA, SHOHMORI, TSUKADA & WOODRUFF: Advances in Dopamine Research

LANGER, TAKAHASHI, SEGAWA & BRILEY: New Vistas in Depression

LECHAT, THESLEFF & BOWMAN: Effects of Aminopyridines & Similarly Acting Drugs on Nerves, Muscles & Synapses

MARUYAMA: Microwave Fixation Symposium

NAMBA & KAIYA: Psychobiology of Schizophrenia (in Memory of C. & O. Vogt & M. Hayashi)

TAKAHASHI & HALBERG: Toward Chronopharmacology

UVNAS & TASAKA: Advances in Histamine Research

Send to your nearest Pergamon office for further details

ADVANCES IN PHARMACOLOGY AND THERAPEUTICS II

Proceedings of the 8th International Congress
of Pharmacology, Tokyo 1981

Volume 5
TOXICOLOGY AND EXPERIMENTAL MODELS

Editors

H. YOSHIDA
Y. HAGIHARA
S. EBASHI
Japan

RM300
I49
1981
Vol. 5

PERGAMON PRESS

OXFORD · NEW YORK · TORONTO · SYDNEY · PARIS · FRANKFURT

U.K.   Pergamon Press Ltd., Headington Hill Hall,
                        Oxford OX3 0BW, England

U.S.A.   Pergamon Press Inc., Maxwell House, Fairview Park,
                        Elmsford, New York 10523, U.S.A.

CANADA   Pergamon Press Canada Ltd., Suite 104,
                        150 Consumers Road, Willowdale, Ontario M2J 1P9,
                        Canada

AUSTRALIA   Pergamon Press (Aust.) Pty. Ltd., P.O. Box 544,
                        Potts Point, N.S.W. 2011, Australia

FRANCE   Pergamon Press SARL, 24 rue des Ecoles,
                        75240 Paris, Cedex 05, France

FEDERAL REPUBLIC   Pergamon Press GmbH, 6242 Kronberg-Taunus,
OF GERMANY   Hammerweg 6, Federal Republic of Germany

First edition 1982

British Library Cataloguing in Publication Data
International Congress of Pharmacology
(8th: 1981: Tokyo)
Advances in pharmacology & therapeutics II.
Vol. 5: Toxicology & experimental models
1. Pharmacology—Congresses 2. Therapeutics
—Congresses
I. Title II. Yoshida, H. III. Hagihara, Y.
IV. Ebashi, S.
615   RM21
ISBN 0-08-028025-0

*In order to make this volume available as economically
and as rapidly as possible the authors' typescripts have
been reproduced in their original forms. This method unfortunately has its typographical limitations but it is
hoped that they in no way distract the reader.*

Printed in Great Britain by A. Wheaton & Co. Ltd., Exeter

Contents

Heme Synthesis and Degradation: Its Role in Predicting Drug Toxicity

Delayed Toxic Effects of Pre- and Perinatal Drug Exposure

Alcohol Intoxication and Withdrawal

Models of Experimental Peptic Ulcers and Therapeutic Agents

Contents

Models and Quality Control of Laboratory Animals

Introduction

This is the fifth volume of a six-volume compilation of the scientific papers of invited speakers of the 8th International Congress of Pharmacology. You will find the real forefront of modern pharmacology presented here in concise form denoting that the 'Era of Pharmacology' has come.

In addition to the invited speakers, more than 2,000 submitted papers were given. It was a noteworthy event that most of these papers, about 1,900, were presented in poster form. We are now convinced that poster presentation is the best means to overcome the language barrier at international meetings. It was impressive to see pharmacologists from nations all over the world enthusiastically discussing their results before orderly lined panels in a brightly lighted hall. We regret that we do not have a means of communicating such a stimulating atmosphere to the readers.

Taking this opportunity, we would like to express our heartfelt thanks to all members of the International Advisory Board and the Executive Committee of IUPHAR for their invaluable suggestions concerning the scientific program. Our sincere thanks are also due to the staff members of Pergamon Press for their unselfish cooperation.

Hiroshi YOSHIDA
Yashiro HAGIHARA
Setsuro EBASHI

SYMPOSIUM

The Rational Interpretation of Species and Strain Differences in Toxicity for the Prediction of Risk to Man

Chairmen: D. S. Davies, H. Frohberg

The Rational Interpretation of Species and Strain Differences for the Prediction of Risk to Man Introduction

D. S. Davies

Department of Clinical Pharmacology, Royal Postgraduate Medical School, London, UK

INTRODUCTION

It is fashionable in reviewing the value of animal toxicology data for the prediction of risk to man to high-light the limitations. However the original approach of the toxicologist was very successful, i.e. the identification of drugs or chemicals which directly caused lesions to major organs.

Zbinden (1981) has stated that in toxicity testing the majority of results are negative suggesting that for most drugs, within reasonable dose limits, deleterious effects are uncommon. This is a realistic prediction of the situation in human therapy where toxic reactions are the exception. Thus toxicity testing usually succeeds in predicting the conditions under which new drugs can be safely administered to man.

However there are failures to predict from animal tests toxic reactions in man. Lesions which are biochemical rather than morphological in nature such as lactic acidosis induced by phenformin may be more difficult to detect in animals. Hypersensitivity reactions seen in man rarely have suitable animal models. In addition it is difficult to predict from studies in animals the likely risk to man of drugs which are toxic through the formation of chemically reactive metabolites. In the latter case it would, at first sight, appear that species differences in toxicity should be of value in predicting human risk. However the species "most like man" will vary with the drug being tested.

Valuable complementary information may be obtained by comparing the capacity of human and animal cells or subcellular organelles to generate toxic metabolites. However the limitations of this approach, particularly when using subcellular preparations devoid of many of the cell's defense mechanisms, must always be borne in mind. The cytochrome P-450 enzyme system catalyses the formation of a large number of toxic metabolites (Davies, 1981). It is now established that there are multiple forms of the cytochrome with differing substrate specificities which further complicates the prediction of human risk from studies in animals.

3

In general human liver microsomes oxidise drugs more slowly than those from rat liver (Table 1).

Table 1   Drug Oxidation by Human or Rat Liver Microsomes

Substrate	Rat Vm (pmoles/mg/min)	Human Vm (pmoles/mg/min)
Ethylmorphine	8500 ± 400	3100 ± 250
Antipyrine		
3-hydroxylase	3540 ± 290	450 ± 100
4-hydroxylase	1630 ± 120	460 ± 50
N-demethylase	840 ± 80	310 ± 130
Ethoxycoumarin	3800 ± 120	770 ± 70

However this is not always true. For example the O-dealkylation of phenacetin (Boobis et al, 1981a) proceeds at similar rates with human and rat liver (Vmax 1.7 and 1.5 nmol/mg/min respectively) whilst the N-hydroxylation of 2-acetylaminofluorene is three times as rapid with human liver microsomes (Boobis et al, 1981b).

There is considerable interspecies variation in the toxicity of paracetamol, a drug which causes severe liver injury through cytochrome P-450 catalysed formation of a toxic metabolite (Mitchell et al, 1973). In the mouse a dose of 500 mg/kg causes liver necrosis in 76% of animals whilst in rats doses of 1500 mg/kg are associated with a very low incidence of toxicity. It has been shown (Mitchell et al, 1974) that the activation of paracetamol to the benzoquinoneimine intermediate is more rapid with mouse than rat liver (Table 2) which is in accord with the species difference in toxicity. Which species is appropriate for man? Paracetamol in a dose of 200 mg/kg

Table 2   Cytochrome P-450 mediated activation of paracetamol
           (acetaminophen) by liver microsomes

Species	Paracetamol Activation[+]
Mouse	420
Rat	5

[+]Covalent binding of paracetamol to microsomes expressed as
Vm (nmol/mg/min)/Km (mM)

commonly causes liver lesions in man suggesting a sensitivity somewhat greater than the mouse. The limited data on the microsomal activation of paracetamol by human liver (von Bahr et al, 1980) suggests that the rate of formation of the benzoquinoneimine may be similar to the mouse. It remains to be established that this alone explains man's sensitivity to paracetamol-induced liver lesions.

Interindividual differences in rates of drug oxidation in vivo in man are commonly encountered. Evidence that this is largely due to differences in enzyme activity is now being accumulated. Studies in this Department have demonstrated wide ranges of activity for a number of substrates including antipyrine, phenacetin, 2-acetylaminofluorene and debrisoquine (Table 3).

Table 3. Inter-individual Variation in Drug Oxidation by Human Liver Microsomes

Substrate	Vm (pmoles/mg/min)		
∧HH	5	-	68
Ethylmorphine	2000	-	8800
Debrisoquine	0	-	157
Antipyrine			
3-hydroxylase	190	-	800
4-hydroxylase	130	-	560
N-demethylase	80	-	690
Phenacetin			
High affinity	0	-	350
Low affinity	347	-	2290
Ethoxycoumarin			
High affinity	22	-	209
Low affinity	154	-	1239
2-AAF			
1-hydroxylase	2	-	11
3-hydroxylase	70	-	418
5-hydroxylase	7	-	97
7-hydroxylase	178	-	754
9-hydroxylase	28	-	112
N-hydroxylase	35	-	263

A genetic polymorphism for the in vivo oxidation of the last drug has been established (Mahgoub et al, 1977). We have recently shown (Davies et al, 1981) that liver from a patient previously phenotyped in vivo as a poor oxidiser of debrisoquine had no measurable debrisoquine 4-hydroxylase activity in vitro (Table 4). This liver had a normal capacity to oxidise antipyrine (Table 5). These data suggest that a single form of cytochrome P-450 may be absent or altered in a small sub-population of people and this

Table 4. In vivo and in vitro formation of 4-hydroxydebrisoquine

Patient number	Metabolic ratio	Phenotype	Hepatic[*] cytochrome P-450 content	Microsomal[**] oxidation
02019	1.3	EM	360	49.6
02035	0.8	EM	380	25.7
02037	1.1	EM	270	39.3
02047	4.5	EM	150	29.9
02031	48	PM	410	0

Ratio of debrisoquine/4-hydroxydebrisoquine in 4 h urine sample following single oral dose of 10 mg debrisoquine

[*] Content expressed as pmol cytochrome P-450 mg^{-1} protein

[**] Expressed as pmol 4-hydroxydebrisoquine formed mg^{-1} protein min^{-1} of incubation

Table 5.   In vitro oxidation of antipyrine (AP) by human liver microsomes

| | AP Metabolite Formation (pmo mg^{-1}min^{-1}) | | |
Patient number	3-Hydroxymethyl AP	4-Hydroxy AP	Norphenazone
Mean (n = 9)			
non-phenotyped	370 (170-560)[*]	390 (130-620)	170 (110-350)
02035 (EM)	200	500	360
02031 (PM)	270	330	200

[*]Values in parenthesis show range of activity

may have toxicological implications. For example failure to oxidise a drug along the usual non-toxic pathway may allow the formation of toxic metabolites. This may explain the observation of Shahidi (1968) that two Swiss females developed severe methaemoglobinaemia following ingestion of phenacetin. The normal O-dealkylation of phenacetin was deficient in the two subjects and as a consequence they formed more of the toxic 2-hydroxy-p-phenetidin. It is now known from studies in vivo and in vitro (Davies et al, 1981) that poor oxidisers of debrisoquine have a reduced capacity to O-dealkylate phenacetin. Thus phenotyping of subjects for ability to oxidise probe drugs such as debrisoquine may be of value in elucidating toxic reactions which occur in a sub-group of patients.

In conclusion species differences in toxicity may be of value in predicting the likely risk to man. It is suggested that comparison of metabolism in vitro by human and animal tissues may provide complimentary data which improve the prediction.

REFERENCES

von Bahr, C., Groth, C-G, Jansson, H., Lundgren, G., Lind, M. and
    Glauman, H. (1980). Clin. Pharmacol. Ther. 27, 711-725
Boobis, A.R., Brodie, M.J., McManus, M.E., Staiano, N., Thorgeirsson, S.S.
    and Davies, D.S. (in press) In: Second International Symposium on
    Biological Reactive Intermediates (R. Snyder, ed). Plenum Publishing
    Corp. N.Y.
Boobis, A.R., Kahn, G.C., Whyte, C., Brodie, M.J. and Davies, D.S. (1981a)
    (in press) Biochem. Pharmacol.
Davies, D.S. (1981) in: Drug Reaction and the Liver (Ed: M Davis,
    L M Tredger & R Williams). pp. 12-18. Pitman Medical, London, UK.
Davies, D.S., Kahn, G.C., Murray, S., Brodie, M.J. and Boobis, A.R. (1981)
    Br. J. clin. Pharmacol. 11, 89-91.
Mahgoub, A., Idle, J.R., Dring, L.G., Lancaster, R. and Smith, R.L. (1977).
    Lancet ii, 584-586.
Mitchell, J.R., Jollow, D.J., Potter, W.Z., Davis, D.C., Gillette, J.R.
    and Brodie, B.B. (1973) J. Pharmacol. Exp. Ther. 187, 185-194.
Mitchell, J.R., Thorgeirsson, S.S., Potter, W.Z., Jollow, D.J. and
    Keiser, H. (1974). Clin. Pharmacol. Ther. 16, 676-687.
Shahidi, N.T. (1968). Annals. N.Y. Acad. Sci. 151, 822-832.
Zbinden, G. (1981) In: Organ-Directed Toxicity: Chemical Indices and
    Mechanisms (Ed: S S Brown & D S Davies). pp. 3-10. Pergamon Press,
    Oxford, UK.

The Potential Value of Immunopathology in Toxicity Studies

E. D. Wachsmuth

Research Department, Pharmaceuticals Division CIBA-GEIGY
Limited, CH-4002 Basle, Switzerland

ABSTRACT

In order to determine immunosuppressive or stimulatory activity of test compounds, a two step procedure appears to be the most sensible approach. Any subacute or chronic toxicity study should be supplemented by a quantitative evaluation of the serum γ-globulin concentration, the absolute counts of blood lymphocytes and the weights of representative lymphatic organs (e.g. thymus and secondary lymph nodes and spleen in rats) accompanied by a standardized histology. It is suggested to determine in addition immunoglobulin (IgG and IgM) and complement (mainly C_3) levels in serum or plasma and in particular cases immune complexes in kidney. If changes are observed, the reason for their occurrence has to be elucidated, possibly by conducting, special, simple tests, i.e. preferentially in vivo experiments.

KEYWORDS

Immunology; Toxicology; Drug Reactions; Thymus; Spleen; Dog; Rat.

PRESENT POSITION

In recent years, the medical profession has become aware of the involvement of the immune system in many diseases. As a result, there has been a growing interest in immunological aspects of pharmacology and toxicology. Moreover, in view of the increasing number of environmental chemicals and pharmacologically highly active drugs, the interest in immunological desired effects and side-reactions has increased (e.g. Seinen and Penninks, 1979; Sterzl, 1980; Ovtcharov and others, 1980; Dean and others, 1981).

In simple terms, the immune status of an individual depends on the relative number and activity of different classes of cells. Disturbance of this status can lead to depression (or suppression) or activation as a consequence of the direct toxic action of a test compound on the afferent limb of the immune system. Depression might impart an increased risk of infection and possibly an enhanced susceptibility towards cancer whereas activation might lead to a greater incidence of autoimmunity. On the other hand, allergies or hypersensitivities are consequences of the immunizing process towards the test-compound and reflect the activity of the effector pathway. Testing for the latter in toxicology has become routine in recent years and schedules for detecting adverse drug reactions have been developed (e.g. Maurer and others, 1978). One major concern today is the detection of changes in the afferent limb, since they might escape detection when investigating only the effector pathway. These changes are not only apparent in functional changes, but are also reflected at the morphological level in lymphatic organs at the cellular level (i.e. lymphocytes, basophilic and eosinophilic granulocytes and monocytes) and in the plasma protein levels (i.e. immunoglobulins, complement-components and lymphokines).

TABLE 1   Immunotoxicological Screening (Dean and others, 1979)

Delayed hypersensitivity to keyhole limpet haemocyanin;
    bovine gamma globulin and tetanus toxoid
Lymphocyte proliferation to: T and B-cell mitogens;
    mixed lymphocyte culture
IgG levels
Antibody titre and plaque assay: T-dependent antigen
Tumour challenge
Clearance by the reticulo-endothelial system
Delayed hypersensitivity to T-independent antigen
Lymphocyte proliferation in response to antigen
Helper cell function
Macrophage function
In vitro production of antibody
Specific antibody titre to T-independent antigen
Cytotoxicity
Bacterial challenge
Virus challenge
Ouchterlony gel diffusion
Specific antibody titration
Reversed passive Arthus reaction
Immediate cutaneous hypersensitivity
Delayed-type cutaneous hypersensitivity

POSSIBLE STRATEGIES

Several proposals have been put forward for testing the functioning of the immune system (Vos, 1977; Speirs and Speirs, 1979; Dean and others, 1979; Bradley and Morahan, 1980). One of the most elaborate is shown in Table 1 and reflects the enormous complexity of the immune system. The suggested tests, therefore, are so many and diverse that it is difficult to carry them all out, yet alone test their validity. The results obtained with this approach for three compounds in mice serve as examples (Dean and others, 1981, Table 2). In all cases, the thymus weight decreases concomitantly with a decrease in T-cell dependent functions and the resistance to infection decreases. Therefore, initially, it might be much easier to use thymus weights or resistance to infection as indicators of immunotoxicity, and avoid other more complex tests.

Bradley and Morahan (1980) have suggested that the host resistance in mice or rats in defined infection models can be determined along these lines using streptococcus pneumoniae for the B-cell system, Listeria monocytogenes for the T-cell system and macrophages and herpes simplex virus for both the B-cell and the T-cell system. However, little experience has been accumulated until now as to how valid and predictive such models would be. Nevertheless, whenever a complex situation has to be analysed, an in vivo test appears to be superior to any in vitro system.

In addition to the complexity of the immune system, the testing of drugs for adverse reactions is further complicated by variable responses of species, age, sex and environmental conditions. This suggests that detailed schedules of testing are not suitable for obtaining the initial information about possible disturbances of the immune system. They might, however, be useful for furthering our knowledge of a particular side effect, if the applicability and validity of the mentioned tests has been demonstrated not only in mice but also in other animal species, particularly in rats and dogs, the standard species used in toxicity studies.

TABLE 2   Assessment of Immunotoxicity in Mice*

Parameter	Tetrachloridi-benzo-p-dioxin	Diethylstilbestrol	Benzo(a)pyrene
Dose (mg/kg)	0.001; 0.005	0.2; 2; 8	50; 200; 400
Thymus weight	↓	↓	↓
Femur marrow cellularity	↓	↓	↑
Bone marrow-progenitors: a) pluripotent (CFU-Spleen) b) Macrophage-granulocyte (CFU-C)	↓ 0	↓ ↓	↓ ↓
IgM a) anti-SRBC PFC b) anti-LPS PFC	ND ND	↓ ↓	↓ ↓
Lymphoproliferative response in vitro PHA (T-cells) ConA (T-cells) LPS (B-cells)	↓ ↓ ↓	↓ ↓ ↓	↓ ↓ ↓
Host resistance (survival) PYB6 Tumour Listeria monocytogenes Endotoxin	↓ ↓ ND	↓ ↓ ↓	(↓) (↓) (↓)

* According to J.H. Dean and others, (1981);
   Much of this data agrees with those reported earlier by Voss and others 1979.

TOXICITY STUDIES IN RATS AND DOGS

Rats and dogs are the main species used for determining possible adverse toxic effects in subchronic and chronic trials of a drug. Let us consider an immuno-suppressive drug as an example: A particular corticosteroid was given daily orally to dogs (one year old) and rats (6 weeks old). The level of γ-globulin (consisting mainly of immunoglobulins) was calculated from the serum protein concentration and an electrophoretic serum analysis. The γ-globulin levels tend to decrease (relative to controls) with dose and time during the course of the steroid treatment (over 3 months) in rats but not in dogs (Fig. 1). The lymphocytes in the peripheral blood tend to decrease similarly in rats and to a lesser, but still significant extent in dogs.

It should be noted, however, that the γ-globulin increases in control rats during the first 9 weeks of this experiment. This is due to the natural maturation of their immune system. Both the γ-globulin levels and the lymphocyte counts return to normal when both animals are left for a further month without treatment indicating that the lymphatic system recovers. The dose dependency of the corticosteroid treatment is reflected in the significant dose dependent reduction in the net weights of the thymus and spleen of rats after 3 months of treatment (Fig. 2). The same corticosteroid reduces the thymus weight in dogs, although some normal involution of the thymus takes place during this time. The weight of the spleen is unaffected. One reason for this finding in dogs might be the physiological role of the spleen in this species: it serves as a major storage organ for erythrocytes and thus the organ weight will represent the leucocyte content only to a minor degree. The involvement of the immune system in the treated dogs is indicated by the increased abnormal number of parasites in their lungs without any significant signs of an inflammatory reaction. Dogs kept for an additional month without treatment suffer severely from extensive inflammation in their lungs because of the restoration of their immunological resistance after the immunosuppressive drug has been withdrawn.

The question then arises as to whether the weight of a lymphatic organ reflects its content of leucocytes and lymphocytes. To answer it, a short-term experiment was carried out on 9-week-old rats with the same corticosteroid as previously. Whereas the erythrocyte counts in the blood increase with increasing doses, they decrease in the spleen concomitantly with the falling weight of this organ (Fig. 3, left). The leucocyte numbers, on the other hand, decrease in blood, spleen and thymus, the decrease being due to the fall in lymphocyte counts (Fig. 3, right). The organ weights and the leucocyte counts in the organs correlate well (Fig. 4; thymus, r = 0.982, p < 0.001; spleen r = 0.952, p < 0.001). Moreover, the leucocyte counts in blood also correlate well with the leucocyte number in the two organs (Fig. 4; thymus r = 0.843, p < 0.001; spleen r = 0.838, p < 0.001). Therefore, the organ weights of rats are a good measure of the lymphocyte numbers in the organs. Since determinations of weight are more easily performed than the counting of cells and the quantification of spleen and thymus histology, they are a more reliable quantitative measure of a dose dependent adverse reaction. In addition, results obtained recently with a number of test compounds indicate that determination of the weight of secondary, and easily obtained lymph nodes (e.g. the popliteal and axillary lymph nodes) have a good predictive value for determining effects on the immune system.

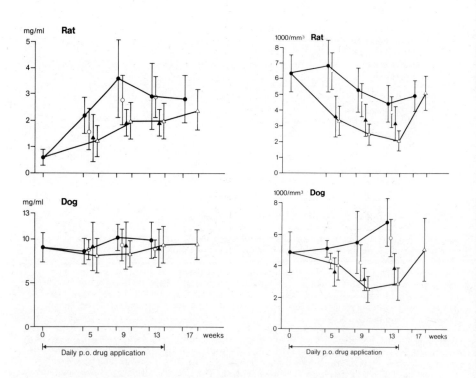

Fig. 1.   Serum γ-globulin concentration (left side) and blood lymphocyte counts (right side) (x̄±s) of rats and dogs treated daily for 3 months with a corticosteroid and, in addition, left for one month without treatment. Daily doses: 0 μg/kg (●), 10 μg/kg (○), 30 μg/kg (▲), 100 μg/kg (△).

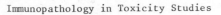

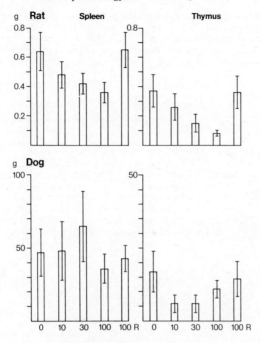

Fig. 2.   Spleen (left side) and thymus (right side) weights of rats
and dogs treated for 3 months with a corticosteroid.
Conditions as in Fig. 1; R = 1 month recovery group,
abscissa gives the daily dose in μg/kg.

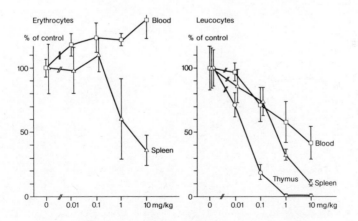

Fig. 3.   Dose response to a corticosteroid (as in Fig. 1) in rats
after 4 oral applications (once daily): effect on erythrocytes
(left side) and leucocytes (right side). Measurements were
done with a Coulter Counter.

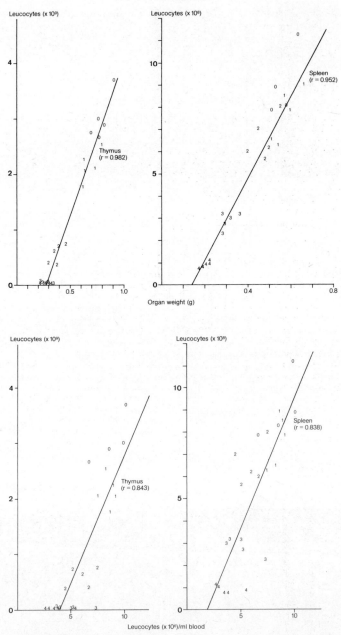

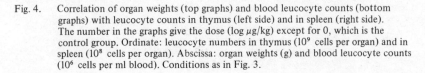

Fig. 4.   Correlation of organ weights (top graphs) and blood leucocyte counts (bottom graphs) with leucocyte counts in thymus (left side) and in spleen (right side). The number in the graphs give the dose (log μg/kg) except for 0, which is the control group. Ordinate: leucocyte numbers in thymus (10^9 cells per organ) and in spleen (10^8 cells per organ). Abscissa: organ weights (g) and blood leucocyte counts (10^6 cells per ml blood). Conditions as in Fig. 3.

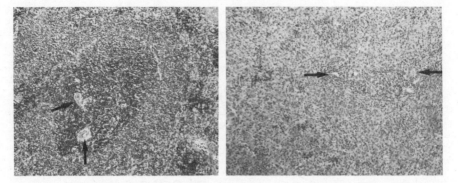

Fig. 5.   Rat spleen after 3 months treatment with a corticosteroid (conditions as in Fig. 1).
Follicle with periarteriolar sheaths. Artery (arrow), control (left side), top dose
(right side). Magnification x 72.

Changes in the morphology of lymphatic organs are another common means of determining effects on the
immune system but quantification is difficult to achieve and minor changes might escape observation.
A 20% reduction of rat spleen weight can just be picked up by histological observations (e.g. the reduction
of the periarteriolar sheaths and a decrease in the size and number of follicles), but the reduction is
significant at larger doses (Fig. 5). Differences in the spleen of treated and non-treated dogs are marginal
and only recognizable to the trained eye. If the thymus is sectioned adequately, preferably neither tangen-
tially nor transversely, but longitudinally, a semiquantitative analysis can be performed and the ratio of
medulla to cortex judged. However, the gain in information is small compared to weight determinations.
On the other hand, lymph node histology yields useful information. This is particularly true for the
secondary lymph nodes, e.g. axillary, cervical and popliteal lymph nodes (Fig. 6) but is much less so for
intestinal lymph nodes which are easily altered by other factors and thus normally show large variations.
To obtain reliable answers from histology, however, it is important to section the lymph nodes in a
standardized plane, preferably transversely through the hilus, in order to allow one to compare sections
from different animals. This is of greatest importance when only minor changes occur and the organ is
morphologically heterogenous, as illustrated in Fig. 7: the longitudinal section may represent the normal
state, a section in plane I might be interpreted as activated state, whereas in plan II an immuno-suppressed
state might be diagnosed. Standardized sections then can serve for a detailed histological diagnosis
(Cottier and coworkers, 1973).

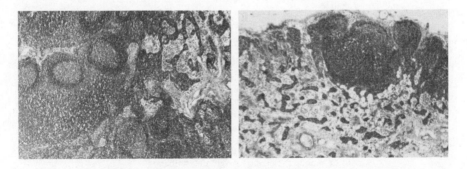

Fig. 6.   Dog cervical lymph node after 3 months treatment with a corticosteroid
(conditions as in Fig. 1). Cortex with follicles and medulla. Control (left side),
top dose (right side, missing paracortex). Magnification x 29.

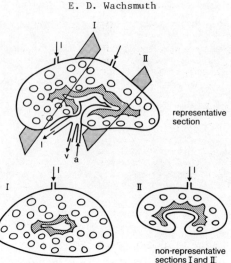

Fig. 7.   Longitudinal section through a lymph node and 2 random
           planes of sectioning. l = lymph vessels, a = artery, v = vein.

TABLE 3   Minimal requirements for detection of toxic effects related
           to the immune apparatus.

Dose dependency of an effect in any tested animals species.

1. Serum analyses
     Total serum protein
     Electrophoresis   } γ-globulin concentration
     (Immunochemical determination of immunoglobulin, total
     or classes, and complement C_3).

2. Blood cell analysis
     Total number of leucocytes } number of lymphocytes,
     Differentials   } monocytes and eosinophiles
                                   per ml blood.

3. At autopsy
     Size of lymph nodes: weight of popliteal, axillary,
                                 cervical and mesenteric lymph node,
                                 both sides (if possible).
     Size of thymus and spleen: weight determination.

4. Histo-pathology
     Spleen, lymph nodes, thymus: Reproducibility of plane
                                  of sectioning should be guaranteed.

MINIMAL REQUIREMENTS FOR IMMUNO-TOXICOLOGY

In order to obtain preliminary information about the effect of a test compound on the immune system, it appears reasonable to investigate the parameters summarized in Table 3. In addition to an adequate evaluation of the parameters investigated in most toxicity studies, it might be helpful to measure immunoglobulin and complement levels. However, it has to be kept in mind that at present only a few specific antisera for carrying out these sorts of measurements are available for dogs and rats and routine screening involving large numbers of animals have not yet been developed. If dose dependent changes with the parameters given in Table 3 do occur, one has to find out whether these changes are due to direct effects on the immune system and thus possibly have to be analyzed further with special tests as discussed by Voss (1977) and Dean and coworkers (1979), or whether they are due to indirect effects such as nutritional deficiencies, pathogenic organisms and changes in the endocrine balance. For subsequent testing it might become worthwhile following up Bradley and Morahan's (1980) suggestion for measuring resistance to infection in animal models as mentioned above.

SPECIFIC IMMUNOPATHOLOGICAL INVESTIGATIONS

In addition to the basic testing of newly developed compounds for their effects on the immune system, it might be interesting to investigate specific immunological phenomena in other species or in man with compounds of similar pharmacological action or chemical configuration, i.e. compounds with a potential immunopathological risk. For example newly developed antibiotics might be particularly antigenic or immunostimulatory. We have recently tested, therefore, a number of new antibiotics in dogs for such effects and found one, which caused a Schönlein-Henoch purpura. This is due to antigen-antibody complexes adsorbed to erythrocytes and platelets and an immune-complex glomerulonephritis, in which the complexes contained lipid-A as one antigen. In view of this finding and the absence of the antibiotic from the immune-complexes, it was thought that the antibiotic might have given rise to an unspecific immune response directed against bacterial constituents as a consequence of its action. Further development of the compound was stopped.

Hydralazine has been reported to cause a drug-induced systemic lupus erythematosus in some patients when given over a prolonged period in large doses. We investigated this phenomenon in rats, which were given the hydralazine analogue dihydralazine orally (dose range $30-300$ mg/kg) for 3 months. Their sera were analysed for anti-nuclear factor (ANF) and other auto-antibodies and their kidneys by means of immunofluorescence for immune-complexes. No immunopathological findings were seen in rats. Moreover, when dihydralazine (doses up to 20 mg/kg) was administered in the same way to dogs for 6 months, neither ANF nor anti-sheep red blood cell antibody are observed in the serum and no immune-complexes found in the kidney. However a dose dependent but slight and reversible increase in immunoglobulin levels (but not complement-C_3 levels) is found. This rise in immunoglobulin is accompanied by a rise in glomerular immunoglobulin (but not complement-C_3) levels, which also occurs after treatment with hydralazine in rats (dose range from $20-200$ mg/kg for 3 months). The missing complement argues against the formation of immune-complexes but points to increased glomerular retention of immunoglobulin when the serum concentrations are raised. Thus, dihydralazine and hydralazine do not provoke a drug-induced SLE in dogs and rats, although hydralazine might do this in certain mice strains (Ten Veen and Feltkamp, 1972). It is feasible that this difference is due to the genetic background of the test animals. Recently, it has been claimed that sex and the HLA-DR locus in this context are determinants for the risk of a drug-induced SLE occurring in man during treatment with hydralazine (Batchelor and coworkers, 1980).

Another example is the β-blocker practolol. This drug produces in man a relatively high incidence of psoriatic rashes, cerato-conjunctivitis and sclerosing peritonitis and pleuritis (Felix and coworkers, 1974), which lead eventually to the drug being withdrawn from the market. However, up to date, it has not been possible to demonstrate these phenomena in any of many animal species investigated in several laboratories. A successful demonstration would have given us the model of a positive control for the testing of the safety of other newly developed β-blockers. Thus one must rely on careful clinical observations in man and an awareness of the practolol syndrome, for assessing any immunopathological adverse reactions of such drugs in man.

CONCLUSION

The rational of a toxicological approach for detecting the effects of any drug on the immune system, requires two steps. In the initial phase, simple and thus manageable, reliable and reproducible tests should be carried out. Slightly extended and careful analyses of routine toxicity studies in rats and dogs have already been carried out in many laboratories. These procedures appear to be sufficient if the investigators are aware of the problems involved. The analyses should consist of a careful quantitative and dose-related evaluation of the serum γ-globulin fractions, absolute lymphocyte numbers, weights and standardized histology of representative lymphatic organs. The aim of such studies must be to detect changes in the immune system. Should changes considered as direct effects on the immune system occur, these studies have to be supplemented with additional specific tests in order to determine the nature of the potential immunopathological risk.

Of course, it is always possible to carry out more detailed investigations for any particular drug. Apart from the sharp increases in the time, cost, and expertise required for doing this extra work, the additional data do not always help one to understand the underlying immunopathological mechanisms much further. On the contrary the more data that become available, the more difficult it often becomes to interpret the potential immunopathological phenomenon. Thus, in the early stages, simple in vivo experiments should be the main hallmark for testing because they are more informative.

REFERENCES

Batchelor, J.R., Welsh, K.I., Tinoco, R.M., Dollery, C.T., Hughes, G.R.V., Bernstein, R., Ryan, P., Naish, P.F., Aber, G.M., Bing, R.F. and Russell, G.I. (1980). Lancet 2, 1107–1109.
Bradley, S.G. and Morahan, P.S. (1980). Meeting on Organ Toxicity: Immune System (sponsored by NIEHS) Arlington, Oct. 1980.
Cottier, H., Rutk, J. and Slobin, L. (1973). J. clin. Path. 26, 317–331.
Dean, J.H., Padarathsingh, M.L. and Jerrels, T.R. (1979). Drug Chem. Toxicol. 2, 5–17.
Dean, J.H., Luster, M.I., Boorman, G.A., Chae, K., Lauer, L.D., Luebke, R.W., Lawson, L.D. and Wilson, R.E. (1981). Adv. in Immunopharmacology (J. Hadden, L. Chedid, P. Mullen, F. Spreafico eds.) Pergamon Press, Oxford, etc. pp 37–55.
Felix, R.H., Ive, F.A. and Dahl, M.G.C. (1974). Brit. Med. J. 4, 321–324.
Maurer, Th., Thomann, P., Weirich, E.G. and Hess, R. (1978). Contact Dermatitis 4, 321–333.
Ovtcharov, R., Gventcheva, G. and Michailova, S. (1980). Arch. Toxicol. Suppl. 4, 120–131.
Seinen, W. and Penninks, A. (1979). N.Y. Acad. Sci. 320, 499–517.
Speirs, R.S. and Speirs, E.E. (1979). Drug Chem. Toxicol. 2, 19–33.
Sterzl, J. (1980). Arch. Toxicol. Suppl. 4, 109–119.
Ten Veen, J.H. and Feltkamp, T.E.W. (1972). Clin. exp. Immunol. 11, 265–276.
Vos, J.G. (1977). Critical Rev. Toxicol. 5, 67–101.
Vos, J.G., van Logten, M.J., Kreeftenberg, J.G., Steerenberg, P.A. and Kruizinga, W. (1979). Drug Chem. Toxicol. 2, 61–76.

Lessons from Studies in Animals for the Evaluation of Human Risk from Teratogenic Agents

F. Beck

Department of Anatomy, The Medical School, University of Leicester,
UK

ABSTRACT

In order to achieve meaningful results a knowledge of the distribution and
fate of potentially teratogenic agents in both man and the experimental
animal model used is essential. Of equal importance is a detailed knowledge
of the stage of embryonic development at which treatment is applied and an
appreciation of the placental system which is functional at the time of
treatment. Before a working placental system involving direct exchange of
solutes between the maternal and embryonic blood streams occurs, a beating
heart must perfuse the extraembryonic membranes of the conceptus. Before
this 'haemotrophic' phase the embryo survives by the uptake and intracellular breakdown of uterine secretions and decidua in the extraembryonic
tissue — the so called stage of histiotrophic nutrition. The switch over
from one to the other mode of embryonic nutrition takes place at different
times in various species and this may lead to an altered teratogenic response.
Whole embryo culture as well as isolated embryonic organ and tissue culture
may therefore be of further help in assessing teratogenicity. It should be
remembered that pharmacologically active agents may act independently on
the mother, fetus, and fetal membranes thus considerably complicating the
in vivo picture.

KEYWORDS

Teratogenesis; animal models for teratogenesis; in vivo teratogenesis;
in vitro teratogenesis.

INTRODUCTION

Theoretically a teratogenic agent may exert its primary toxic effects on
the mother, the embryo or the extraembryonic membranes. Indeed there is no
reason why it should not act to some extent at all three sites. In a
limited presentation such as this I do not propose to dwell upon teratogenic
effects which are primarily maternal in origin since, important as they are,
they illustrate problems which in some ways are basically matters of general
toxicology. The suitability of animals for the evaluation of human risk in

this respect clearly involves basic parameters of drug excretion,
distribution and metabolism as well as the relevant physiology and biochemistry of the species concerned. It is when we begin to look at possible
primary or secondary action sites involving the embryo or extraembryonic
membranes that the reproductive principles which fundamentally distinguish
teratology from the remainder of toxicology are involved.

A basic requirement for any animal study in teratology is a thorough knowledge of development in the species concerned for there often is a remarkable variation in developmental timing between species examined in the
organogenetic period. This knowledge is required because of the well known
phenomenon of 'critical periods' whereby individual organs pass through one
or more 'critical times' with respect to their susceptibility to specific
teratogenic agents. This is illustrated in Figs. 1 and 2.

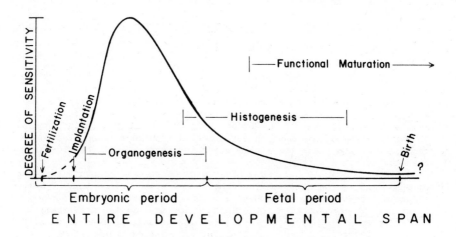

Fig. 1. A theoretical curve depicting the susceptibility
of the human embryo to teratogenesis. Organogenesis (about
18-60 days) marks the period of maximal sensitivity to
morphological defect from teratogens. After this the
incidence of anatomical defect diminishes but it is likely
that minor structural effects (often very important in
nervous system development, etc) can be generated in
certain instances until after birth. Defects generated
during the late fetal and neonatal period are more likely
to involve growth and function because these factors pre-
dominate at this time (after Wilson 1972).

Thorough documentation of the developmental stages equivalent to those of
man exist for many monkeys (especially the Macaque and baboon, Heuser &
Streeter 1941, Hendrickx and co-workers 1971), as well as for the pig
(Keibel 1897), rat (Henneberg 1937), mouse (Otis & Brent 1954), many other
rodents and the rabbit (Minot & Taylor 1905). All of these have been used
in teratogenic studies but, apart from rodents and rabbits, their cost is
great. Ideally a good experimental animal is one which is cheap, easy to
keep and breed, in which timed matings are reliable, pseudopregnancy rare
and delayed implantation unknown. Many rodents, as well as the rabbit,
belong to this category but because of their similarity in placental structure

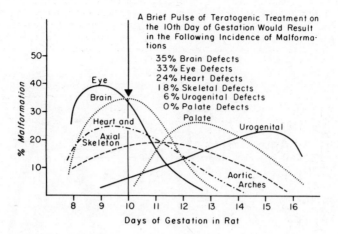

Fig. 2. A group of curves illustrating the maximal susceptibility of different organs in the rat at various stages of gestation. A simplistic approach to this concept should be viewed with caution because the organs affected represent a 'final common pathway' and the origin of their maximal susceptibility may vary with the teratogen (after Wilson 1965).

it is desirable to identify an additional species which is neither rodent nor lagomorph. The Ferret (Symposium, Teratology in press) is presently commanding some interest because, being a carnivore it has a different placentology (see below) and also a different embryonic and fetal developmental timetable and metabolism to that of rodents and lagomorphs (Gulamhusein & Beck 1981). This may make it a useful alternative species for testing when both rodents and lagomorphs are suspected of an atypical reaction due to their inverted yolk sac placenta (see below).

EMBRYONIC NUTRITION

In the early stages of embryonic development of Eutherian mammals, the embryo will be entirely dependent upon intracellular degradation of intra-uterine biopolymers for its development, a phenomenon known as histio-trophic nutrition. This is because the heart has not yet developed sufficiently to perfuse the embryonic side of the placenta. Early embryonic nutrition of the rodent embryo is typified by the rat (Fig. 3) from which it is clear that a very special system quite unlike that of man is involved. When a beating embryonic heart adequately perfuses the chorio-allantoic placenta embryonic nutrition changes from being predominantly histiotrophic to a stage when solutes can pass across the placental membrane from the maternal to the embryonic circulations. This is the period of haemo-trophic nutrition. The system is further complicated by the fact that histiotrophic nutrition may persist for a time as the principal form of placentation after the development of the embryonic heart as in the chorio vitelline placenta of the ferret (Gulamhusein and Beck 1975) and also by the fact that the histology and possibly the physiological permeability

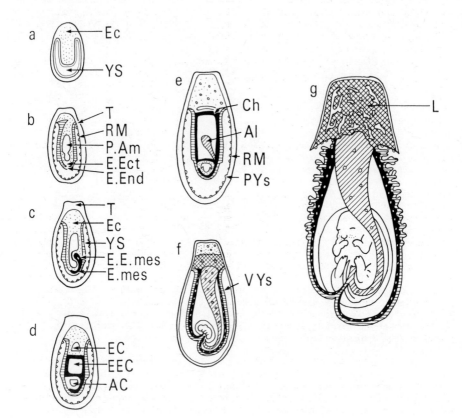

Fig. 3. Development of the extraembryonic membranes of the rat. (a) At 6½
days postfertilization. The ectoplacental cone has grown so that the inner
cell mass has become invaginated into the yolk-sac cavity. The latter is now
horseshoe shaped. (b) At 8 days; formation of the proamniotic cavity. A
proamniotic cavity has appeared in the inner cell mass extending into the
ectoplacental cone. The endoderm covering the sides of the ectoplacental
cone is called the visceral layer of the yolk-sac endoderm and in contrast
to the parietal layer that is separated from the trophoblast only by an
acellular layer known as Reichert's membrane, is highly pinocytic. The ectoplacental cone and the embryonic region at its apex are together known as the
egg cylinder. (c) At 9¼ days, gastrulation is well advanced. Mesoderm has
migrated from the embryonic area into the region of the ectoplacental cone
where ("pushing" the extraembryonic ectoderm ahead of it) it begins to sub-
divide the proamniotic cavity. A small extraembryonic coelom continuous with
the embryonic coelom has developed. (d) At 9½ days; division of the proamniotic cavity into three. The extraembryonic mesoderm with its contained
extraembryonic coelom has grown right across the proamniotic cavity, and
three cavities are apparent in the egg cylinder. They are an upper epamniotic cavity, a middle extraembryonic coelom, and a lower amniotic cavity.

(e) At 10 days; development of the allantoic bud. The embryo has begun to
form head and tail folds. The allantois, an outgrowth of the endoderm in the
tail fold covered by allantoic mesoderm, is growing into the extraembryonic
coelom. The epamniotic cavity has collapsed; its original lower wall
consists of extraembryonic ectoderm and nonvascularised mesoderm, thus forming
the chorion. (f) At 11¼ days; early chorioallantoic placenta. The allantois
has fused with the chorion, and a labyrinthine chorioallantoic hemochorial
placenta is established. The embryo has turned so that it is now convex
dorsally and has become invaginated into the extraembryonic coelom (this is
sometimes incorrectly referred to as the yolk-sac cavity). (g) At 16 days to
full term; disappearance of parietal yolk-sac and Reichert's membrane. The
parietal layer of the yolk-sac, Reichert's membrane, the adjacent trophoblast, and attenuated decidua capsularis are resorbed, and the visceral
layer of the yolk-sac is exposed to the cavity of the uterus. Ec ectoplacental cone; Ys yolk-sac cavity; T trophoblast; P. Am. proamniotic
cavity; E.Ect embryonic ectoderm; E.End, embryonic endoderm; E.mes,
embryonic mesoderm; EC epamniotic cavity; EEC extraembryonic coelom; AC,
amniotic cavity; Ch, chorion; Al allantois; R.M. Reichert's membrane;
PYs parietal yolk-sac wall; VYs, visceral yolk-sac wall; L, chorioallantoic placental labyrinth. The visceral yolk-sac endoderm is essentially
the organ responsible for histiotrophic nutrition in the rat and in all other
rodents so far examined. It's cells absorb biopolymers in solution which
have passed through the parietal yolk-sac wall (or are secreted directly
into the uterine lumen after 16½ days of pregnancy). Haemotrophic nutrition
possibly begins to function at 11½ days when the allantois has established
the beginnings of a labyrinthine haemochorial placenta.

of the chorio allantoic placenta in various Eutherian mammals differs
(Grosser 1927, Steven 1975).

IN VIVO TERATOGENESIS

Table 1 shows the somite number at which the 'switch over' from histiotrophic to haemotrophic nutrition occurs in various species and Table 2
clearly indicates the significance of this in relation to teratogenesis.

TABLE 1

Species	Onset of haemotrophic nutrition (somites)	Chorio vitelline placentation	Inverted yolk sac placentation	Chorio allantoic placenta
Rat	20 +	-	+	Haemochorial
Guinea Pig	20 +	-	+	Haemochorial
Rabbit	20 +	+	+	Haemochorial
Ferret	35	+	-	Endothelio chorial
Pig	35-50	+	-	Epithelio chorial
Man	1-5	-	-	Haemochorial
Rhesus	5 +	-	-	Haemochorial

It illustrates that a teratogen (trypan blue) which acts, at least in part,
on the histiotrophic nutritional capacity of the extraembryonic membranes
(Williams and co-workers 1976) is teratogenic at equivalent developmental

TABLE 2   *Effects of s.c. injection of trypan blue or saline into rats and ferrets*

Day of injection	No. of females treated	No. of implantations	No. (%) resorption	Average fetal wt. of survivors (gms.)	External abnormalities			No. of fetuses sectioned	No. (%) of sectioned fetuses showing external or internal anomalies	No. of fetuses stained with alizarin	No. (%) of stained fetuses showing external or internal anomalies
					No.	% of fetuses surviving to term	% of total implantations				
Rats 100 mg/kg trypan blue 8.5 days	9	83	36 (43)	3.24	17	36	20	32	11 (34)	15	7 (50)
Rats 100 mg/kg trypan blue 11.5 days	9	82	3 (4)	3.81	0	—	—	54	3 (6)¹	25	0
Rats 5 ml/kg saline 8.5 days	7	57	0	3.65	0	—	—	38	0	19	0
Rats 5 ml/kg saline 11.5 days	5	51	0	3.78	0	—	—	34	0	17	0
Ferrets 50 mg/kg trypan blue 13 days	10	65	33 (51)	3.04	12	38	18	22	11 (50)	10	3 (33)
Ferrets 50 mg/kg trypan blue 18 days	9	52	44 (85)	3.28	6	86	12	6	5 (83)	2	1 (50)
Ferrets 25 mg/kg 13 days	10	76	45 (59)	3.29	7	23	1	21	6 (29)	10	4 (40)
Ferrets 25 mg/kg 18 days	10	53	38 (72)	2.93	5	33	9	11	4 (36)	4	1 (25)
Ferrets 5 ml/kg saline 13 days	10	64	14 (22)²	3.10	1	2	2	35	1 (3)	15	0
Ferrets 5 ml/kg saline 18 days	16	117	51 (44)³	3.40	0	—	—	46	0	20	0

All hydronephrosis with enlarged ureter.
Including one mother with total resorption of the litter.
Including six mothers with total resorption of the litter.

stages (Table 3) in both rat and ferret when the embryos of both species depend upon histiotroph. At a later stage when the ferret is still using histiotroph to maintain the embryo while the rat has already switched to haemotrophic nutrition, it is clear that trypan blue has ceased to be teratogenic in the rat but that its action persists in the ferret. The method

TABLE 3 Equivalent Stages in the Development of the Rat and Ferret

Rat	Ferret	Stage	
$6\frac{1}{2}$–$7\frac{1}{2}$ days	11–12 days	1	Before the full establishment of gastrulation
$8\frac{1}{2}$ days	13 days	2	Primitive streak established
$9\frac{1}{2}$ days	14–15 days	3	Head process. Paraxial mesoderm differentiating to form earliest somites
$10\frac{1}{2}$ days	16–17 days	4	Between 9 and 20+ somites. Neural folds fused at diencephalic–mesencephalic junction in earliest specimens; anterior neuropore closed in a few of the more mature examples
$12\frac{1}{2}$ days	19 days	5	Ferret embryos on average a little more advanced than rat embryos. 33–39 somites. Paddleshaped enlargement of the distal part of forelimb bud beginning to develop. Maxillary process has met lateral nasal process.
$13\frac{1}{2}$ days	22 days	6	Paddleshaped distal part of forelimb well formed. Tubercles on contiguous sides of mandibular and hyoid arches. 40–47 somites

used for assessing resorption and congenital malformation in this experiment is that described by Wilson (1965) and modified by Barrow & Taylor (1969). Ferret offspring may be examined at 35 days of a 42 day gestation period when both the freehand razor blade sections and the alizarin stained skeletons obtained are quite similar in both rat and ferret (Beck 1977). Wilson's (1965) method has become standard for examining the fetus in many laboratories; after sacrifice, uterine resorption sites are noted on a preprepared examination sheet often after specific staining to localise early resorptions(Kopf and others,1964).Subsequently fetuses are fixed in Bouin's fluid and two out of every three are razor sectioned by hand at about 1mm intervals (Fig. 4). Every third survivor is eviscerated and stained with alizarin in order to examine the skeleton (Fig. 5). Many laboratories carry out microdissection rather than razor section examination (Sterz 1977) and the more expensive the animal in question the more widely this is practised (Wilson and co-workers 1970). Examination after alizarin staining on the other hand yields maximal information about bony structures and is thus widely practised even in monkeys. More thought is perhaps required concerning the best way to examine aborted human material (spontaneous or elective). Often there is considerable maceration or traumatic destruction of such material resulting from the circumstances of the abortion but, surprisingly, a considerable amount of information is often still available. The reader is referred to the Eurocat guide to a service in Fetal and Perinatal Pathology (Emery & Weatherall 1981) which suggests varying

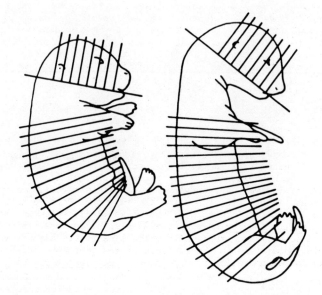

Fig. 4. Diagram of 21 day rat and 35 day
ferret embryos to show sites of freehand
razor sections which yield most information.

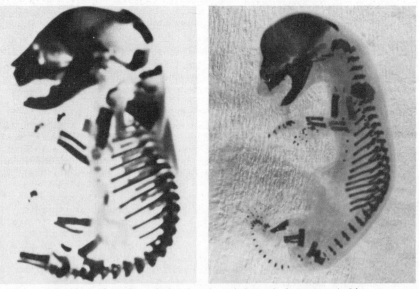

Fig. 5. Alizarin stained rat and ferret fetuses at 21
and 35 days respectively.

procedures depending upon the age of the specimen concerned. To some extent
it is against this background that a fuller meaning of the relevance of
animal experiments and in particular the antenatal diagnosis of congenital
defect should be viewed.

Before turning to more sophisticated in vitro experiments and their value in
the evaluation of potential teratogens, a word may be said about the feas-
ability of complete elimination of human defect; an oft quoted objective
even among the most eminent paediatricians. Clearly this is a highly unlikely - even perhaps undesirable - objective. It has been postulated that
the majority of congenital defects are both polygenic and multifactorial.
Variety is the stuff of evolution both biological and social, and inevitably
the distribution of phenotypes will be such that certain combinations will be
classified as defective. This is particularly clear where a 'threshold'
exists beyond which frank malformation occurs such as in cleft palate (Carter
1969) but on the other side of which stigmata which relate to a malformation
(such as cleft lip) may be recognised by careful observation (Fraser &
Pashayan 1970). The aim of the clinician must therefore be to reduce the
incidence of frank malformation without essentially affecting the extent of
the genetic pool. In vivo animal studies will be designed to inform the
experimental scientist whether, within the constraints already referred to,
environmental conditions in the presence of the substance being tested are
essentially normal and allow reproduction to proceed at the same level as in
controls.

IN VITRO TERATOGENESIS

Various in vitro systems allow us to tease out whether a putative teratogenic
agent has a direct action on the conceptus and in some cases even to begin
to define the site of such action. New (1978) has perfected a method whereby
rat embryos may be grown inside the inverted yolk sac in vitro on a medium
of specially prepared rat serum. Under such conditions the embryo grows and
differentiates at normal rates between the primitive streak and the 25-30
somite stages; its extraembryonic membranes break down the proteins of its
histiotroph into amino acids and build them up again on the embryonic side
into protein at the same rate as in vivo (Freeman and co-workers in press,
Gupta and co-workers (1980), Gupta & Beck in press) so that it may reason-
ably be inferred that the in vitro system is physiologically sound. Glucose
is the only source of energy and only certain vitamins are required
(Cockcroft 1979). Since New's pioneer experiments, the growth of mouse
embryos has also been achieved in vitro at the same level of efficiency
(Sadler 1979). In an elegant experiment (Fantel and co-workers 1979) it was
shown that cyclophosphamide was not teratogenic in such systems without the
prior addition of the S9 fraction of activated rat liver homogenates and a
source of energy. This drug therefore needs processing by maternal liver
before the production of teratogenic metabolites. In direct contrast,
McGarrity and co-workers (in press) have shown that sodium salicylate has
similar morphological effects if it is added to the culture serum or if rat
embryos are grown in sera derived from mothers which have partially metabolised the drug but whose serum still contains levels of undegraded
salicylate similar to those added in the first experiment. This together
with the observation that the metabolites in rat are without effect in vivo
indicates a direct action of the drug on the conceptus. The whole embryo
culture model is capable of yielding still further information, for both in
the case of trypan blue (Williams and co-workers 1976) and leupeptin (Lowy
1981) the drugs can be shown to have a direct inhibitory effect upon the
rate of breakdown of histiotroph by the inverted yolk sac and this is pre-

sumed to play a major (though not necessarily complete) part in the genesis
of congenital defects. Unfortunately centrally implanting embryos such as
in the macaque, ferret or rabbit have not been successfully cultured in
vitro in a consistent way and it is therefore only with caution that the
results of experiments involving embryo culture inside an inverted yolk sac
can be extrapolated to man. Further simplification of model systems involve
the culture of mouse (Kochhar 1975) or ferret (Gulamhusein and co-workers
1980) limb buds in the presence of teratogens. Here the results require even
more cautious interpretation for many of the checks and balances of the whole
embryo-'placental' unit have now been eliminated with the possibility that
even more error may be introduced. This is even more true of embryonal cell
culture for, although the systems allow greater probing at the cellular
level, they may easily demonstrate effects which do not occur in vivo.

Recently it has become possible to grow rat embryos on human serum (Chatot
and co-workers 1980). In our hands normal growth has only occured if 10%
rat serum prepared by New's method is added to the culture medium but Al-
Alousi (personal communication) has shown that 10% rat serum diluted only
with buffered salt solution and supplemented by the appropriate addition of
vitamins and glucose does not sustain rat embryo growth while 20% rat serum
under similar conditions does. It is likely therefore that the addition of
10% rat serum to the human serum supplies some vital trace factors but is
not the main source of histiotrophic nutrition in the system. Using human
serum preliminary results indicate a significant (p$<$.05) deficiency in
weight of embryos grown in the serum of smokers when compared with the serum
of non-smokers. No abnormal development was observed but in order to be
comprehensive this investigation will have to be completed by investigating
the effects of sera from individuals who give up smoking during the course
of the experiment.

The importance of the possibility of growing rat embryos on human sera is
great. The method is presently being exploited by Dr. Klein at Storrs,
Connecticut, as well as by ourselves and could lead to the isolation not only
of potential teratogens in human serum but to other factors which lead to
sterility or poor reproductive performance in some individuals.

CONCLUSION

In summary, therefore, it should be stressed that the use of studies in
animals for the evaluation of human risk from teratogenic agents is not only
a question of in vivo drug screening. A considerable amount of experimental
toxicological information may be obtained by selection of the appropriate
in vitro animal model provided always that proper caution in the extrapolation
of results is exercised and that the limitations of the model (based upon our
knowledge of its functional capacity) is available.

REFERENCES

Barrow, M. W., and W. J. Taylor (1969). A rapid method for detecting mal-
    formations in rat fetuses. J. Morph., 127, 291-306.
Beck, F. (1977). Evaluation of organs (Gross organ pathology) In D. Neubert,
    J. H. Merker and T. E. Kwasigroch (eds) Methods in Prenatal Toxicology,
    103-112.
Carter, C. O. (1969). Genetics of common disorders. Br. Med. Bull., 25, 52.
Chatot, C. L., N. W. Klein, J. Piatek and L. J. Pierro (1980). Successful
    culture of rat embryos on human serum: Use in the detection of Teratogens.
    Science, 207, 1471-1473.
Cockcroft, D. L. (1979). Nutrient requirements of rat embryos undergoing
    organogenesis in vitro. J. Reprod. Fert., 57, 505-510.

Conference on the Ferret as an alternative species in Teratology and Toxicology (Teratology, in press).

Emery, J. L. and J. A. C. Weatherall (1981). Eurocat guide to a service in fetal and Perinatal pathology. Eurocat. Brussels.

Fantel, A.G., Jean, C. Greenaway, Mont. R. Judian and Thomas H. Shepard (1979). Teratogenic activation of cyclophosphamide in vitro. Life Sci., 25, 67-72.

Fraser, F. C. and H. Pashayan. (1970). Relation of face shape to susceptibility to congenital cleft lip. A preliminary report. J. Med. Genet., 7, 112.

Freeman, S. J., F. Beck and J. B. Lloyd. The role of the visceral yolk sac in mediating protein utilization by rat embryos cultured in vitro. J. Embryol. Exp. Morph. (in press).

Grosser, O. (1927). Frühentwicklung, Eihautbildung und Placentation des Menschen und der Säugetiere. München.

Gulamhusein, A. P. and F. Beck (1975). Development and structure of the extra-embryonic membranes of the ferret: A light microscopic and ultrastructural study. J. Anat., 120, 349-365.

Gulamhusein, A. P. and F. Beck (1981). External features of the developing ferret embryo. Biblithca. Anat., 19, 234-246.

Gulamhusein, A. P., F. Beck and B. Zimmerman (1980). Development of ferret limbs in organ culture. J. Anat., 131, 347-354.

Gupta, M., A. P. Gulamhusein and F. Beck (1980). Studies of endocytosis in the yolk sac endoderm of post implantation rat embryos in vivo and in vitro. J. Anat., 131, 761-62.

Gupta, M. and F. Beck. Uptake of colloidal gold by the rat visceral yolk sac in vitro. J. Anat. (in press).

Hendrickx, A. G., M. L. Houston, D. C. Kraemar, R.F. Gasser and A. J. Bollert (1971). Embryology of the Baboon. Univ. of Chicago Press, Chicago, Ill.

Henneberg, B. (1937). Normentafeln zur Entwicklungsgeschichte der Wanderatte (Rattus norwegicus Erxleben) F. Keibel (ed) Normentafeln zur Entwicklungsgeschichte der Wirbeltiere. Vol. 15, Gustav Fischer Verlag, Jena.

Heuser, C. H. and G. L. Streeter (1941). Development of the Macaque embryo. Carnegie Contrib. embryol., 29, 15-55.

Keibel, F. (1897) Normaltafel zur Entwicklungsgeschichte des Schweines (Sus Scrofa domesticus). Normaltafeln zur Entwicklungsgeschichte der Wirbeltiere. Vol. 1, Gustav Fischer Verlag, Jena.

Kochhar, D. (1975). The use of in vitro procedures in teratology. Teratology, 7, 289-98.

Kopf, R., D. Lorenz, and E. Salewski (1964). Der einfluss von Thalidomid auf die Fertilität von Ratten im Generation versuch uber zwei Generationen. Arch. Exp. Path u Pharm. 247, 121-135.

Lowy, A. (1981). The effect of an inhibitor of lysosomal proteolysis on early development in the rat. J. Anat., 449-450.

Minot, C. S. and E. Taylor (1905). Normal plates of the development of the rabbit (Lepus cuniculus). F. Keibel (ed) Normentafeln zur Entwicklungsgeschichte der Wirbeltiere. Vol. 5, Gustav Fischer Verlag, Jena.

McGarrity, C., N. Samani., F. Beck and A. P. Gulamhusein. The effect of sodium salicylate on the rat embryo in culture: an in vitro model for the morphological assessment of teratogenicity. J. Anat. (in press).

New, D. A. T. (1978). Whole-embryo culture and the study of mammalian embryos during organogenesis. Biol. Rev., 53, 81-122.

Otis, E.M. and R. Brent (1954). Equivalent ages in mouse and human embryos. Anat. Rec., 120, 33-63.

Sadler, T. W. (1979). Culture of early somite mouse embryos during organo-

genesis. J. Embryol. exp. Morph., 49, 17-25.
Sterz, H. (1977). Routine examination of rat and rabbit fetuses for mal-
formation of internal organs. Combination of Barrow's and Wilson's
methods in D. Neubert, J-H Merker and T. E. Kwasigroch (eds) Methods in
Prenatal Toxicology, 113-122.
Steven, D. H. (1975). Comparative Placentation. Academic Press, New York
and London.
Williams, K. E., G. Roberts, E. M. Kidston, F. Beck and J. B. Lloyd (1976).
Inhibition of pinocytosis in the rat yolk sac by trypan blue. Teratology,
14, 343-354.
Wilson, J. G. (1965). Methods for administering agents and detecting mal-
formations in experimental animals in J. G. Wilson and J. Warkany (eds)
Teratology, Principles and techniques, 262-277.
Wilson, J. G., R. Fradkin and A. Hardman (1970). Breeding and pregnancy
in Rhesus monkeys used for teratological testing. Teratology, 3, 59-71.

ACKNOWLEDGEMENTS

The author wishes to thank Dr. A.J. Beck and Dr. J. Wakely for helpful
comments in the preparation of the manuscript and for checking the final
production. Mrs. C.S. Gibson rapidly and carefully typed the manuscript
and I am grateful for her usual high standards.

I am grateful also to the MRC for a grant in aid of research.

Genetic Variability in Man as a Complicating Factor in the Extrapolation of Toxicological Data from Animals

F. Sjöqvist, C. von Bahr and L. Bertilsson

Department of Clinical Pharmacology at the Karolinska Institute,
Huddinge Hospital, S-141 86 Huddinge, Sweden

ABSTRACT

It is well established that pathways and especially rates of drug
metabolism vary not only between but also within species,
particularly in humans. This paper discusses the implications
of interindividual variability in drug metabolism for the clinical
evaluation of drugs. Recent pharmacogenetic research strongly
suggests the occurrence of polymorphisms in the oxidation of
certain drugs, a few percent in the population being slow oxidizers.

The clinical pharmacologist must thus be prepared to encounter slow
oxidizers during clinical trials. Preliminary appraisal of the
extent of interindividual variability in drug oxidation in man may
be obtained from *in vitro* studies using human tissue from a liver
bank containing specimens with vastly different rates of metabolism
of various "prototype" drugs. Further information may be obtained
by studying the fate of a new drug in a panel of subjects who have
been phenotyped with regard to those oxidative pathways that appear
to be under monogenic control. An important task for clinical
pharmacology is to develop simple tests by which the activity of
individual drug metabolic processes can be assessed in man.

Equally important is to perform detailed drug metabolic studies
in subjects who develop unique adverse drug reactions during
phases III and IV of clinical drug evaluation. Increased cooperation between drug epidemiologists and experts in drug
metabolism may lead to an early identification of "phenotypes at
risk" to develop severe concentration-dependent side effects of
various drugs.

KEYWORDS

Pharmacogenetics, polymorphism, tricyclic antidepressants,
debrisoquine, antipyrine, cytochrome P-450, adverse reactions.

INTRODUCTION

Species and strain differences in pathways and rates of drug
metabolism must be considered in the extrapolation of toxicological
data from animals to man (Brodie, 1964). Recent advances in drug
analysis and pharmacokinetics have helped to overcome some of these
difficulties. It is reasonable today that a clinical pharmacologist who is designing a phase I-trial requests information on the

range of steady-state plasma concentrations (preferably the unbound concentration) that produce the effects in animals which are believed to be most relevant for the expected clinical action(s). On the basis of kinetic studies of small doses in volunteers it is usually possible to calculate the dose required to yield plasma concentrations of unbound drug in the expected effective range. This is much more difficult if the drug has concentration-dependent metabolism and binding. Although conceptionally attractive there are at least two major problems with this approach.

Firstly, marked species differences may also occur in drug-receptor interactions or at "second messenger" levels. Secondly, a limited number of subjects, usually healthy young volunteers, are used in early phase I studies. Thus the extent of interindividual differences in the metabolism of the drug occurring in the population at large may be much greater than that demonstrated in the test subjects. In fact, the biochemical individuality of man and the heterogeneity in environment of different members of the human species invalidate the extrapolation of drug metabolism data obtained in a small sample of volunteers to the population with the target disease. This paper deals with this problem.

INTER-SUBJECT VARIABILITY IN DRUG METABOLISM

It is now well established that there is marked interindividual variability in pharmacokinetics, particularly in drug metabolic processes. Research on drug acetylation provided clinicians with the first simple tool (isoniazid half-life) by which patients could be classified into clearly disctinct metabolic phenotypes, fast and slow acetylators (Price Evans & White, 1964). Subsequent studies have shown that slow acetylators are at considerably higher risk to develop adverse reactions on standard doses of several drugs such as isoniazid, hydralazine and procainamide which seem to be acetylated by similar enzymatic mechanisms (cf Sjöqvist & co-workers, 1980b). It is obviously of great help to be able to "diagnose" the phenotype at risk to develop side effects, particularly those which are not readily detected, but very few drugs are acetylated and the isoniazid test is seldom used for this purpose in clinical medicine. In fact most clinically useful drugs are metabolized by oxidation.

Early studies of the kinetics of drugs that are oxidized showed marked interindividual variability in composite kinetic variables such as plasma half-life, clearance and steady-state concentrations. In general, the distribution of these variables in the population seemed to indicate a polygenic control, although hints of non-normal distribution of steady-state plasma concentrations of phenytoin (Kutt & co-workers, 1964) and monomethylated tricyclic antidepressants (Hammer & Sjöqvist, 1967) were reported. Twin and family studies established a genetic control of the steady-state plasma concentrations and plasma clearance of nortriptyline, possibly mediated by a small number of allelic genes (Alexanderson & co-workers, 1969; Åsberg & co-workers, 1971; Alexanderson, 1973). Using antipyrine as a probe drug Vesell and co-workers were able to identify a number of environmental factors that tended to modify the preexisting genetically determined variability in kinetics (Vesell, 1979).

Comparing the kinetics of different drugs in the same individuals investigators found examples of strong correlations. Thus the plasma clearances and steady-state plasma concentrations of nortriptyline (NT) and desmethylimipramine (both being hydroxylated) correlated significantly (n = 8-11; r = 0.90 and 0.97) and so did the reciprocal plasma levels (reflecting clearance by demethylation) of amitriptyline and chlorimipramine (n =15, r = 0.87). In other words slow (or rapid) hydroxylators of NT were also slow (or rapid) hydroxylators of desmethylimipramine, while slow (or rapid) demethylators of amitriptyline also were slow (or rapid) demethylators of chlorimipramine (cf Sjöqvist & co-workers, 1980a). Significant correlations were also found between the half-lives of antipyrine and phenylbutazone on one hand and amobarbital and phenytoin on the other (for ref. see Kalow & Inaba, 1976). For the majority of drug pairs that were compared low and non-significant intraindividual correlations were found between kinetic parameters reflecting metabolism (loc. cit). These observations are consistent with the occurence of multiple forms of cytochrome P-450, each preferentially oxidizing a family of drug substrates.

PHARMACOGENETICS - RECENT FINDINGS

During the last few years increasing evidence has accumulated that polymorphisms also exist in drug oxidation. The clinical pharmacologist must therefore be prepared to encounter slow oxidizers during clinical drug trials. Independent studies strongly suggested the occurrence of polymorphic N-oxidation of sparteine (Eichelbaum & co-workers, 1979) and C-hydroxylation of debrisoquine (Mahgoub & co-workers, 1977). Possibly these two enzymatic reactions are under similar monogenic control - in any case indices of these two oxidative reactions are strongly correlated in a small sample of human volunteers (Bertilsson & co-workers, 1980a). The ratio between debrisoquine and 4-hydroxydebrisoquine in urine (sampled for 6 hours) after a 10 mg oral dose separates humans into extensive and poor oxidizers of both compounds.

The frequency of poor oxidizers may vary geographically but is generally about a few percent of the population. Price Evans and co-workers (1980) reported that 8.9% of 258 white British volunteers belonged to the poor hydroxylator phenotype (debrisoquine ratios above 12.6) compared to 3.2% (5/155) in a Swedish population (unpublished data). The debrisoquine phenotype seems to be an accurate prediction of the rate of oxidation of some other drugs, i.e. phenformin (Shah & co-workers, 1980), phenacetine (Smith & Idle, 1981) and phenytoin (Sloan & co-workers, 1981).

We have studied the metabolism of two pharmacogenetic probe drugs, nortriptyline (NT) and antipyrine (Fig. 1), in volunteers who have been phenotyped with a debrisoquine test. Eight Swedish subjects, covering a wide range in the ability to hydroxylate debrisoquine were given a single oral dose of NT. The total plasma clearance of NT in these 8 subjects varied from 0.30 to 0.90 L x kg^{-1} x hr^{-1}. There was a fairly close relationship (Spearman rank correlation coefficient r_s = -0.83; p = 0.01) between the urinary debrisoquine/ 4-hydroxydebrisoquine ratio and the NT clearance (Fig. 2), which is determined largely by the capacity of the liver to 10-hydroxylate NT (Alexanderson, 1973).

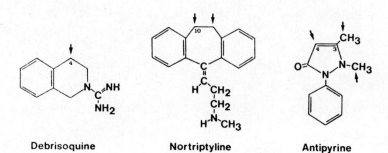

Debrisoquine   Nortriptyline   Antipyrine

FIGURE 1

Structural formulae of three pharmacogenetic probe drugs.
Arrows indicate positions where oxidations occur.

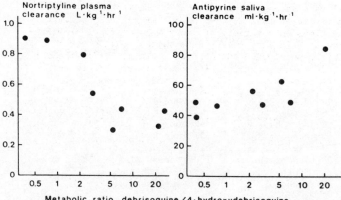

FIGURE 2

Relationship between the metabolic ratio debrisoquine/4-hydroxy-
debrisoquine and the plasma clearance of nortriptyline (left;
Spearman r_s = -0.83; n = 8; p = 0.01) and the clearance of
antipyrine in saliva (right; Spearman r_s = 0.65; n = 8; p < 0.05).
From Bertilsson et al., 1980b.

Further analysis showed that the urinary debrisoquine/4-hydroxy-debrisoquine ratio was significantly correlated to the plasma clearance of NT by E-10-hydroxylation (r_s = -0.88; p < 0.01) but not to the clearance by Z-10-hydroxylation (r_s = -0.48; N.S.). As E-10-OH-NT is a major metabolite of NT, there was a strong correlation (r = 0.96; p < 0.001) between the total plasma clearance of NT and the metabolic clearance by E-10-hydroxylation. These results suggest that the major metabolic pathway, the E-10-hydroxylation of NT, is controlled by similar genetic factors as the hydroxylation of debrisoquine (cf Mellström et al., 1981). A considerably larger sample of subjects has to be examined to clarify the genetic mechanisms involved.

By contrast, there was no meaningful correlation between the debrisoquine/4-hydroxydebrisoquine ratio and the salivary clearance of antipyrine (Fig. 2), nor did the clearance of antipyrine through the various pathways indicated in Fig. 1 correlate to the debrisoquine ratio (Eichelbaum, Bertilsson & Säwe, unpublished data). The 8 subjects were also given an oral dose of amitriptyline. Its plasma clearance by demethylation was not significantly correlated to the debrisoquine metabolic ratio (Spearman r_s = -0.38) or NT clearance (unpublished data). Similarly demethylation of amitriptyline and hydroxylation of nortriptyline *in vitro* by human liver microsomes seem to be independently regulated (von Bahr & Mellström, unpublished). Thus, although one form of cytochrome P-450 may be deficient in a small subpopulation, other forms involved in the metabolism of the same group of drugs may have normal activity.

The overall data strongly suggest that a small proportion of the population may be at risk to develop concentration-dependent adverse reactions on a variety of drugs being oxidized similarly to debrisoquine. In fact recent data suggest that adverse reactions after phenformin (Oates & co-workers, 1981; Wiholm & co-workers, 1981) and nortriptyline (Bertilsson & co-workers, 1981) are, at least partly, related to this hydroxylation deficiency. It may thus be of interest to examine the oxidation of new drugs in volunteers who have been characterized previously with regard to the oxidation of certain "model" drugs (Smith, 1980). Using a phenotyped panel of volunteers, however, implies difficult ethical problems in view of the repeated exposure to various drugs.

It may be more acceptable to study the clinical significance of interindividual differences in drug metabolism in subjects who develop unique adverse drug reactions during long-term therapy. Increased cooperation between drug epidemiologists and experts in drug metabolism may help identifying "phenotypes at risk" to develop severe concentration-dependent side effects. In the case of phenformin this approach was never tried before the drug was removed from the market, because it induced lactic acidosis in a minority of patients. It is an important aspect of clinical pharmacology to develop simple clinical tests by which impairment of various drug metabolic processes can be ascertained. Perhaps in the future some of us will carry a card informing the prescribing physician about our drug metabolic deficiencies!

IN VITRO STUDIES OF HUMAN DRUG METABOLISM

During the late sixties several research groups studied the
oxidation of xenobiotics in human liver tissue *in vitro* (for
references see von Bahr & co-workers, 1980). Up till now a large
variety of different oxidations have been demonstrated including
the formation of potentially toxic and mutagenic metabolites.

It is important to standardize the procedures involved in
obtaining and preparing human liver microsomes. This has been
accomplished in a recent study from our group making use of a
"liver bank" (von Bahr & co-workers, 1980). The liver tissue is
obtained shortly after circulatory arrest from cadaveric (cerebral
infarction) kidney transplant donors. Postmortem changes are
minimal. Subcellular liver fractions are prepared immediately and
part of this is used directly for assay. Intact pieces and subcellular fractions are stored in different media at -80°. Each
liver is characterized by light and electron microscopy.

Several enzymes, including cytochromes P-450 and b_5, NADPH-
cytochrome c reductase, demethylation of aminopyrine and
amitriptyline, epoxidation of carbamazepine, oxidation of
acetaminophen and benzo(a)pyrene, were tested with freshly prepared
fractions giving each liver a "drug metabolic profile". This
"test battery" was repeated after storing to evaluate the effect
of storage.

The preparation technique gave a well preserved microsomal fraction
with minimal contamination. In freshly prepared microsomes the
following activities (levels) were observed (n = 13): cytochrome
P-450, 0.13 to 0.73 nmole/mg protein; NADPH-cytochrome c reductase,
70 to 426 nmole/mg protein; demethylation of aminopyrine, 0.9 to
4.1 and of amitriptyline, 0.11 to 0.92 nmole/mg protein; carba-
mazepine-10,11 epoxidation, 0.03 to 0.46 nmole/mg protein; oxidation
of acetaminophen, 0.48 to 2.11 and of benzo(a)pyrene, 0.04 to 0.11
nmole/mg. Thus, there is a very marked interindividual variability
in rates of drug metabolism matching that found in patients.
Similar observations have previously been reported using liver
biopsy material (Davies & Thorgeirsson, 1971). Attempts are now
made to phenotype the specimens *in vitro* using debrisoquine and
nortriptyline.

The various metabolic activities obtained in freshly prepared
microsomes from different livers have been compared. There was
a correlation between demethylation of aminopyrine and the oxidation
of acetaminophen (n = 7; r = 0.91) and between amitriptyline
demethylation and carbamazepine epoxidation (n = 8, r = 0.72).
Correlations were also found between cytochrome P-450 and b_5 levels;
between cytochrome P-450 on the one hand and NADPH-cytochrome c
reductase, demethylation of aminopyrine and AT, and acetaminophen
oxidation on the other. Furthermore, a significant correlation
of high degree was found between NADPH-cytochrome c reductase and
demethylation of amitriptyline (to nortriptyline). This approach
may be useful in identifying reactions that correlate with the
metabolism of genetic probe drugs. Inhibition experiments may also

be useful to screen for oxidations dependent on components involved
in e.g. debrisoquine hydroxylation.

Further work in this area may lead to the establishment of a bank
of livers with a spectrum of drug metabolic profiles, hopefully
also some with deficient oxidations of certain drugs. Using
this material Warholm & co-workers (1981) have purified a new
glutathione-S-transferase, previously not found in animals. An
intriguing feature of this enzyme was that it occurred only in some
of the livers suggesting qualitative interindividual differences in
man. We have utilized our material for preliminary studies of
pathways and rates of metabolism of new drugs and drug metabolites
not given to man previously. As an example the metabolism of
carbamazepine-10,11-epoxide was studied *in vitro* before it was
given to our first human volunteer - the *in vitro* findings predicted
efficient metabolism to the trans-diol (Fig. 3) and this was later
confirmed *in vivo* (Bertilsson, unpublished data).

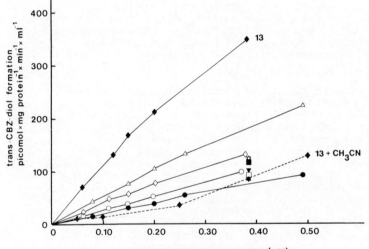

FIGURE 3

Metabolism of carbamazepine-epoxide in human liver microsomes. The
formation of trans-CBZ-diol from various concentrations of the
epoxide by human liver microsomes obtained from ten different
subjects. In five livers only one concentration (0.38 mM) was used.
The substrate was added in water solution to all incubations.
Microsomes from liver no 13 were also incubated with the epoxide
added in 50 μl acetonitrile (CH_3CN). Tybring & co-workers
(unpublished).

Comparing humans with other species profound differences have been
found which have helped to explain differences between animals and
man in pharmacokinetics. One example may suffice. When racemic
propranolol (d,l-P), consisting of two optical isomers (d and l)
is given to dogs d-P reaches higher plasma concentrations than
l-P which has been considered to be a result of a more marked
presystemic glucuronidation of l-P than of d-P (Walle & Walle,
1979). However, in man we have found opposite *in vivo* kinetics
(Fig. 4) - after oral administration of d,l-P, l-P reaches the
highest concentrations (Hermansson & von Bahr, 1980).

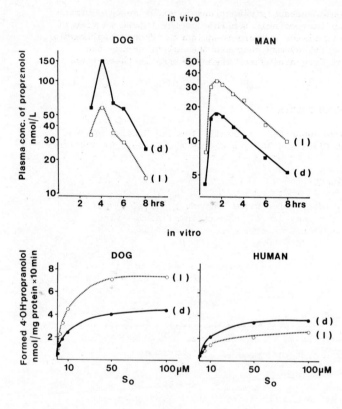

FIGURE 4

In vivo (above) and *in vitro* kinetics of d-l-propranolol in dog
(left) and man (right). Human subjects and dogs got d,l-propranolol.
d- and l-propranolol plasma levels were quantitated separately.
The dog data stem from Walle & Walle (1979).
The formation of 4-hydroxy-propranolol from d- and l-propranolol was
studied in human and dog liver microsomes.
S_0 = initial propranolol concentration. Indubation performed at
37°C for 10 min. Protein concentration 1 mg/ml.

To elucidate the mechanisms behind these differences we incubated
d- and l-P separately with human and dog liver microsomes. Fig. 4
shows that d-P is more rapidly 4-hydroxylated than l-P in human
liver and that the opposite can be seen in dog liver microsomes.
In both human and dog microsomes l-P is more rapidly glucuronidated
than d-P but this reaction proceeds slower than the oxidation of P.
The *in vitro* studies show that it is the oxidation of d-P which is
the main determinant for the species differences observed *in vivo*.
This species difference in stereoselective metabolism is pharmacologically relevant when extrapolating dog data to humans because
the l-isomer mainly accounts for the β-blockade.

Utilization of human tissue preparations in experimental pharmacology may become increasingly feasible in the future in view of
recent advances in tissue culture techniques. Proper application
of such *in vitro* methods may increase the safety during the
critical phase of drug evaluation when the step is taken from
animals to man.

ACKNOWLEDGEMENTS

These studies were supported by grants from the Swedish Medical
Research Council (3902 and 5677) and from the Karolinska Institute.

REFERENCES

Alexanderson, B., D.A. Price Evans, and F. Sjöqvist (1969).
Steady-state plasma levels of nortriptyline in twins:
Influence of genetic factors and drug therapy.
Br. Med. J., 2, 764-768

Alexanderson, B. (1973). Prediction of steady-state plasma levels
of nortriptyline from single oral dose kinetics - A study
in twins. Europ. J. clin. Pharmacol., 6, 44-53

Åsberg, M., D.A. Price Evans, and F. Sjöqvist (1971). Genetic
control of nortriptyline kinetics in man - A study of the
relatives of propositi with high plasma concentrations.
J. Med. Gen. 8, 129-135

von Bahr, C., C.-G. Groth, H. Jansson, G. Lundgren, M. Lind, and
H. Glaumann (1980). Drug metabolism in human liver in vitro.
Establishment of a human liver bank. Clin. Pharmacol. Ther.
27, 711-725

Bertilsson, L., H.J. Dengler, M. Eichelbaum, and H.-U. Schulz
(1980a). Pharmacogenetic covariation of defective N-oxidation
of sparteine and 4-hydroxylation of debrisoquine. Europ. J.
clin. Pharmacol., 17, 153-155

38   F. Sjöqvist, C. Von Bahr and L. Bertilsson

Bertilsson, L., M. Eichelbaum, B. Mellström, J. Säwe, H.-U. Schulz,
    and F. Sjöqvist (1980b). Nortriptyline and antipyrine
    clearance in relation to debrisoquine hydroxylation in man.
    Life Sci., 27, 1673-1677

Bertilsson, L., B. Mellström, F. Sjöqvist, B. Mårtensson, and
    M. Åsberg (1981). Slow hydroxylation of nortriptyline and
    concomitant poor debrisoquine hydroxylation: clinical
    implications. The Lancet, I, 560-561

Brodie, B.B. (1964). Of mice, microsomes and man. Pharmacologist,
    6, 12-26

Davies, D.S., and S.S. Thorgeirsson (1971). Mechanism of hepatic
    drug oxidation and its relationship to individual differences
    in rates of oxidation in man. Ann. N.Y. Acad. Sci., 179,
    411-420

Eichelbaum, M., N. Spannbrucker, B. Steinecke, and H.J. Dengler
    (1979). Defective N-oxidation of sparteine in man: A new
    pharmacogenetic defect. Europ. J. clin. Pharmacol., 16,
    183-187

Hammer, W., and F. Sjöqvist (1967). Plasma levels of monomethylated
    tricyclic antidepressants during treatment with imipramine-
    like compounds. Life Sci., 6, 1895-1903

Hermansson, J., and C. von Bahr (1980). Simultaneous determination
    of d- and l-propranolol in human plasma by high-performance
    liquid chromatography. J. Chromatogr., 221, 109-117

Kalow, W., and T. Inaba (1976). Genetic factors in hepatic drug
    oxidations. Prog. Liver Dis., 5, 246-258

Kutt, H., M. Wolk, R. Scherman, and F. McDowell (1964). Insufficient
    para-hydroxylation as a cause of diphenylhydantoin toxicity.
    Neurology, 14, 542-548

Mahgoub, A., J.R. Idle, L.G. Dring, R. Lancaster, and R.L. Smith
    (1977). Polymorphic hydroxylation of debrisoquine in man.
    The Lancet, II, 584-586

Mellström, B., L. Bertilsson, J. Säwe, H.-U. Schulz, and F. Sjöqvist
    (1981). E- and Z-10-hydroxylation of nortriptyline in man -
    Relationship to polymorphic hydroxylation of debrisoquine.
    Clin. Pharmacol. Ther., in press

Oates, N.S., R.R. Shah, J.R. Idle, and R.L. Smith (1981).
    Phenformin-induced lacticacidosis associated with impaired
    debrisoquine hydroxylation. The Lancet, I, 837

Price Evans, D.A., A. Mahgoub, T.P. Sloan, J.R. Idle, and R.L. Smith
(1980). A family and population study of the genetic polymorphism of debrisoquine oxidation in a white British population.
J. Med. Gen. 17, 102–105

Price Evans, D.A., and T.A. White (1964). Human acetylation polymorphism. J. Lab. Clin. Med., 63, 394–403

Shah, R.R., N.S. Oates, J.R. Idle and R.L. Smith (1980). Genetic
impairment phenformin metabolism. The Lancet, II, 1147

Sjöqvist, F., L. Bertilsson, and M. Åsberg (1980a). Monitoring
tricyclic antidepressants. Ther. Drug Monitoring, 2, 85–93

Sjöqvist, F., O. Borgå, and M.L'E. Orme (1980b). Fundamentals of
clinical pharmacology. In Drug Treatment, pp. 1–61, ed. by
G.S. Avery, Adis Press, Sydney

Sloan, T.P., J.R. Idle, and R.L. Smith (1981). Influence of
D^H/D^L alleles regulating debrisoquine oxidation on phenytoin
hydroxylation. Clin. Pharmacol. Ther. 29, 493–497

Smith, R.L. (1980). Some clinical and toxicological implications
of polymorphic drug oxidation. Workshop "Polymorphism of
drug oxidation in man", October 11–12, 1980, Bonn, FRG

Smith, R.L., and J.R. Idle (1981, in press). The debrisoquine
hydroxylation gene: A gene of multiple application.
In: Davis, M., J.M. Tredgar and R. Williams (eds). Drug
reactions and the liver. Tunbridge Wells, Pitman Medical

Walle, T., and K. Walle (1979). Stereoselective oral bioavailability
of (±)-propranolol in the dog. Res. Comm. Chem. Pathol.
Pharmacol., 23, 453–464

Warholm, M., C. Guthenberg, B. Mannervik, and C. von Bahr (1981).
Purification of a new glutathione s-transferase (transferase
μ) from human liver having high activity with benzo(a)pyrene-
4,5-oxide. Biochem. Biophys. Res. Commun. 98, 512–519

Vesell, E. (1979). Pharmacogenetics: Multiple interactions
between genes and environment as determinants of drug
response. Am. J. Med., 66, 183–190

Wiholm, B., G. Alvan, L. Bertilsson, J. Säwe, and F. Sjöqvist
(1981). Hydroxylation of debrisoquine in patients with
lacticacidosis after phenformin. The Lancet, I, 1098–1099

The Rational Interpretation of Species and Strain Differences in Toxicity for the Prediction of Risk to Man: Review and Concluding Remarks

H. Frohberg

Hauptleitung Medizin, E. Merck, Frankfurter Str. 250, 6100
Darmstadt 1, Federal Republic of Germany

ABSTRACT

The problems of the predictability of toxicity studies from
animals to man, and the possibilities for improvement are
discussed.

KEYWORDS

Metabolic activation, metabolic inactivation, reproductive
toxicology, immunotoxicology.

When we look at the outcome of toxicological experiments,
we can distinguish between:

    true positive results,
    true negative results,
    false positive results, and
    false negative results.

False positive and, even more so, false negative results are
a serious problem for the toxicologist. Factors which can
lead to a false positive or false negative outcome when extrapolating the results of short- and longterm, reproductive toxicity, mutagenicity and carcinogenicity studies to humans are:

-   species differences in metabolism and kinetic behavior,
-   enzyme inhibition leading to an increase in suscep-
    tibility or tolerance,
-   enzyme induction leading to tolerance or an increase in
    susceptability, if a toxic metabolite is formed,
-   different receptor sensitivities,
-   anatomic and physiologic differences,
-   absence of pre-existing pathologic conditions,
-   lack of appropriate assays, and
-   failure to use appropriate methods.

Lesions which are directly caused locally and systemically
and especially morphological lesions are predictable from
animal experiments, if they are caused by substances requiring
neither metabolic activation nor inactivation. All these
effects are strictly dose-dependent. For risk estimation
linear extrapolation from species to species and from high
to low doses is possible.

Species differences in metabolic activation

Apparent species differences in the system of metabolic
activation have to be considered in connection with all
compounds which do not have a toxic effect themselves, but
whose reactive metabolites present the toxic principle.

The classical example is 2-acetylaminofluorene (2-AAF)
which is hepatocarcinogenic in all species besides guinea
pigs. 2-AAF requires aromatic N-hydroxylation to form the
N-hydroxy-2-AAF. Since guinea pigs do not have this enzyme,
they are insensitive. The higher sensitivity of male rats
to 2-AAF in comparison to females is correlated to the high
sulfotransferase activity of males, as the rate of carcinogenicity is also dependent on the formation of a sulfo-
derivative.

Not only the qualitative but also the quantitative differences in the metabolizing rate can affect the response of
the different species to toxic compounds.

Generally the human liver metabolizes chemicals much more
slowly than rodents (Buchter and co-workers, 1978; Davies,
1981). Examples thereof are chloroform, vinyl chloride, trichloroethylene, and 1,1-dichloroethylene. There exist, however,
exceptions to this rule, such as phenacetin or 2-AAF. Such
cases where the metabolizing rate in the human liver is
equal to or even quicker than in rodents can have important
toxicological implications.

The mechanisms that metabolically activate a chemical can be
saturated at high doses. This explains why beyond a certain
level of exposure to vinyl chloride e.g. no further increase
in metabolites is observed (Bolt and co-workers, 1980).

Species differences in metabolic inactivation

There is evidence, too, that the presence of a metabolically
inactivating mechanism modifies adverse effects of chemicals.
The hepatotoxic and carcinogenic effects of aflatoxin B1, for
example, are attributed to the formation of an epoxide.

The lower susceptibility to aflatoxin B1 carcinogenicity of
mice in comparison to rats is due to a more effective inactivation of the reactive aflatoxin B1 intermediate owing to the formation of glutathione conjugates. All halogenated ethylenes are
activated to reactive epoxides as well. However only the asym-
metrically halogenated ethylenes which cannot be quickly re-
arranged to harmless compounds are mutagenic and carcinogenic.

An exception to this rule is trichloroethylene which is quickly detoxified to the less reactive and therefore harmless chloral under the condition prevailing in eukaryotic cells (Henschler, 1977).

According to Oesch the microsomal epoxide hydratase activity plays an important role in the inactivation of many aromatic and olefinic chemicals. Since man has a much higher hydratase activity than most laboratory animal species (Oesch and co-workers, 1977; Oesch, 1980), one can expect that man is the species the least sensitive to such compounds.

The very low hydratase concentration found in certain strains of mice is certainly one of the reasons for the hepatocarcinogenic effect of phenobarbitone which is specific to mice. The assumption that phenobarbitone is not carcinogenic for humans was confirmed by the epidemiologic studies of Clemmesen and Hjalgrim-Jensen (1978 and 1980). The results of these long-term epidemiologic studies in epileptic patients showed that phenobarbitone should not be suspect of being a human carcinogen.

Overwhelmed metabolic inactivation

When high doses of a chemical are administered, it is possible that these high doses overwhelm inactivation mechanisms.

In toxicology threshold levels on the basis of overwhelming inactivation have long been established.

Furosamide is excreted predominantly unaltered in the urine when therapeutic doses are given. Administration of high doses, however, overwhelms renal clearance and causes a disproportionate increase in toxic metabolites reacting with macromolecules. Following investigations with dioxane (Young, J.D. and co-workers, 1975, 1976a, 1976b), 2,4,5-trichlorophenoxy acetic acid (Sauerhoff and co-workers, 1976; Koschier and Berndt, 1976), chloroform (Reitz and co-workers, 1979) and vinyl chloride (Gehring and co-workers, 1978, 1979), Gehring, Ramsey and Watanabe concluded that threshold doses exist below which the metabolic detoxification proceeds normally (1981).

On condition that the human metabolism of a compound under investigation corresponds to the metabolism in laboratory animals and that threshold values are much higher than the concentrations in the work room environment or the therapeutic doses of drugs, such an exposition represents a negligible hazard to humans.

Some guidelines for teratology experiments require that the pregnant mother shows toxicity from the administered compound regardless of the dose level essential to achieve this goal and of the blood and tissue concentrations that are reached in these experiments.

This can also lead to overwhelmed metabolic inactivation or to saturation of a transport process. The thus secondarily mediated impairment of the embryonal development can not be considered an indication of true embryotoxicity.

All efforts should be made that regulatory bodies acknowledge
the existance of non-linear kinetics at high dose levels
which may lead to erroneous toxicological results.

Reproductive toxicology

Despite all efforts there will never be an absolutely safe
teratogenicity trial (Beck, 1981). In many cases the physician
will be forced to carry out a benefit/risk evaluation. But
when all described parameters are considered in the performance of trials, the extrapolation has certainly become more
reliable than a few years ago. On the other hand one must
point out that a therapeutic nihilism during pregnancy is not
right, and studies involving humans will always only be possible to a limited extent. Therefore it is important to examine the mechanism of teratogenic effects.

Certain in vitro techniques using mammalian embryonic tissues
are very suitable tools for elucidating the mode of action of
teratogenic agents, and they may serve as a model for several
basic processes, also for the situation probably existing in
humans. Such in vitro methods provide little, if any, advantage over in vivo experiments, if a mass screening of a possible teratogenic potential of chemicals is attempted. But
such in vitro trials can only be extrapolated to the in vivo
conditions to a limited extent, as the kinetics and metabolism in the mother and the placental membranes are excluded.

The studies performed so far have shown that it is possible
to supplement the in vitro culture of embryonic tissue with a
drug metabolizing capacity. All these approaches must be considered preliminary and much more work is needed to arrive at
reliable and versatile systems that can be used routinely with
a high degree of reproducibility (Barrach and Neubert, 1980).

In teratogenicity trials it is important to consider the compartments mother, embryo and placental membranes. Therefore
dose comparisons with regard to teratogenic effects in different species should only be drawn on the basis of comparative
kinetic studies.

As differences in the pharmacokinetics of a substance - and
especially in the half-life - are frequently observed among
different animal species and in the comparison to man, species
differences in teratology may well be due to different half-
lives in the species concerned. The fact, for instance, that
in the rat, even under continuous infusion, a low dose of
chloramphenicol does not have an embryolethal effect, and that
such an effect only occurs at doses of 300 to 1000 mg/kg, does
not lead to the conclusion that a therapeutic dose of about
30 mg/kg in humans does not involve a risk for the fetus. This
is due to the different half-lives of chloramphenicol which
are about 30 minutes in the rat, but 3 hours in man. It follows that much higher doses are required in the rat to reach
the same serum and tissue concentrations as in man. Therefore,
when a substance is concerned which has a very short half-
life, it must be made sure that it acts long enough on the
embryo or fetus under the chosen mode of administration
(Neubert, 1978).

Numerous substances induce their own metabolisation. The serum and tissue concentrations of the administered substance are reduced, the concentration of the metabolites is increased. In the case of an accelerated inactivation, embryotoxic effects can be overlooked after repeated administration.

A cumulation in the fetal compartment can explain why some teratogenic substances require either high single doses or many small doses in long-term treatment.

Proposals to improve the predictability of toxicological experiments

In order to improve the predictability of toxicological long-term and special tests, e.g. of reproductive toxicological studies with regard to man, Brodie suggested as early as 1962 to use animal species absorbing, metabolizing and excreting the potential new drug in a way similar to man. This requires to study the kinetic behavior and the metabolic pattern in man during phase I studies.

In vitro studies are performed much more easily and quickly than in vivo experiments. Therefore the approach of Davies (1981), Sjöqvist (1981) and Sugimura (1981), i.e. to compare in vitro the capacity of human and animal liver cells or subcellular liver fractions to metabolically activate or inactivate substances, is to be considered a major advance.

Intact cell systems are superior to cell-free fractions and freshly isolated hepatocytes are said to be the best defined of all cellular in vitro systems (Greim, 1979).

There is now increasing evidence that genetic polymorphisms exist, not only in acetylation but also in oxydation in man. Examples are debrisoquine, sparteine, phenacetin (Davies, 1981; Sjöqvist, 1981). These observations further decrease the rate of predictability of toxicological experiments of compounds requiring metabolic activation and/or inactivation.

By establishing many more human liver banks similar to that in Stockholm (von Bahr and co-workers, 1980), where livers of different biochemical profiles are available and can be used for in vitro metabolic studies, the knowledge of the genetically caused polymorphisms in the metabolic pathway of foreign substances is deepened and more signs pointing to such genetically caused side effects are detected.

Sjöqvist's suggestion to perform metabolic studies in people who develop the unique side effect during chronic treatment seems to be important, too. For such investigations the cooperation between epidemiologists and biochemical pharmacologists is essential.

As far as special tests are available to detect a distinct enzyme polymorphism in man, these tests should be performed in order to exclude subjects having a certain enzyme polymorphism. An example might be the determination of the low-Km-acetaldehydedehydrogenase phenotype in hair roots of man (Goedde and co-workers, 1980). By such a screening all chronic alcoholics

in Asia who possess an abnormal low-Km-acetaldehydedehydrogenase could be excluded from treatment with alcoholaversive
agents like disulfiram and cyanimide so that severe side
effects can be avoided.

Clinical experience indicates, however, that functional side
effects are much more frequent than the toxic reactions due to
morphological and biochemical lesions. It is, thus, highly desirable that the toxicological evaluation of new drugs includes experimental procedures which can detect disturbances
of physiological functions. These will be based on techniques
developed for the assessment of pharmacodynamic drug actions.

This approach involves repeated pharmacological measurements
in chronically treated animals. But for such studies only noninvasive techniques can be used. Examples of noninvasive pharmacological techniques in the course of chronic toxicity experiments are measurements of blood pressure, body temperature
and locomotor activity, recordings of the electrocardiogram,
evaluations of the sensory, neuromuscular and pulmonary functions, gastrointestinal motility, appetite, and behavior.

The decision on the methods to be included in the experimental
design of a long-term toxicity study, largely depends on the
pharmacodynamic properties of the compound to be tested.

In man adverse reactions in the cardiovascular system concern
mainly the heart. Methods are available which allow to predict
morphological as well as functional side effects which will
occur in this organ.

After chronic daily treatment of rats with maximally tolerated
doses of 5 antidepressants, 3 phenothiazines and 5 butyrophe-
none neuroleptics, the same ECG changes were induced as those
seen in patients treated with therapeutic doses (Zbinden and
co-workers, 1980).

Adriamycin-induced cardiotoxicity similar to that observed in
humans (Buja and co-workers, 1973; Lefrak and co-workers, 1973)
was produced in New Zealand Black rats (Olson and Capen, 1978)
as well as in mice and rabbits (Jaenke, 1974; Olson and co-
workers, 1974; Young, D.M., 1975). In chronic rat experiments
it was possible to monitor the development of ECG changes induced by anthracycline antibiotics (Zbinden and Brändle, 1975).

In reproductive toxicity studies, excess pharmacodynamic
effects in the dams can lead to a secondary impairment of the
embryonal development. For example, major tranquilizers as
well as anticonvulsants and hypnotics can have a secondary embryotoxic effect. In pregnant Wistar rats chlorpromazine led
to a reduced body weight gain as well as many abortions and
resorptions in daily doses of 30 and 100 mg/kg. The same
effect was observed with phenobarbitone in 3 daily doses of
120 mg/kg administered from days 9 to 11 p.c. This embryolethal effect is primarily due to the strongly reduced food consumption following the sedation of the dams (Frohberg, 1978).

As the human embryonic development is not as much influenced
by a limited food intake as is that of laboratory animals,
embryotoxic effects by phenothiazines or barbiturates are not

expected to occur in man. This assumption is substantiated by clinical experience, for extensive clinical studies did not give any indication of an influence of these drugs on pre- and postnatal development, except for a few positive single case descriptions (Nishimura and Tanimura, 1976; Tuchmann-Duplessis, 1978).

Species differences caused by different receptor sensitivities

A well known example of a false positive result due to different receptor sensitivities is the occurrence of mammary gland tumors in the dog caused by different gestagens.

This induction of mammary gland nodules in dogs must be considered a species-specific effect related to the high progestational activity of these compounds in the dog and their stimulatory effect on the highly mammatropic canine growth hormone (Etreby and Gräf, 1979).

19-nortestosterone derivatives seem to be less tumorigenic in the canine mammary gland than 17α-hydroxy-progesterone derivatives. This difference is caused by the hormonal potency of the latter compound in Beagle dogs which is 30 to over 100 times higher than that of the 19-nortestosterone derivatives (Hill and co-workers, 1970; Neumann and Gräf, 1979).

If one compares these data with the corresponding situation in human females, one finds an inverse relationship. Most of the 19-nortestosterone derivatives are more active with respect to the endometrial transformatory potency than the 17α-hydroxy-progesterone derivatives (Neumann and Gräf, 1979).

The 10 to 25-fold therapeutic human daily dose of chlormadinone acetate administered to dogs in long-term trials, equalled - concerning the gestagen activity - the 450 and 1125-fold pharmacodynamically effective dose.

As opposed to the dog, an enhanced risk to develop mammary gland tumors could not be substantiated for women using oral contraceptives for long periods of time. On the contrary, progestagen-estrogen combinations were even thought to be protective against the development of proliferative breast diseases.

This example shows that species-specific differences in receptor sensitivities, and the neurohumal control mechanisms have also to be taken into account when toxicological findings are extrapolated from one species to another, especially to man.

Species differences in anatomy and physiology

Species differences in anatomy and physiology can also be the cause of false positive or false negative results of long-term as well as reproductive toxicity studies.

Some antibiotics, e.g. cephalosporins, can have an embryotoxic effect in certain species as a consequence of insufficient specificity. The cephalosporins such as cefazedone do not have a teratogenic action in mice and rats. In rabbits, on

the other hand, cefazedone produces abortions and fetal resorptions already in human therapeutic daily doses (50 mg/kg).
These are caused by the typhlitis following the displacement
of the mainly gram-positive intestinal flora in rabbits by
gram-negative coliform bacteriae.

It is impossible to reproduce these effects of cephalosporins
in man with his physiologically gram-negative intestinal
flora. One must conclude that rabbits are not suitable for
reproduction toxicological studies of cephalosporins (Fritz,
1978; Frohberg and co-workers, 1979).

Species differences due to the absence of preexisting pathologic conditions

Studies with antidiabetics during pregnancy may serve as
an example for species differences due to the absence of
preexisting pathologic conditions.

The fact that on the one hand embryonic damage was prevented
by giving insulin and oral antidiabetics to pregnant diabetics
and that on the other hand malformations were caused in pregnant schizophrenics by insulin shock therapy lead to the assumption that hypoglycemic states may be embryotoxic themselves. For this reason the many positive teratogenicity
trials performed with compounds lowering the blood sugar in
healthy laboratory animals are not relevant for the clinical
use of such drugs in diabetic women, as it is the aim of an
insulin or oral antidiabetics therapy to put the patient into
a euglycemic state and maintain him/her there (Baeder, 1978).

Immunotoxicology

Chronic exposure to certain environmental chemicals or drugs
can affect the immune system and lead to immunodeficiency or
immunosuppression, systemic immunostimulation or autoimmune
diseases. Allergic or sensitization reactions occur only in a
few of all the people exposed to a drug, independent of the
dose. But on the whole they present the largest group of drug-
related side effects, as several hundred drugs are known to
possess the potential of producing hypersensitivity reactions
in specially disposed cases. Strong reactive skin sensitizing
compounds, such as phenylhydrazine, paraphenyldiamine, dini-
trochlorophenol, dinitrotoluol can be recognized as such in
animal experiments. Weak skin sensitizers like ethyl- and
isopropyl alcohol which in very few cases produce an allergic
contact dermatitis, cannot be recorded in animal experiments.

Specific immunotoxicity testing was performed only rarely (Vos,
1977; Seinen and Penninks, 1979). To the present day it has
only been possible in individual cases to establish the causal
relationship of immunogically induced side effects of drugs.

Agents used in cancer chemotherapy like alkylating compounds,
antimetabolites and actinomycin have immunosuppressive properties. Chemicals with known immunotoxic effects include dioxin,
PCB, PBB, heavy metals, organometals. In addition, many drugs
are incriminated in producing blood dyscrasia through an al-
leged immunologic mechanism. Examples are aplastic anemia by

chloramphenicol, gold salts, phenylbutazone, phenothiazines, penicillin, PAS, sulfonamides and sulfonylureas and the different groups of immune drug-induced hemolytic anemiae, namely the immune complex type by PAS, INH, sulfonamides, phenacetin and rifampicine, the passive hemagglutination type caused by penicillin, cephalosporins, and the autoimmune type caused by methyldopa, chlorpromazine, and perhaps captoprile (Dean and co-workers, 1979; Miescher and Miescher, 1978).

How difficult it can be to establish the causal relationship of immunologically induced side effects is shown by the example of practolol. To this day it has not been possible to say with certainty whether the immunologic changes observed in individual patients given practolol are a secondary effect of the organ changes produced by this compound or whether these organ changes were caused primarily by a change in the immune status induced by practolol.

This situation demonstrates that one should watch out for possible immunologic dysfunction when performing toxicity trials. This might become feasible by the tier approach of Wachsmuth (1981).

First indications of possible immunotoxic reactions are changes in organ weight and histological alterations of the lymphatic tissue, changes in the absolute number of leukocytes and increase in the absolute ß- and γ-globulin concentrations.

If this tier 1 gives any indication of an immunological dysfunction, in tier 2 special immunological investigations in serum and red blood cells as well as special histochemical investigations in the potential target organs (lymph nodes, kidney and liver) are essential.

As the number of immunologic changes in man caused by exogenic factors is ever increasing, the tier approach proposed by Wachsmuth (1981) should be applied on a broad basis with all chemicals suspected to cause such changes, because an intensification of the immunotoxicological research with the objective of recording immunologic changes by relatively simple methods at an early stage in the performance of toxicity studies seems to be urgently required.

REFERENCES

Baeder, C. (1978). Einfluß der Hypoglykämie auf die Embryonal-
    entwicklung. In. B. Schnieders, G. Stille, and
    P. Grosdanoff (Eds.), Embryotoxikologische Probleme in
    der Arzneimittelforschung, AMI-Berichte 1/1978, Dietrich
    Reimer Verlag, Berlin. pp. 133-136.
von Bahr, C., C.-G. Groth, H. Jansson, G. Lundgren, M. Lind,
    and H. Glaumann (1980). Drug metabolism in human liver
    in vitro: Establishment of a human liver bank.
    Clin. Pharmacol. Ther., 27, 711-725.
Barrach, H.-J., and D. Neubert (1980). Significance of organ
    culture techniques for evaluation of prenatal toxicology.
    Arch. Toxicol., 45, 161-187.

Beck, F. (1981). Lessons from studies in animals for the evalu-
ation of human risk from teratogenic agents. In S. Ebashi
(Ed.), 8th International Congress of Pharmacology,
Pergamon Press, Oxford.
Bolt, H.M., J.G. Filser, R.J. Laib, and H. Ottenwälder (1980).
Binding kinetics of vinyl chloride and vinyl bromide at
very low doses. Arch. Toxicol., Suppl. 3, 129-142.
Brodie, B.B. (1962). Difficulties in extrapolating data on
metabolism of drugs from animal to man.
Clin. Pharmacol. Ther., 3, 374.
Buchter, A., H.M. Bolt, J. Filser, H.W. Görgens, R.J. Laib,
W. Bolt (1978). Pharmakokinetik und Karzinogenese von
Vinylchlorid: Arbeitsmedizinische Risikobeurteilung.
Verh. Dtsch. Ges. Arbeitsmedizin, 18, 111-124.
Buja, L.M., V.J. Ferrans, R.J. Mayer, W.C. Roberts, and
E.S. Henderson (1973). Cardiac ultrastructural changes
induced by daunorubicin therapy. Cancer, 32, 771-788.
Clemessen, J., and S. Hjalgrim-Jensen (1978). Is phenobarbital
carcinogenic? A follow-up of 3078 epileptics.
Ecotoxicol. Environm. Safety, 1, 457-470.
Clemessen, J., and S. Hjalgrim-Jensen (1980). Epidemiological
studies of medically used drugs. Arch. Toxicol.,
Suppl. 3, 19-25.
Davies, D.S. (1981). The rational interpretation of species
and strain differences in toxicity for the prediction of
risk to man: Introduction. In S. Ebashi (Ed.), 8th International Congress of Pharmacology, Pergamon Press, Oxford.
Dean, J.H., M.L. Padarathsingh, and T.R. Jerrells (1979). Assessment of immunobiological effects induced by chemicals,
drugs or food additives. I. Tier testing and screening
approach. Drug Chem. Toxicol., 2 (162), 5-17.
El Etreby, M.F., and K.-J. Gräf (1979). Effect of contracep-
tive steroids on mammary gland of beagle dog and its
relevance to human carcinogenicity.
Pharmac. Ther., 5, 369-402.
Fritz, H. (1978). Antibiotische Wirkung und teratogene Eigen-
schaften. In B. Schnieders, G. Stille, and P. Grosdanoff
(Eds.), Embryotoxikologische Probleme in der Arzneimittel-
forschung, AMI-Berichte 1/1978, Dietrich Reimer Verlag,
Berlin. pp. 141-144.
Frohberg, H. (1978). Embryotoxizität und Pharmakodynamie. In
B. Schnieders, G. Stille, and P. Grosdanoff (Eds.),
Embryotoxikologische Probleme in der Arzneimittel-
forschung, AMI-Berichte 1/1978, Dierich Reimer Verlag,
Berlin. pp. 115-126.
Frohberg, H., J. Gleich, H.D. Unkelbach (1979). Reproduction
toxicological studies on cefazedone.
Arzneim.-Forsch./Drug Res., 29(I), 2a, 419-423.
Gehring, P.J., P.G. Watanabe, and C.N. Park (1978). Resolu-
tion of dose-response toxicity for chemicals requiring
metabolic activation: Example - vinyl chloride.
Toxicol. Appl. Pharmacol. 44, 581-591.
Gehring, P.J., P.G. Watanabe, and C.N. Park (1979). Risk of
angiosarcoma in workers exposed to vinyl chloride as
predicted from studies in rats.
Toxicol. Appl. Pharmacol., 49, 15-21.

Gehring, P.J., J.C. Ramsey, and P.G. Watanabe (1981). Application of pharmacokinetics and metabolism in extrapolation of toxicological data from animals to man. Tokyo, 8th International Congress of Pharmacology, July 19-24, 1981. Japanese Pharmacological Society and Science Council of Japan, Abstracts, p. 27.

Goedde, H.W., D.P. Agarwal, and S. Harada (1980). Genetic studies on alcohol-metabolizing enzymes: Detection of isozymes in human hair roots. Enzyme, 25, 281-286.

Greim, H. (1979). Personal communication.

Henschler, D. (1977). Mechanismen der Aktivierung chlorierter aliphatischer Verbindungen - experimentelle Zugänge und klinische Bedeutung. Arzneim.-Forsch./Drug Res., 27(II), 9b, 1827-1832.

Hill, R., E. Averkin, W. Brown, W.E. Gagne, E. Segre (1970). Progestational potency of chlormadinone acetate in the immature beagle bitch: Preliminary report. Contraception, 2, 381-390.

Jaenke, R.S. (1974). An anthracycline antibiotic-induced cardiomyopathy in rabbits. Lab. Invest., 30, 292-304.

Koschier, F., and W.O. Berndt (1976). In vitro uptake of organic ions by renal cortical tissue of rats treated acutely with 2,4,5-trichlorophenoxyacetic acid. Toxicol. Appl. Pharmacol., 35, 355-364.

Lefrak, E.A., J. Pitha, S. Rosenheim, and J.A. Gottlieb (1973). A clinicopathologic analysis of adriamycin cardiotoxicity. Cancer, 32, 302-314.

Miescher, P.A., and A. Miescher (1978). Immunologic drug-induced blood dyscrasias. Klin. Wschr., 56, 1-5.

Neubert, D. (1978). Bedeutung pharmakokinetischer Parameter für die Teratologie. In B. Schnieders, G. Stille, and P. Grosdanoff (Eds.), Embryotoxikologische Probleme in der Arzneimittelforschung, AMI-Berichte 1/1978, Dietrich Reimer Verlag, Berlin. pp. 83-88.

Neumann, F., and K.J. Gräf (1979). Some comparative endocrine-pharmacological aspects and their relevance in the interpretation of adverse drug effects. Pharmac.Ther., 5, 271-286.

Nishimura, H., and T. Tanimura (1976). Clinical aspects of the teratogenicity of drugs. Excerpta Medica, Amsterdam, Oxford.

Oesch, F., D. Raphael, H. Schwind, and H.R. Glatt (1977). Species differences in activating and inactivating enzymes related to the control of mutagenic metabolites. Arch. Toxicol., 39, 97-108.

Oesch, F. (1980). Species differences in activating and inactivating enzymes related to in vitro mutagenicity mediated by tissue preparations from these species. Arch. Toxicol., Suppl. 3, 179-194.

Olson, H.M., and C.C. Capen (1978). Chronic cardiotoxicity of doxorubicin (adriamycin) in the rat: Morphologic and biochemical investigations. Toxicol. Appl. Pharmacol., 44, 605-616.

Olson, H.M., D.M. Young, D.J. Prieur, A.F. Leroy, and R.L. Reagan (1974). Electrolyte and morphologic alterations of myocardium in adriamycin-treated rabbits. Amer. J. Pathol., 77, 439-450.

52   H. Frohberg

Reitz, R.H., P.J. Gehring, P.G. Watanabe, and C.N. Park (1979).
Carcinogenic risk estimation for chloroform: Incorpora-
tion of pharmacokinetic data.
Toxicol. Appl. Pharmacol., 48, A 148.

Sauerhoff, M.W., W.H. Braun, G.E. Blau, and P.J. Gehring
(1976). The dose-dependent pharmacokinetic profile of
2,4,5-trichlorophenoxy acetic acid following intravenous
administration to rats. Toxicol. Appl. Pharmacol., 36,
491-501.

Sjöqvist, F., C. von Bahr, and L. Bertilsson (1981). Genetic
variability in man as a complicating factor in the extrapolation of toxicological data from animals. In S. Ebashi
(Ed.), 8th International Congress of Pharmacology,
Pergamon Press, Oxford.

Seinen, W., and A. Penninks (1979). Immune suppression as a
consequence of a selective cytotoxic activity of certain
organometallic compounds on thymus and thymus-dependent
lymphocytes. N.Y. Acad. Sci., 320, 499-517.

Sugimura, T. (1981). The rationalization of the interpretation
of animal carcinogenesis experiments. In S. Ebashi (Ed.),
8th International Congress of Pharmacology, Pergamon
Press, Oxford.

Tuchmann-Duplessis (1978). Embryotoxische Eigenschaften zen-
tralwirksamer Pharmaka. In B. Schnieders, G. Stille, and
P. Grosdanoff (Eds.), Embryotoxikologische Probleme in
der Arzneimittelforschung, AMI-Berichte 1/1978, Dierich
Reimer Verlag, Berlin. pp. 137-140.

Vos, J.G. (1977). Immune suppression as related to toxicology.
Crit. Rev. Toxicol., 5, 67-101.

Wachsmuth, E.D. (1981). The potential value of immunopathology
in toxicity studies. In S. Ebashi (Ed.), 8th International
Congress of Pharmacology, Pergamon Press, Oxford.

Young, J.D., and P.J. Gehring (1975). The dose-dependent fate
of 1,4-dioxane in male rats.
Toxicol. Appl. Pharmacol., 33, 183.

Young, J.D., W.H. Braun, J.E. LeBeau, and P.J. Gehring (1976a).
Saturated metabolism as the mechanism for the dose-depen-
dent fate of 1,4-dioxane in rats.
Toxicol. Appl. Pharmacol., 37, 138

Young, J.D., W.H. Braun, P.J. Gehring, B.S. Horvath, and
R.L. Daniel (1976b). 1,4-Dioxane and ß-hydroxyethoxy-
acetic acid excretion in urine of humans exposed to
dioxane vapors. Toxicol. Appl. Pharmacol., 38, 643-646.

Young, D.M. (1975). Pathologic effects of adriamycin
(NSC-123127) in experimental systems. Cancer
Chemother. Rep., 6, 159-175.

Zbinden, G., and E. Brändle (1975). Toxicological screening
of daunorubicin (NSC-82151), adriamycin (NSC-123127),
and their derivatives in rats. Cancer Chemother. Rep.,
59, 707-715.

Zbinden, G., R. Ettlin, and E. Bachmann (1980). Electro=
cardiographic changes in rats during chronic treatment
with antidepressant and neuroleptic drugs. Arzneim.-
Forsch./Drug Res., 30(II), 10, 1709-1715.

SYMPOSIUM

Chemical Interactions Resulting in Liver and Kidney Injury

Chairmen: J. B. Hook, G. L. Plaa

Ethanol Potentiation of Liver Injury

O. Strubelt

Institut für Toxikologie der Medizinischen Hochschule Lübeck,
D-2400 Lübeck, Federal Republic of Germany

ABSTRACT

Our present knowledge concerning the interactions between ethanol and other hepatotoxic agents is reviewed. Ethanol potentiates the effects of many but not of all hepatotoxic substances. Not only high doses of ethanol but also the moderate amounts commonly consumed today by many people are active in this respect. An induction, or activation, of the microsomal drug metabolizing system is the main cause of ethanol-induced potentiation of liver injury. In the case of CCl_4, a hypermetabolism-induced hepatic hypoxia may also be implicated in the enhanced hepatotoxic response after ethanol treatment. Changes in the overall pharmacokinetics of the hepatotoxins, depletion of hepatic glutathione and metabolization of ethanol to acetaldehyde are not implicated in ethanol potentiation of liver injury. Ethanol-consuming persons run a higher risk in being injured by hepatotoxic agents than abstinent persons, and interactions with other hepatotoxic agents should be envisaged as a possible additional factor in ethanol-induced human liver damage.

KEYWORDS

Alcohol, ethyl; hepatitis, toxic; poisons; carbon tetrachloride; acetaminophen; biotransformation; mixed function oxidases; glutathione; hypoxia.

INTRODUCTION

Carbon tetrachloride

In the twenties, carbon tetrachloride (CCl_4) was commonly used for treatment of hookworm infestations, especially in the United States. Already the first reports on CCl_4 intoxication drew attention to the fact that CCl_4 was extremely toxic both for chronic alcoholic addicts and for those who drank ethanol immediately before or after treatment with the drug. Since then many experimental investigations in dogs, rabbits, rats and mice have confirmed the ability of ethanol to potentiate the hepatotoxic effects of CCl_4 (reviewed by Strubelt, 1980).

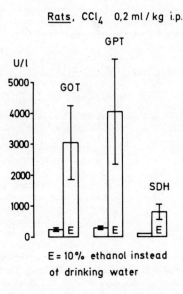

Rats, CCl₄ 0,2 ml / kg i.p.

E = 10 % ethanol instead
of drinking water

Fig. 1. Serum enzyme concentrations in rats 24 hr after treatment with CCl4.
Means ± S.E.M. from 4 animals each.

Ethanol potentiation of CCl4-induced liver injury can be easily and repro-
ducibly demonstrated by treating rats or mice 16 hr before CCl4 with a single
ethanol load ranging between 3 and 5 g/kg. Maximum blood ethanol levels produced by such doses in rats or mice do not exceed 2 mg/ml (Strubelt, Siegers
and Breining, 1974; Strubelt, Obermeier and Siegers, 1978) and thus are quite
within the range of blood ethanol levels reached in man after drinking sprees.
Furthermore, exposure of rats to 5 % or 10 % ethanol instead of drinking
water for only one week is also sufficient to potentiate the hepatotoxic response to CCl4 as evidenced by higher serum enzym levels 24 hr after CCl4
treatment (Fig. 1). In both the acute and the subacute treatment pattern ethanol alone does not display hepatotoxic effects (Strubelt, Obermeier and
Siegers, 1978; Strubelt and co-workers, 1978).

Other hepatotoxic agents

Ethanol-induced potentiation of liver injury is not only observed with CCl4,
but with many other hepatotoxic agents (Table 1). Ethanol, however, does not
produce a general hypersensitivity of the liver to toxic injury but a specific
one concerning many but not all hepatotoxic agents. The hepatotoxic activity
of α-amanitin even was found to be attenuated after pretreatment with ethanol
(Table 1).

TABLE 1   Influence on Hepatotoxicity of Pretreatment with Ethanol
(Animal Experiments)

Hepatotoxic Agent	Effect	First Reference
Carbon tetrachloride	+	Gardner and co-workers (1925)
Chloroform	+	Rosenthal (1930)
Trichloroethane	+	Klaassen and Plaa (1966)
Trichloroethylene	+	Cornish and Adefuin (1966)
Thioacetamide	+	Maling and co-workers (1975)
Dimethylnitrosamine	+	Maling and co-workers (1975)
Paracetamol	+	Strubelt, Obermeier and Siegers (1978)
Aflatoxin B_1	+	Glinsukon and co-workers (1978)
Chlorpromazine	+	Teschke, Stutz and Moreno (1980)
Cocaine	+	Smith, Freeman and Harbison (1981)
Galactosamine	(+)	Strubelt, Obermeier and Siegers (1978)
Allyl alcohol	(+)	Strubelt, Obermeier and Siegers (1978)
	Ø	Maling and co-workers (1975)
Bromobenzene	Ø	Maling and co-workers (1975)
Phalloidin	Ø	Strubelt, Obermeier and Siegers (1978)
Praseodymium	Ø	Strubelt, Obermeier and Siegers (1978)
α-Amanitin	-	Strubelt, Obermeier and Siegers (1978)

+ Increase   (+) Moderate Increase   Ø No Effect   - Decrease

MECHANISM(S) OF ACTION

Changes in the overall pharmacokinetics of the hepatotoxins

The concentrations in liver of CCl_4 and its metabolite, $CHCl_3$, were not affected significantly by pretreatment with 4 doses of 5 g/kg ethanol (measured
in rats 1 hr after treatment with CCl_4; Maling and co-workers, 1975). In own
experiments, no differences in the hepatic concentrations of CCl_4 and $CHCl_3$
were seen between rats provided with 10 % ethanol and the tap-water provided
controls (Table 2). A comparable result concerning the hepatic concentrations
of CCl_4 and $CHCl_3$ was gained in mice pretreated with an oral load of 4.8 g/kg
ethanol 16 hr before (not demonstrated). Furthermore, we measured the concentrations of ^{14}C derived from i.p. administered $^{14}CCl_4$ in 6 organs of the
rat and again did not find any changes induced by pretreatment with 10 %
ethanol in exchange for tap water (not demonstrated). The hepatic concentrations of paracetamol were even found to be lower in ethanol-fed rats than
controls (Sato, Matsuda and Lieber, 1981). All these pretreatment schemes,
however, were able to potentiate the hepatotoxic effects of CCl_4 or paracetamol. Thus there is no support for the hypothesis that changes in the over-
all-pharmacokinetics (i. e. absorption, distribution, elimination) of the
hepatotoxic agents might account for ethanol potentiation of liver injury.

Enhanced microsomal production of reactive metabolites

An increased activity of the microsomal mixed-function oxidase system was
seen repeatedly after acute or chronic ethanol administration (for references
cf. Strubelt, 1980). This seems to be the main cause of ethanol-induced potentiation of liver injury since most of the hepatotoxic agents the action of
which is potentiated by ethanol are known to be metabolized in the liver to
toxic metabolites. A direct confirmation of this hypothesis has been

TABLE 2   Hepatic Concentrations of CCl_4 and $CHCl_3$ [1]

Pretreatment [2]	Time [3] (h)	CCl_4 [4] μg/g	$CHCl_3$ [4] μg/g
Water	1	53.1 ± 19.8	6.87 ± 1.42
Ethanol 10 %	1	32.0 ± 9.7	4.08 ± 1.32
Water	2	36.5 ± 7.1	4.24 ± 0.69
Ethanol 10 %	2	30.1 ± 12.1	3.64 ± 0.62
Water	4	6.3 ± 1.0	1.06 ± 0.16
Ethanol 10 %	4	5.1 ± 1.6	1.18 ± 0.33

[1] GC/MS-head space analysis with 13-C compounds as internal standard (Pentz and co-workers, unpublished).

[2] Male Wistar rats were provided with 10 % ethanol in exchange for tap water for 7 - 9 days.

[3] After administration of 0.2 ml/kg CCl_4 i.p.

[4] Means ± S.E.M. of 6 investigations each.

established for CCl_4 and paracetamol by the following results:

1. Chronic ethanol feeding in rats (36 % of total calories) increased the in vitro-covalent binding of [14]CCl_4 metabolites to hepatic microsomal protein, accelerated the in vitro-biotransformation of CCl_4 to CO_2 (Hasumura, Teschke and Lieber, 1974) and enhanced the covalent binding of paracetamol to microsomal protein both in vitro and in vivo (Sato, Matsuda and Lieber, 1981).

2. Subacute pretreatment of rats with four doses of ethanol increased the in vitro-covalent binding of [14]CCl_4 to liver microsomal protein and the in vivo-binding of [14]CCl_4 to liver lipid and protein (Maling and co-workers, 1975).

3. 30 % ethanol in the drinking water for 6 - 8 weeks enhanced the cytochrome P-450 dependent activation of paracetamol (measured as glutathione conjugate formation) in isolated hepatocytes threefold (Moldeus and co-workers, 1980); 10 % ethanol in the drinking water for 3 weeks increased the in vitro-covalent binding of reactive metabolites of paracetamol to hepatic microsomal protein (Peterson and co-workers, 1980).

4. Pretreatment of mice with one oral dose of 4.8 g/kg ethanol even suffices to enhance the in vivo-covalent binding of [14]CCl_4 and ^{3}H-paracetamol to liver microsomal protein by 110 and 50 %, respectively (Table 3).

Depletion of hepatic glutathione

High doses of ethanol may decrease the concentration of hepatic glutathione (Estler and Ammon, 1966; MacDonald, Dow and Moore, 1977; Vina and co-workers, 1980). This effect, however, only lasts for 6 - 8 hr (Videla and co-workers, 1980) and thus has vanished when ethanol-induced potentiation of liver injury is maximal (18 hr after ethanol; Traiger and Plaa, 1971). Furthermore, we did

TABLE 3   Effect of Pretreatment with Ethanol[1] on the _in vivo_ Covalent
Binding of [14]CCl$_4$ and ^{3}H-Paracetamol to Liver Microsomal Protein
in Mice

Hepatotoxic Agent	Protein Binding[4] (nmoles/g liver)	
	Water-pretreatment	Ethanol-pretreatment
[14]CCl$_4$ [2]	9.72 ± 0.89	20.37 ± 3.0 *
[3]H-Paracetamol [3]	2.20 ± 0.02	3.30 ± 0.06 *

[1] 4.8 g/kg p.o., 16 hr before administration of the hepatotoxic agent.

[2] 0.02 ml/kg (10 µCi/mouse), 4 hr prior to sacrifice.

[3] 300 mg/kg (15 µCi/mouse), 4 hr prior to sacrifice.

[4] Covalently bound radioactive material to total liver protein.

* $P < 0.05$.

not find any decrease of liver GSH in mice 16 hr after 4.8 g/kg ethanol
though there was a clearcut increase in the hepatotoxic response to CCl$_4$ and
other agents (Strubelt, Obermeier and Siegers, 1978).

As shown in Fig. 1, exposition of rats to 10 % ethanol instead of drinking
water strongly enhances CCl$_4$ hepatotoxicity. Hepatic glutathione levels,
however, were the same in control and ethanol-treated rats before CCl$_4$ administration (Fig. 2). After treatment with CCl$_4$ some decrease in hepatic
GSH was noted in the ethanol-treated mice; however, this is not the cause
but the consequence of ethanol-induced potentiation of liver injury. Comparable results in mice were reported recently by Peterson and co-workers
(1980).

GSH-depletion therefore cannot be the cause of ethanol-induced potentiation
of liver injury.

Hepatic hypermetabolism and hypoxia

Treatment with ethanol was shown to produce an increase in the oxygen consumption of rat liver (Israel and co-workers, 1975a). This hypermetabolic
state was suggested to produce oxygen deficiency thereby explaining the development of ethanol-induced hepatic injury (Israel and co-workers, 1975b).
We have supposed that hepatic hypermetabolism might also be involved in ethanol potentiation of liver injury since hypoxemia or hepatic hypermetabolism
were shown to increase CCl$_4$ hepatotoxicity (Strubelt and Breining, 1980). To
test this hypothesis, the influence of hypermetabolism (induced by administration of 2,4-dinitrophenol) and hypoxia (induced by exposure to a reduced
oxygen tension) on the hepatotoxic effects of 5 agents was investigated in
rats (Table 4). No general correlation, however, was found between the
changes in hepatotoxicity induced by ethanol on the one hand and those observed after DNP or hypoxia on the other hand. Hepatic hypermetabolism or
hepatic hypoxia therefore cannot be the general pathogenic mechanism responsible for ethanol potentiation of liver injury although they may be implicated in the increased response to CCl$_4$ (presumably due to an enhanced
metabolic activation of CCl$_4$; Reiner and co-workers, 1972).

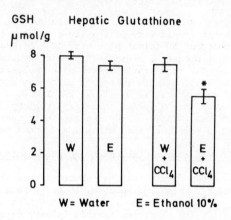

Fig. 2. Hepatic glutathione in rats provided with water (W) or 10 % ethanol
(E) instead of drinking water. CCl$_4$ (0.2 ml/kg i.p.) was given 2 hr
prior to determinations. Means ± S.E.M. from 6 animals each.
* P < 0.05.

TABLE 4   Influence on Hepatotoxicity [a]

Hepatotoxic Agent	Additional Treatment [b]		
	Ethanol	6 % O$_2$	DNP
CCl$_4$	+	+	+
Paracetamol	+	∅	+
Thioacetamide	+	−	∅
Allylalcohol	(+)	∅	∅
Brombenzene	∅	∅	∅

+ Increase   (+) Moderate Increase   ∅ No Effect
− Decrease

[a] According to Strubelt, Obermeier and Siegers (1978),
   Strubelt and Breining (1980) and Strubelt (1981)

[b] 2,4-Dinitrophenol 20 mg/kg s.c.

Lipid peroxidation

As shown independently in two investigations, pretreatment with ethanol does
not consistently augment CCl$_4$-induced hepatic lipid peroxidation (Maling and
co-workers, 1975; Lindstrom and Anders, 1978). Unpublished work done in our
laboratory confirmed these findings. Bromotrichloromethan, on the other hand,
was found to promote malondialdehyde production in hepatocytes from ethanol-
drinking rats to a higher extent than in cells from control animals (Remmer,
Albrecht and Kappus, 1977).

Interrelations between hepatotoxic agents and ethanol

On account of our present knowledge it can be taken for granted that ethanol consumption increases the sensitivity of the liver to many toxic agents. On the other hand, pretreatment of guinea pigs with CCl_4 or D-galactosamine enhances the hepatotoxic response to ethanol (Strubelt, Buettner and Siegers, 1975). Furthermore, hepatic regeneration after both D-galactosamine intoxication and partial hepatectomy is inhibited by acute and chronic ethanol intoxication (Wands and co-workers, 1979). These results show that ethanol may be more toxic for a previously diseased than for a healthy liver. Thus a mutual exacerbation of hepatotoxicity may contribute to the hepatic damage occurring after combined treatment with ethanol and other hepatotoxic agents.

The latency period between ethanol treatment and potentiation of liver injury

Potentiation of CCl_4 hepatotoxicity was not observed when ethanol was given only two hr before CCl_4 (Cornish and Adefuin, 1966). A peak potentiating response occurs when the ethanol treatment preceeds the CCl_4 challenge by 18 hr (Traiger and Plaa, 1971). The existence of this latency period led to the suggestion that the metabolization of ethanol to acetaldehyde might be involved in the potentiation of CCl_4 liver injury (Traiger and Plaa, 1971). This hypothesis, however, cannot be held on account of the fact that inhibition of ethanol metabolism by treatment with pyrazol did not decrease but enhanced ethanol-induced potentiation of CCl_4 hepatotoxicity and that acetaldehyde itself did not influence CCl_4-induced liver damage (Traiger and Plaa, 1971).

As shown by Pennington, Smith and Tapscott (1978), the increase in liver cytochrome P-450 content after a single ethanol dose does not occur immediately but after a latency period of 6 hr. Furthermore, the maximum increase in aniline hydroxylation after an acute dose of ethanol occurred at 24 hr (Powis, 1975). The time lag between ethanol treatment and potentiation of liver injury can thus be taken as a further proof for the thesis that an induction of the microsomal drug-metabolizing system accounts for ethanol potentiation of liver injury.

In this context it must be mentioned that the simultaneous administration of ethanol and a hepatotoxic agent may even decrease liver injury. This was demonstrated for paracetamol by Wong and co-workers (1980) and for vinylidene chloride by Heidbüchel and Younes (1981). In both investigations the decrease in hepatotoxicity was accompanied by an inhibition of the biotransformation of the hepatotoxic substances which is due to the fact that the acute action of ethanol on the hepatic microsomal drug-metabolism system is an inhibitory one (Rubin and co-workers, 1970). Thus the ingestion of ethanol may acutely eliminate an accelerated drug metabolism and also an enhancement of hepatotoxicity resulting from chronic ethanol consumption.

CLINICAL IMPLICATIONS

These are twofold. First, chronic ethanol consumption can increase the liver injury induced by many hepatotoxic agents. Thus chronic alcoholics have developed severe liver failure after ingesting paracetamol in doses which are innocuous for "non-induced" persons not drinking ethanol (Wright and Prescott, 1973; Barker, de Carle and Anuras, 1977; Goldfinger and co-workers, 1978; McClain and co-workers, 1980). It must be stressed that in most of these cases hepatotoxicity was the consequence of ingesting paracetamol for therapeutic reasons and not as a suicide attempt: this must be borne in mind when prescribing potential hepatotoxic drugs to persons regularly abusing (or only

consuming) ethanol. Second, since alcoholism is often accompanied by drug abuse and many drugs possess a hepatotoxic potential, an enhanced hepatotoxic
response to those agents may, at least partially, contribute to ethanol-induced liver damage.

ACKNOWLEDGEMENTS

The unpublished experimental results from our laboratory mentioned in this
paper were gained in cooperation with R. Pentz, M. Younes, Uta Preuß and
J. G. Dreckmann. In am very much indebted to Mrs. Edith Strelow for excellent
preparation of the manuscript.

REFERENCES

Barker, J. D., jr., D. J. de Carle and S. Anuras (1977). Chronic excessive
acetaminophen use and liver damage. Ann. Intern. Med., 87, 299-301.
Cornish, H. H., and J. Adefuin (1966). Ethanol potentiation of halogenated
aliphatic solvent toxicity. Amer. industr. Hyg. Ass. J. 27, 57-61.
Estler, C.-J., and H. P. T. Ammon (1966). Glutathion und SH-gruppenhaltige
Enzyme in der Leber weißer Mäuse nach einmaliger Alkoholgabe.
Med. Pharmacol. exp. 15, 299-306.
Gardner, G., R. Grove, R. Gustafson, E. Maire, M. Thompson, H. Wells and
P. Lamson (1925). Studies on the pathological histology of experimental
carbon tetrachloride poisoning. Bull. Johns Hopk. Hosp. 36, 107-133.
Glinsukon, T., S. Taycharpirpranai and C. Toskulkao (1978). Aflatoxin B$_1$
hepatotoxicity in rats pretreated with ethanol. Experientia (Basel) 34,
869-870.
Goldfinger, R., K. S. Ahmed, C. S. Pitchumoni and S. A. Weseley (1978).
Concomitant alcohol and drug abuse enhancing acetaminophen toxicity.
Amer. J. Gastroenterol. 70, 385-388.
Hasumura, Y., R. Teschke and C. Lieber (1974). Increased carbon tetrachloride
hepatotoxicity, and its mechanism, after chronic ethanol consumption.
Gastroenterol. 66, 415-422.
Heidbüchel, K., and M. Younes (1981). Altered hepatotoxicity and metabolism
of vinylidene chloride in rats following treatment with ethanol, dithio-
carb or (+)-catechin. Arch. Pharmacol. 316, Suppl., R 22.
Israel, Y., L. Videla, V. Fernandez-Videla and J. Bernstein (1975a). Effects
of chronic ethanol treatment and thyroxine administration on ethanol metabolism and liver oxidative capacity. J. Pharmacol. exp. Ther. 192, 565-574).
Israel, Y., H. Kalant, H. Orrego, J. M. Khanna, L. Videla and J. M. Phillips
(1975b). Experimental alcohol-induced hepatic necrosis: supression by
propylthiouracil. Proc. nat. Acad. Sci. (Wash.) 72, 1137-1141.
Klaassen, C. D., and G. L. Plaa (1966). Relative effects of various chlorinated hydrocarbons on liver and kidney function in mice. Toxicol. appl.
Pharmacol. 9, 139-151 .
Lindstrom, T. D., and M. W. Anders (1978). Effect of agents known to alter
carbon tetrachloride hepatotoxicity and cytochrome p-450 levels on carbon
tetrachloride-stimulated lipid peroxidation and ethane expiration in the
intact rat. Biochem. Pharmacol. 27, 563-567.
MacDonald, C. M., J. Dow and M. R. Moore (1977). A possible protective role
for sulphydryl compounds in acute alcoholic liver injury.
Biochem. Pharmacol. 26, 1529-1531.
Maling, H. M., B. Stripp, I. G. Sipes, B. Highman, W. Saul and M. A. Williams
(1975). Enhanced hepatotoxicity of carbon tetrachloride, thioacetamide, and
dimethylnitrosamine by pretreatment of rats with ethanol and some comparisons with potentiation by isopropanol. Toxicol. appl. Pharmacol. 33, 291-308.

McClain, C. J., J. P. Kromhout, F. J. Peterson and J. L. Holtzman (1980).
Potentiation of acetaminophen hepatotoxicity by alcohol.
J. Amer. Med. Ass. 244, 251-253 (1980).

Moldeus, P., B. Andersson, A. Norling and K. Ormstad (1980). Effect of
chronic ethanol administration on drug metabolism in isolated hepatocytes
with emphasis on paracetamol activation. Biochem. Pharmacol. 29, 1741-1745.

Pennington, S. N., C. P. Smith and E. B. Tapscott (1978). Effect of an acute
dose of ethanol on rat liver microsomal mixed function oxygenase components
and membrane lipid composition. Alcoholism 2, 311-316.

Peterson, F. J., D. E. Holloway, R. R. Erickson, P. H. Duquette,
C. J. McClain and J. L. Holtzman (1980). Ethanol induction of acetaminophen
toxicity and metabolism. Life Sciences 27, 1705-1711.

Powis, G. (1975). Effect of a single oral dose of methanol, ethanol and
propan-2-ol on the hepatic microsomal metabolism of foreign compounds in
the rat. Biochem. J. 148, 269-277.

Reiner, O., S. Athanassopoulos, K. H. Hellmer, R. E. Murray and H. Uehleke
(1972). Bildung von Chloroform aus Tetrachlorkohlenstoff in Lebermikro-
somen, Lipidperoxidation und Zerstörung von Cytochrom P-450.
Arch. Toxikol. 29, 219-233 (1972).

Remmer, H., D. Albrecht and H. Kappus (1977). Lipid peroxidation in isolated
hepatocytes from rats ingesting ethanol chronically.
Arch. Pharmacol. 298, 107-113.

Rosenthal, S. M. (1930). Some effects of alcohol on the normal and damaged
liver. J. Pharmacol. exp. Ther. 38, 291-301.

Rubin, E., H. Gang, P. S. Misra and C. S. Lieber (1970). Inhibition of drug
metabolism by acute ethanol intoxication. Amer. J. Med. 49, 801-806.

Sato, C., Y. Matsuda and C. S. Lieber (1981). Increased hepatotoxicity of
acetaminophen after chronic ethanol consumption in the rat.
Gastroenterol. 80, 140-148.

Smith, A. C., R. W. Freeman and R. D. Harbison (1981). Ethanol enhancement
of cocaine-induced hepatotoxicity. Biochem. Pharmacol. 30, 453-458.

Strubelt, O. (1980). Interactions between ethanol and other hepatotoxic
agents. Biochem. Pharmacol. 29, 1445-1449 (1980).

Strubelt, O. (1981). Influence of 2,4-dinitrophenol on the susceptibility
of rats to hepatotoxic injury. Toxicol. Lett., in press.

Strubelt, O., and H. Breining (1980). Influence of hypoxia on the hepatotoxic effects of carbon tetrachloride, paracetamol, allyl alcohol,
bromobenzene and thioacetamide. Toxicol. Lett. 6, 109-113.

Strubelt, O., F. Buettner and C.-P. Siegers (1975). The hepatotoxic effect
of ethanol after pretreatment with carbon tetrachloride, allyl alcohol,
or d-galactosamine. Arch. Pharmacol. 287, Suppl., R 102.

Strubelt, O., F. Obermeier and C.-P. Siegers (1978). The influence of ethanol
pretreatment on the effects of nine hepatotoxic agents.
Acta pharmacol. (Kbh.) 43, 211-218.

Strubelt, O., F. Obermeier, C.-P. Siegers and M. Völpel (1978). Increased
carbon tetrachloride hepatotoxicity after low-level ethanol-consumption.
Toxicology 10, 261-270.

Strubelt, O., C.-P. Siegers and H. Breining (1974). Comparative study of the
absorption, elimination and acute hepatotoxic action of ethanol in guinea
pigs and rats. Arch. Toxicol. 32, 83-95.

Teschke, R., G. Stutz and F. Moreno (1980). Cholestasis following chronic
alcohol consumption. Enhancement after an acute dose of chlorpromazine.
Biochem. Biophys. Res. Commun. 49, 1013-1019.

Traiger, G. J., and G. L. Plaa (1971). Differences in the potentiation of
carbon tetrachloride in rats by ethanol and isopropanol pretreatment.
Toxicol. appl. Pharmacol. 20, 105-112.

Videla, L. A., V. Fernandez, G. Ugarte, A. Valenzuela and A. Vellanueva
    (1980). Effect of acute ethanol intoxication on the content of reduced
    glutathione of the liver in relation to its lipoperoxidative capacity in
    the rat. FEBS Lett. 111, 6-10.
Vina, J., J. M. Estrela, C. Guerri and F. J. Romero (1980). Effect of
    ethanol on glutathione concentration in isolated hepatocytes.
    Biochem. J. 188, 549-552.
Wands, J. R., E. A. Carter, N. L. R. Bucher and K. J. Isselbacher (1979).
    Inhibition of hepatic regeneration in rats by acute and chronic ethanol
    intoxication. Gastroenterol. 77, 528-531.
Wong, L. T., L. W. Whitehouse, G. Solomonraj and C. J. Paul (1980). Effect
    of a concomitant single dose of ethanol on the hepatotoxicity and metabo-
    lism of acetaminophen in mice. Toxicology 17, 297-309.
Wright, N., and L. F. Prescott (1973). Potentiation by previous drug therapy
    of hepatotoxicity following paracetamol overdosage. Scot. med. J. 18,
    56-58.

Potentiation of Liver and Kidney Injury by Ketones and Ketogenic Substances

G. L. Plaa* and W. R. Hewitt**

*Département de pharmacologie, Faculté de médecine et Faculté des
études supérieures, Université de Montréal, Montréal, Québec,
Canada
**Department of Veterinary Anatomy-Physiology, College of
Veterinary Medicine, University of Missouri-Columbia, Columbia,
Missouri, USA

ABSTRACT

Various facets of the potentiation of haloalkane-induced liver and kidney injury by ketones or ketogenic chemicals have been pursued in mice and rats.
Chlordecone pretreatment produces a lateral shift in the dose-response curve
for $CHCl_3$ hepatotoxicity. With acetone, a threshold dosage for potentiation
is observed. The peak blood concentration values of acetone correlate well
with the degree of potentiation, whereas area-under-curve values are less satisfactory. Increasing the chain-length of a series of ketones (3 to 7 carbons) results in enhanced potentiation. The time interval between pretreatment and haloalkane challenge during which potentiation occurs is lengthened
with the following compounds: acetone < methyl ethyl ketone < methyl n-butyl ketone < 2,5-hexanedione. Chlordecone and acetone potentiate the liver
injury induced by some brominated methane derivatives. Cholestatic, as well
as necrogenic, liver injury can be potentiated. Acetone, methyl n-butyl ketone, 2,5-hexanedione, n-hexane and chlordecone can potentiate the nephrotoxic effect of $CHCl_3$. Increasing the chain-length of a series of ketones (3 to
7 carbons) results in enhanced potentiation. $^{14}CHCl_3$ binding data in liver
indicate that increased bioactivation plays an important role in the potentiation due to chlordecone, but other mechanisms may be involved.

KEYWORDS

Liver injury, kidney injury, chemical potentiation, ketones, haloalkanes,
chlordecone, chloroform, carbon tetrachloride.

INTRODUCTION

Many chemicals potentiate haloalkane hepatotoxicity (Zimmerman, 1978). Recent studies indicate that ketones (acetone, methyl n-butyl ketone, 2,5-hex-
anedione, chlordecone) and ketogenic chemicals (isopropanol, 2-butanol, n-hexane, 1,3-butanediol, alloxan) potentiate the acute necrogenic effects of
CCl_4 or $CHCl_3$ in mice or rats (Curtis and Mehendale, 1980; Curtis, Williams
and Mehendale, 1979; Hanasono, Côté and Plaa, 1975; Hewitt and Plaa, 1979;
Hewitt and co-workers, 1979, 1980a, 1980b; Traiger and Bruckner, 1976; Trai-

65

ger and Plaa, 1971, 1972).

Potentiation of haloalkane-induced nephrotoxicity has been less successful. Klaassen and Plaa (1966) showed that ethanol can increase $CHCl_3$ and 1,1,2-trichloroethane renal dysfunction in mice. Isobutyl and isoamyl alcohol potentiated $CHCl_3$ kidney injury, but isopropanol, n-propanol, sec-butanol and tert-butanol were devoid of activity (Watrous and Plaa, 1971). Mice fed polybrominated biphenyls were shown to be more susceptible to the nephrotoxic effects of $CHCl_3$, CCl_4, trichloroethylene and 1,1,2-trichloroethane (Kluwe and Hook, 1978; Kluwe, Herman and Hook, 1979). In mice, chlordecone exhibited a slight potentiating effect (Hewitt and co-workers, 1979). Potentiation of nephrotoxicity was observed with acetone, n-hexane, methyl n-butyl ketone and 2,5-hexanedione when these agents were given 18 hr before $CHCl_3$ (Hewitt and co-workers, 1980a). Thus, ketones appear to be able to potentiate nephrotoxicity as well as hepatotoxicity.

DOSE-RESPONSE CONSIDERATIONS

Theoretically, potentiation of CCl_4 or $CHCl_3$ hepatotoxicity could manifest itself in several different ways: (1) the dose-response curve is shifted to the left, but remains parallel; (2) the curve is not shifted laterally, but the slope becomes steeper; (3) the curve is shifted to the left and the slope is altered. Of course, more complex dose-response relationships are feasible (biphasic, curvilinear, etc.).

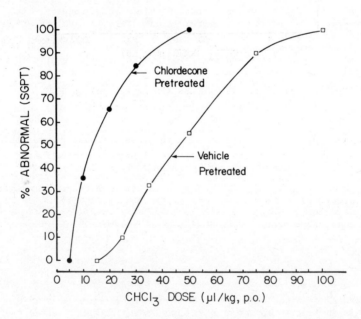

Fig. 1.   Percentage of mice exhibiting $CHCl_3$-induced hepatotoxicity following pretreatment with vehicle or chlordecone (50 mg/kg, po).

In mice, chlordecone pretreatment (50 mg/kg, po) shifts the $CHCl_3$ dose-response curve laterally (Fig. 1), when one uses elevation in plasma GPT or OCT activity as the index of liver injury. Analysis of the log dose-probit curves indicated that they were parallel to each other. We have calculated ED50 values for $CHCl_3$ under these conditions. Using GPT as the index, the following ED50 values were obtained: vehicle-treated, 43 (35-50) μl/kg; chlordecone-treated, 13 (10-17) μl/kg; potency ratio, 3.2 (1.3-7.8). Using OCT as the index, the ED50 values were: vehicle-treated 235 (184-301) μl/kg; chlordecone-treated, 28 (20-43) μl/kg; potency ratio, 8.3 (5.3-12.8).

The same type of relationship is observed if the elevation of GPT enzyme activity is plotted versus the $CHCl_3$ dosage in mice (Fig. 2). The dose-response curve was shifted to the left in the chlordecone-treated animals.

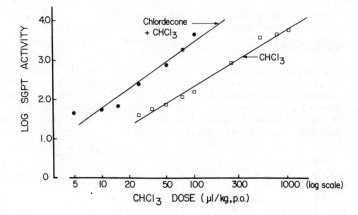

Fig. 2.   Effect of chlordecone (50 mg/kg, po) on SGPT dose-response curves for $CHCl_3$ in mice.

Up to now, the discussion has dealt with the dose-response relationship associated with the haloalkane component of the interacting pair of chemicals. Dose-response relationships can also be established for the potentiating agent. In this situation the dosages of the agent are varied and a fixed challenge dosage of the haloalkane is administered. A clear dose-response relationship has been observed with 1,3-butanediol potentiation of CCl_4 (Hewitt and co-workers, 1980b). With isopropanol-CCl_4 and acetone-CCl_4, these characteristics have been described (Plaa and Traiger, 1973).

Using acetone-CCl_4 we demonstrated that a minimally effective dosage and a noneffective dosage could be established in laboratory animals (Plaa and co-workers, 1981). This permitted us to demonstrate that a threshold blood concentration of acetone does exist, below which potentiation of CCl_4 does not occur. Pharmacokinetic data determined with acetone and CCl_4 support the threshold concept and indicate that the maximal blood concentration (Cpmax), rather than the area-under-the-curve (AUC), is a critical parameter. The data summarized in Table 1 illustrate this situation when the acetone pretreatment regimen was varied. The hepatotoxic response to the CCl_4 challenge was compared to the Cpmax and AUC values.

G. L. Plaa and W. R. Hewitt

TABLE 1   Effect of Various Acetone Pretreatment Regimens
on CCl_4 Hepatotoxicity: Cpmax and AUC Values[*]

Treatment Regimen	GPT	Cpmax	AUC
1.5 ml/kg (infused over 3 days)	65	130	9346
2.5 ml/kg (infused over 3 days)	90	158	11347
1.5 ml/kg (12 divided doses over 3 days)	144	148	4989
1.5 ml/kg (6 divided doses over 3 days)	247	194	6884
6.5 ml/kg (infused over 3 days)	707	763	62122
1.5 ml/kg (single bolus dose)	2588	853	9609

[*]Rats were given CCl_4 (0.1 ml/kg, ip) 18 hr after termination of pretreatment regimen. Rats were killed 24 hr after CCl_4. Units: GPT, U/ml; Cpmax, µg/ml; AUC, µg. hr/ml.

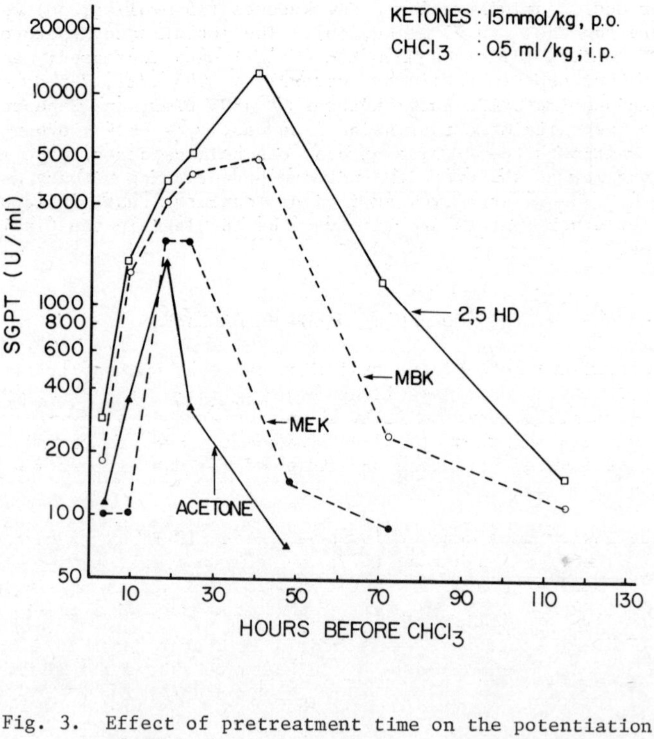

Fig. 3.   Effect of pretreatment time on the potentiation of $CHCl_3$ hepatotoxicity by various ketones in rats.

TIME INTERVAL AND POTENTIATION

The interval of time between the pretreatment and the haloalkane challenge
is another parameter that merits consideration. Unfortunately it has not
been established with all the potentiating agents that we have studied.
Traiger and Plaa (1971) did characterize this parameter with isopropanol-
CCl_4. More recently we investigated this relationship in rats with acetone,
methyl ethyl ketone, methyl n-butyl ketone and 2,5-hexanedione, using $CHCl_3$
as the haloalkane. The data in Fig.3 indicate that the time interval during
which the potentiating interaction could occur increased as the chain-length
increased. It is particularly striking that with 2,5-hexanedione pretreatment, the animals remained more susceptible to $CHCl_3$ hepatotoxicity for up
to 4 days.

CHAIN-LENGTH AND POTENTIATION

The relative potentiating potency of a series of ketones, three to seven carbons in length, was evaluated in rats, with $CHCl_3$ as the haloalkane (Hewitt,
Brown and Plaa, 1981). Hepatotoxicity (elevated SGPT activity) was assessed
24 hr after $CHCl_3$ administration. The ketones (15 mmol/kg, po) were given
18 hr before the $CHCl_3$ (0.75 ml/kg, ip). The potentiated hepatotoxic response (SGPT activity) increased as the chain-length increased: acetone $\sim$
2000 U/ml; 2-butanone (methyl ethyl ketone), $\sim$ 3000 U/ml; 2-pentanone, $\sim$ 4000
U/ml; 2-hexanone (methyl n-butyl ketone), $\sim$ 4800 U/ml; and 2-heptanone, $\sim$
5500 U/ml. The calculated regression line was: y = -636 + 876 x (r = 0.44;
p < 0.05). Although the r-value at best can be considered to be moderate, a
positive correlation was exhibited between potentiating potency and increased
chain-length. The relatively weak r-value indicates that, while chain-length
plays a role, other factors are likely to be involved in the final potentiated response.

HEPATOTOXICITY INDUCED BY OTHER HALOALKANES

In mice, isopropanol potentiates trichloroethylene, but not 1,1,1-trichloro-
ethane or 1,1,2-trichloroethane liver injury (Traiger and Plaa, 1974). However, 1,1,2-trichloroethane toxicity is potentiated in alloxan-diabetic rats
(Hanasono, Witschi and Plaa, 1975). Consequently, we are currently investigating the possible potentiating abilities of various ketones and ketogenic
substances on other haloalkanes.

Male Sprague-Dawley rats were orally pretreated (18-24 hr) with acetone
(3.75 and 7.5 mmol/kg), n-hexane (3.75 and 7.5 mmol/kg), methyl ethyl ketone
(3.75 and 7.5 mmol/kg), methyl n-butyl ketone (7.5 and 15 mmol/kg), or 2,5-
hexanedione (1.88 and 3.75 mmol/kg); 18 hr later they were orally challenged
with trichloroethylene (2.5 ml/kg), tetrachloroethylene (2.5 ml/kg), 1,1,1-
trichloroethane (2.5 ml/kg) or 1,1,2-trichloroethane (2.5 ml/kg). Hepatotoxicity was assessed 24 hr later using elevated plasma transaminase (GPT) activity. 1,1,2-Trichloroethane-induced hepatotoxicity was enhanced in rats
pretreated with n-hexane, methyl ethyl ketone or 2,5-hexanedione, but not
acetone or methyl n-butyl ketone. The hepatotoxic response to the other
three haloalkanes was unaffected by the pretreatments. Chlordecone pretreatment (50 mg/kg) did not potentiate these haloalkanes. Thus, with these haloalkanes, potentiation is relatively minimal.

With the brominated methanes, quite interesting results were obtained. Only
acetone and chlordecone have been tested. However, with both ketones, poten-

tiation of hepatotoxicity was observed (Table 2). This interaction is particularly striking since these haloalkanes (bromoform, dibromochloromethane and
bromodichloromethane) are weak hepatotoxicants; they are devoid of activity
when given acutely at near-lethal dosages to rats. The relative ranking of
the potentiations (bromodichloromethane > dibromochloromethane > bromoform)
that one sees in terms of GPT values also appears to be contrary to what one
would predict on the basis of relative potency as correlated with molecular
characteristics (Zimmerman, 1978). Klingensmith and Mehendale (1981) reported a similar observation after feeding chlordecone to rats. This observation warrants further investigation.

It has been suggested (Traiger and Plaa, 1974) that the degree of potentiation seems to be related to the hepatotoxic properties of the haloalkane involved. Our more recent results indicate that while this appears reasonable
for the chlorinated ethanes and ethylenes, one needs to be cautious in making a more widely applicable generalization.

TABLE 2   Potentiation of Brominated Trihalomethanes[*]

Pretreatment	Challenge Dose (ml/kg)		GPT Activity (U/ml)	
Vehicle	$BrCHCl_2$	(1.00)	72 ±	9
Acetone	$BrCHCl_2$	(0.25)	4398 ±	618
Acetone	$BrCHCl_2$	(0.50)	5154 ±	1428
Acetone	$BrCHCl_2$	(1.00)	2775 ±	888
Vehicle	Br_2CHCl	(1.00)	201 ±	86
Acetone	Br_2CHCl	(0.25)	1506 ±	721
Acetone	Br_2CHCl	(0.50)	521 ±	174
Acetone	Br_2CHCl	(1.00)	1511 ±	607
Vehicle	$BrCHCl_2$	(0.50)	76 ±	18
Chlordecone	$BrCHCl_2$	(0.10)	728 ±	187
Chlordecone	$BrCHCl_2$	(0.50)	2393 ±	610
Chlordecone (3x)	$BrCHCl_2$	(0.10)	1132 ±	556
Chlordecone (3x)	$BrCHCl_2$	(0.50)	3429 ±	953
Vehicle	Br_2CHCl	(0.50)	42 ±	9
Chlordecone	Br_2CHCl	(0.10)	347 ±	119
Chlordecone	Br_2CHCl	(0.50)	888 ±	125
Chlordecone (3x)	Br_2CHCl	(0.10)	103 ±	25
Chlordecone (3x)	Br_2CHCl	(0.50)	2500 ±	1421
Vehicle	Br_3CH	(0.50)	45 ±	6
Chlordecone	Br_3CH	(0.10)	70 ±	13
Chlordecone	Br_3CH	(0.50)	66 ±	7
Chlordecone (3x)	Br_3CH	(0.10)	52 ±	5
Chlordecone (3x)	Br_3CH	(0.50)	400 ±	128

[*]Rats received the haloalkane (po) 18 hr after the pretreatment. Animals were killed 24 hr later. Pretreatment (po) doses: acetone, 15 mmol/kg; chlordecone, 50
mg/kg; chlordecone (3x), 10 mg/kg/day for 3 days. Values are means ± SE.

POTENTIATION OF CHOLESTATIC REACTIONS

Recently, Curtis, Williams and Mehendale (1979) demonstrated that small dosages of CCl_4 (0.1 and 0.2 ml/kg, ip) caused a profound decrease in bile
flow, in addition to necrosis, in rats fed chlordecone (10 ppm) for 15 days.
This result is particularly striking since large dosages of CCl_4, given alone, do not exhibit marked cholestatic effects. This finding suggests that
such potentiating agents might possibly increase the sensitivity of laboratory animals, not only to necrotic, but also to cholestatic lesions. Using
1,3-butanediol-pretreated rats (10% 1,3-butanediol in drinking water for 7
days), de Lamirande and Plaa (1981) showed that the cholestatic properties
of taurolithocholic acid and a manganese-bilirubin combination were potentiated; neither of these cholestatic treatments resulted in necrosis. It was
also shown (de Lamirande and Plaa, 1981) that CCl_4 (0.10 ml/kg, ip) produced
a marked diminution in bile flow in rats pretreated with isopropanol (2.5
ml/kg, po, 18 hr before CCl_4); a large dosage of CCl_4 (1.0 ml/kg, ip), given
alone, failed to affect bile flow; the bile flows were as follows: Control,
11.24 ± 0.72; CCl_4 (0.1 ml/kg), 9.73 ± 0.61; CCl_4 (1.0 ml/kg), 9.24 ± 0.88;
and isopropanol ± CCl_4 (0.1 ml/kg), 4.32 ± 0.73 ml/kg. There are other indirect indications in the literature that cholestatic reactions can be potentiated following pretreatment with ketones or ketogenic substances. Plaa
and co-workers (1975) observed that the hyperbilirubinemic response to α-
naphthylisothiocyanate was enhanced after pretreatment with isopropanol or
acetone. Isopropanol pretreatment was also capable of elevating plasma bilirubin concentrations after CCl_4 (Traiger and Plaa, 1971); 1,3-butanediol pretreatment enhanced the hyperbilirubinemia seen after α-naphthylisothiocyanate (de Lamirande and Plaa, 1981). These data indicate that ketones or ketogenic chemicals can enhance cholestatic, as well as necrogenic, liver injury.

POTENTIATION OF NEPHROTOXICITY

In rats, chlordecone pretreatment 18 hr before the $CHCl_3$ challenge results in
potentiated nephrotoxicity 24 hr after $CHCl_3$, but mirex pretreatment does not
(Table 3). In these experiments (Hewitt and co-workers, 1981), kidney injury
was assessed using various parameters (depression of lactate-stimulated accumulation of p-aminohippurate by renal cortical slices, elevation of blood
urea nitrogen, and histologic evaluation). Table 3 also summarizes the
degree of potentiation of $CHCl_3$-induced nephrotoxicity observed after pretreatment with acetone, n-hexane, methyl n-butyl ketone and 2,5-hexanedione
previously reported by Hewitt and co-workers (1980a).

These data show that ketones and ketogenic chemicals can potentiate $CHCl_3$-
induced nephrotoxicity as well as hepatotoxicity. The relative potency of a
series of ketones, three to seven carbons in length, for the potentiation of
$CHCl_3$ kidney injury was evaluated in rats (Hewitt, Brown and Plaa, 1981).
The ketones (15 mmol/kg, po) were given 18 hr before a $CHCl_3$ challenge (0.75
ml/kg, ip). Nephrotoxicity was assessed on the basis of depressed p-aminohippurate tissue accumulation by renal cortical slices. The potentiated $CHCl_3$
nephrotoxic response (depressed PAH slice-to-medium ratio) increased as the
chain-length increased: acetone, ∿ 22; 2-butanone (methyl ethyl ketone), ∿
19; 2-pentanone, ∿ 16; 2-hexanone (methyl n-butyl ketone), ∿ 15; and 2-hepta-
none, ∿ 13. The calculated regression line was: $y = 28.3 - 2.28x$ ($r = 0.47$;
$p < 0.05$). A positive correlation between potentiating potency and increased
chain-length was exhibited. However, the relatively weak r-value indicates
that, while chain-length plays a role, other factors are likely to be involved in the final potentiated response.

TABLE 3　Effects of Various Pretreatments on $CHCl_3$-
Induced Nephrotoxicity in Rats[*]

Pretreatment	PAH S/M Ratio	BUN (mg/100 ml)	Abnormal Tubules (%)
Vehicle	26.2 ± 1.8	23 ± 2	42.4 ± 9.8
Mirex	25.8 ± 0.9	22 ± 2	49.8 ± 7.3
Chlordecone	15.8 ± 1.9	42 ± 3	74.4 ± 2.3
Vehicle	22.9 ± 1.1	16 ± 1	1.2 ± 0.6
Acetone	13.7 ± 1.6	30 ± 3	18.0 ± 2.6
n-Hexane	17.5 ± 2.2	24 ± 4	13.2 ± 3.2
Methyl n-butyl ketone	14.2 ± 3.1	71 ± 15	27.4 ± 5.5
2,5-Hexanedione	11.8 ± 3.1	47 ± 14	38.8 ± 11.2

[*]Rats received $CHCl_3$ (0.5 ml/kg, po) 18 hr after the pretreatment. Animals were killed 24 hr later. Pretreatment dosages: mirex and chlordecone (50 mg/kg, po);
acetone, n-hexane, methyl n-butyl ketone, and 2,5-hexan-
edione (15 mmol/kg, po).

MECHANISMS INVOLVED

The actual mechanisms of action involved in these various potentiations are
yet to be established. Since a considerable body of evidence indicates that
CCl_4 and $CHCl_3$ are bioactivated to toxic reactive metabolites (Cresteil and
co-workers, 1979; Pohl and co-workers, 1977; Recknagel and Glende, 1973; Zimmerman 1978), it has been natural to suppose that increased bioactivation is
the reason for the potentiation phenomenon; the increased bioactivation is
presumably linked to enhanced mixed function oxidase activity. With isopropanol and acetone potentiation, data exist that are consistent with such an
explanation (Côté, Traiger and Plaa, 1974; Maling and co-workers, 1974, 1975;
Sipes and co-workers, 1973; Traiger and Plaa, 1973). Using chlordecone,
Cianflone and co-workers (1980) demonstrated that in mice the potentiation
of $CHCl_3$ liver injury occurred under conditions in which the irreversible
binding of $^{14}CHCl_3$ to hepatic constituents was enhanced; in these same experiments, chlordecone did not alter hepatic glutathione content, nor did it
increase hepatic cytochrome P-450 concentrations. More recently Hewitt,
Hewitt and Plaa (1981) showed that in rats, chlordecone increased the irreversible binding of $^{14}CHCl_3$ to hepatic constituents, in a manner similar to
that observed in mice. Davis and Mehendale (1980), working with chlordecone-
pretreated rats, showed that hepatic and renal glutathione concentrations
were unaffected at varying times after chlordecone administration as well.
However, in their experiments chlordecone pretreatment did not enhance the
irreversible binding of $^{14}CCl_4$ to hepatic proteins and lipids, although potentiation of hepatotoxicity did occur.

The bulk of the evidence indicates that increased bioactivation of the haloalkane is a major element in the potentiation phenomenon. However, increased
reactivity of subcellular organelles to toxic metabolites remains as an additional possible mechanism of action. We have invoked this possibility to explain certain quantitative differences in the histologic evaluation of the
hepatotoxic lesions observed in potentiated animals versus nonpotentiated

animals (Côté, Traiger and Plaa, 1974; Hewitt and co-workers, 1979, 1980a, 1980b). Other investigators have recognized such a possibility (Curtis, Williams and Mehendale, 1979; Curtis and Mehendale 1980; Davis and Mehendale, 1980). The effect of chlordecone on CCl_4-affected biliary excretory function (Curtis, Williams and Mehendale, 1979; Curtis and Mehendale, 1980) and the effect of isopropanol on CCl_4-affected bile flow (de Lamirande and Plaa, 1981) might be explanable on this basis. Furthermore, the potentiation of taurolithocholate by 1,3-butanediol (de Lamirande and Plaa, 1981) appears to be unrelated to bioactivation. We are presently looking into this phase as an additional mechanism of action.

ACKNOWLEDGEMENT

We gratefully acknowledge the expert technical assistance provided by Johanne Couture, Thérèse Vaillancourt and Monique Morisset. The work reported herein was supported by contracts from the Environmental Research Directorate (Health and Welfare Canada) and research grants from the Natural Sciences and Engineering Council Canada, the National Health Research and Development Program (Health and Welfare Canada), the Commission de la santé et de la sécurité du travail du Québec, the Medical Research Council of Canada, and Grant No. OH00986-01 from the U.S. Public Health Service.

REFERENCES

Cianflone, D.J., W.R. Hewitt, D.C. Villeneuve, and G.L. Plaa (1980). Role of biotransformation in the alterations of chloroform hepatotoxicity produced by Kepone an mirex. Toxicol. Appl. Pharmacol, 53, 140-149.
Côté, M.G., G.J. Traiger, and G.L. Plaa (1974). Effect of isopropanol-induced potentiation of carbon tetrachloride on rat hepatic ultrastructure. Toxicol. Appl. Pharmacol., 30, 14-25.
Cresteil, T., P. Beaune, J.P. Leroux, M. Lange, and D. Mansuy (1979). Biotransformation of chloroform by rat and human microsomes. Chem.-Biol. Interact., 24, 153-165.
Curtis, L.R., and H.M. Mehendale (1980). Specificity of chlordecone-induced potentiation of carbon tetrachloride hepatotoxicity. Drug Metab. Dispos., 8, 23-27.
Curtis, L.R., W.L. Williams, and H.M. Mehendale (1979). Potentiation of the hepatotoxicity of carbon tetrachloride following preexposure to chlordecone (Kepone) in the male rat. Toxicol. Appl. Pharmacol., 51, 283-293.
Davis, M.E., and H.M. Mehendale (1980). Functional and biochemical correlates of chlordecone exposure and its enhancement of CCl_4 hepatotoxicity. Toxicology, 15, 91-103.
De Lamirande, E., and G.L. Plaa (1981). 1,3-Butanediol pretreatment on the cholestasis induced in rats by manganese-bilirubin combination, taurolithocholic acid, or α-naphthylisothiocyanate. Toxicol. Appl. Pharmacol, 59, (in press).
Hanasono, G.K., M.G. Côté, and G.L. Plaa (1975). Potentiation of carbon tetrachloride-induced hepatotoxicity in alloxan- or streptozotocin-diabetic rats. J. Pharmacol. Exp. Ther., 192, 592-604.
Hanasono, G.K. H. Witschi, and G.L. Plaa (1975). Potentiation of the hepatotoxic responses to chemicals in alloxan-diabetic rats. Proc. Soc. Exp. Biol. Med., 149, 903-907.
Hewitt, W.R., E.M. Brown, and G.L. Plaa (1981). Potentiation of $CHCl_3$-induced hepato- and nephrotoxicity by ketones. Toxicologist, 1, 99.
Hewitt, W.R., E.M. Brown, M.G. Côté, H. Miyajima, and G.L. Plaa (1981). Alteration on chloroform-induced nephrotoxicity by exogenous ketones. In Por-

74 G. L. Plaa and W. R. Hewitt

ter, G. (Ed.), Nephrotoxic Mechanisms of Drugs and Environmental Toxins, Plenum, New York, (in press).

Hewitt, L.A. W.R. Hewitt, and G.L. Plaa (1981). Fractional hepatic distribution of CHCl$_3$ in mice and rats treated with Kepone or mirex. Pharmacologist. (in press).

Hewitt, W.R., H. Miyajima, M.G. Côté, and G.L. Plaa (1979). Acute alteration of chloroform-induced hepato- and nephrotoxicity by mirex and Kepone. Toxicol. Appl. Pharmacol. 48, 509-527.

Hewitt, W.R., H. Miyajima, M.G. Côté, and G.L. Plaa (1980a). Acute alteration of chloroform-induced hepato- and nephrotoxicity by n-hexane, methyl n-butyl ketone, and 2,5-hexanedione. Toxicol. Appl. Pharmacol., 53, 230-248.

Hewitt, W.R., H. Miyajima, M.G. Côté, and G.L. Plaa (1980b). Modification of haloalkane-induced hepatotoxicity by exogenous ketones and metabolic ketosis. Federation Proc., 39, 3118-3123.

Hewitt, W.R., and G.L. Plaa (1979). Potentiation of carbon tetrachloride-induced hepatotoxicity by 1,3-butanediol. Toxicol. Appl. Pharmacol. 47, 177-180.

Klaassen, C.D., and G.L. Plaa (1966). Relative effects of various chlorinated hydrocarbons on liver and kidney function in mice. Toxicol. Appl. Pharmacol. 9, 139-151.

Klingensmith, J.S., and H.M. Mehendale (1981). Potentiation of haloalkane hepatotoxicity of brominated analogs of CCl$_4$ by chlordecone and phenobarbital. Toxicologist, 1, 99.

Kluwe, W.M., C.L. Hermann, and J.B. Hook (1979). Effects of dietary polychlorinated biphenyls and polybrominated biphenyls on the renal and hepatic toxicities of several chlorinated hydrocarbon solvents in mice. J. Toxicol. Environ. Health, 5, 605-615.

Kluwe, W.M., and J.B. Hook (1978). Polybrominated biphenyl-induced potentiation of chloroform toxicity. Toxicol. Appl. Pharmacol., 45, 861-869.

Maling, H.M., F.M. Eichelbaum, W. Saul, I.G. Sipes, E.A.B. Brown, and J.R. Gillette (1974). Nature of the protection against carbon tetrachloride-induced hepatotoxicity produced by pretreatment with dibenamine [N-(2-chloroethyl) dibenzylamine]. Biochem. Pharmacol., 23, 1479-1491.

Maling, H.M., B. Stripp, I.G. Sipes, B. Highman, W. Saul, and M.A. Williams (1975). Enhanced hepatotoxicity of carbon tetrachloride, thioacetamide, and dimethylnitrosamine by pretreatment of rats with ethanol and some comparisons with potentiation by isopropanol. Toxicol. Appl. Pharmacol., 33, 291-308.

Plaa, G.L., W.R. Hewitt, P. du Souich, G. Caillé, and S. Lock (1981). Isopropanol and acetone potentiation of carbon tetrachloride-induced hepatotoxicity: single versus repetitive pretreatments in rats. J. Toxicol. Environ. Health, (in press).

Plaa, G.L., and G.J. Traiger (1973). Mechanism of potentiation of CCl$_4$-induced hepatotoxicity. In Loomis, T.A. (Ed.), Pharmacology and the Future of Man, Vol. 2, Karger, Basle, pp. 100-113.

Plaa, G.L., G.J. Traiger, G.K. Hanasono, and H. Witschi (1975). Effect of alcohols on various forms of chemically induced liver injury. In Khanna, J.M., Y. Israel, and H. Kalant (Eds.), Alcoholic Liver Pathology, Addition Research Foundation, Ontario, pp. 225-244.

Pohl, L.R., B. Booshan, N.F. Whittaker, and G. Krishna (1977). Phosgene: a metabolite of chloroform. Biochem. Biophys. Res. Commun., 79, 684-691.

Recknagel, R.O., and E.A. Glende, Jr. (1973). Carbon tetrachloride hepatotoxicity: an example of lethal cleavage. C.R.C. Crit. Rev. Toxicol. 2, 263-297.

Sipes, I.G., B. Stripp, G. Krishna, H.M. Maling, and J.R. Gillette (1973). Enhanced hepatic microsomal activity by pretreatment of rats with acetone or isopropanol. Proc. Soc. Exp. Biol. Med., 142, 237-240.

Traiger, G.J., and J.W. Bruckner (1976). The participation of 2-butanone in 2-butanol-induced potentiation of carbon tetrachloride hepatotoxicity. J. Pharmacol. Exp. Ther., 196, 493-500.

Traiger, G.J., and G.L. Plaa (1971). Differences in the potentiation of carbon tetrachloride in rats by ethanol and isopropanol pretreatment. Toxicol. Appl. Pharmacol., 20, 105-112.

Traiger, G.J., and G.L. Plaa (1972). Relationship of alcohol metabolism to the potentiation of CCl_4 hepatotoxicity induced by aliphatic alcohols. J. Pharmacol. Exp. Ther., 183, 481-488.

Traiger, G.J., and G.L. Plaa (1973). Effect of aminotriazole on isopropanol- and acetone-induced potentiation of CCl_4 hepatotoxicity. Canad. J. Physiol. Pharmacol., 51, 291-296.

Traiger, G.J., and G.L. Plaa (1974). Chlorinated hydrocarbon toxicity: potentiation by isopropyl alcohol and acetone. Arch. Environ. Health, 28, 276-278.

Watrous, W.M., and G.L. Plaa (1971). The potentiation of $CHCl_3$-induced nephrototoxicity by some aliphatic alcohols in mice. Pharmacologist, 13, 227.

Zimmerman, H.J. (1978). Hepatotoxicity, Appleton-Century-Crofts, New-York, pp. 198-219.

Biochemical Mechanisms of Acetaminophen (Paracetamol) Induced Hepatic and Renal Toxicity

G. G. Duggin and J. Mohandas

Toxicology and Renal Units, Royal Prince Alfred Hospital, Sydney, N.S.W., Australia

ABSTRACT

Acute toxicity of acetaminophen in the liver is mediated by cytochrome P450 mixed function oxidase and toxicity is enhanced by compounds which induce the enzyme.   Acute renal cortical toxicity is mediated by two or three enzyme systems: cytochrome P450 m.f.o., prostaglandin endoperoxide synthetase and possibly deacetylase.   Chronic toxicity manifested by analgesic nephropathy with renal inner medullary necrosis is mediated by prostaglandin endoperoxide synthetase and toxicity is enhanced by salicylates.

KEY WORDS

Acetaminophen, paracetamol, hepatotoxicity, cytochrome P450, interactions, prostaglandin endoperoxide synthetase, nephrotoxicity, analgesic nephropathy, salicylate.

Acetaminophen (paracetamol) is one of the most widely consumed antipyretic analgesics and is usually thought to have low toxicity.   However there are four clinical problems recognized as a result of acetaminophen ingestion: acute hepatic necrosis (Prescott and others, 1976), following a significant single (> 150 mg/kg) dose of the drug.   This is often associated with acute renal failure as a result of acute tubular necrosis (Boyer and Rouff, 1971). A third complication of the drug is a chronic active hepatitis like syndrome associated with a high therapeutic intake in a susceptible individual (Bonkowsky and others, 1978).   The fourth syndrome, of analgesic nephropathy, occurs in patients chronically consuming combination analgesics containing acetaminophen and salicylate (Duggin, 1980).

Cytochrome P450 mixed function oxidase (m.f.o.) has been associated with the toxic metabolic activation of acetaminophen through a minor but important pathway in the liver (Mitchell and others, 1973a; 1973b, Jollow and others, 1973; 1974; Potter and others, 1973; 1974).   After a low nontoxic dose of acetaminophen, its reactive intermediate is efficiently detoxified by

conjugation with hepatic glutathione. However after a massive dose of
acetaminophen, glutathione is depleted beyond a critical level and then the
reactive metabolite binds irreversibly to cellular macromolecules leading to
tissue necrosis (Mitchell and others, 1973b). Hepatic necrosis produced by
acetaminophen has been demonstrated to be dose dependent and correlated with
the extent of covalent binding of the reactive metabolite to cellular macromolecules as well as with the depletion of hepatic glutathione (Potter and
others, 1974). Acute acetaminophen toxicity causes hepatic and renal
cortical damage, but the renal papilla is left intact (McMurtry and others,
1978). In analgesic nephropathy chronic papillary damage is due to
combination analgesics containing acetaminophen (Duggin, 1980).

FACTORS INTERACTING TO ENHANCE OR DECREASE
ACUTE ACETAMINOPHEN TOXICITY.

There are multiple factors which can influence the toxicity of acetaminophen
and they can be linked to the proportional metabolic conversion of
acetaminophen into toxic and nontoxic metabolites. The nontoxic major
metabolite pathways producing glucuronide and sulphate are potentially
capacity limited, particularly the sulphate, and therefore an increase in
the availability of acetaminophen could favour the toxic metabolic
activation of acetaminophen.

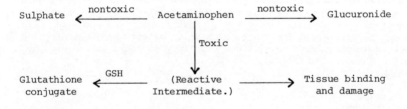

Compounds which Induce Drug Metabolism

Pretreatment of animals with inducers of microsomal cyt. P450 m.f.o. such as
phenobarbital, 3-methyl-cholanthrene and polyhalogenated biphenyls show
differential effects on liver and kidney. Induction of m.f.o. activity
need not necessarily lead to increased toxicity. Prior ingestion of
phenobarbital increases the toxic metabolism of acetaminophen in man,
(Wright and Prescott, 1973), in mice and Sprague-Dawley rats (Mitchell and
others, 1973a). Phenobarbital pretreatment showed alteration only in the
in vitro hepatic microsomal activation in Fischer rats (McMurtry and others,
1978) and provided protective effect to hamsters from liver damage (Potter
and others, 1974). Detoxification of acetaminophen through glucuronidation
is increased in hamsters by phenobarbital pretreatment resulting in decreased
metabolic activation (Potter and others, 1974; Jollow and others, 1974).
The varied effects of acetaminophen in different species has hence been
suggested to be due to differential activation of toxic and nontoxic pathways.
Phenobarbital pretreatment does not alter in vivo kidney protein covalent
binding in Fischer rats (McMurtry and others, 1978), CD-1 mice, Sprague-
Dawley rats (Mudge and others, 1978) or renal tissue necrosis in Fischer
rats (McMurtry and others, 1978) following acetaminophen administration.
Phenobarbital pretreatment in Fischer rats does not alter in vitro
metabolic activation of acetaminophen by kidney microsomes (McMurtry and
others, 1978).

Prior administration of 3-methylcholanthrene in Fischer rats potentiated

acetaminophen mediated hepatic tissue necrosis and in vitro metabolic
activation by hepatic microsomes but showed no influence on the development
of necrosis and protein covalent binding in the kidney in vivo or on protein
covalent binding in vitro by microsomal activation (McMurtry and others,
1978). Pretreatment with 3-methylcholanthrene increased hepatic metabolic
activation of acetaminophen in CD-1 mice and Sprague-Dawley rats but not in
the renal activation of acetaminophen (Mudge and others, 1978). The
effective induction of hepatic activation and lack of induction of renal
activation of acetaminophen by 3-methylcholanthrene suggests that the active
metabolite of acetaminophen was formed in situ in the kidney and not transported from the liver (McMurtry and others, 1978) and that the active
metabolite of acetaminophen may be formed by a different mechanism (Mudge
and others, 1978). Polybrominated biphenyls have been demonstrated to
enhance the activation of acetaminophen in the kidney (Kluwe and Hook, 1980).

Glutathione Depletion and Dietary Factors

Support for the protective role of glutathione comes from studies showing
enhanced toxicity and covalent binding of acetaminophen following depletion
of glutathione by pretreatment with diethylmaleate (Mitchell and others,
1973b). Starvation and low protein diets enhance the hepatotoxicity of
acetaminophen due to a substantial reduction in the levels of cellular
glutathione, in spite of a reduction in cytochrome P450 m.f.o. (McLean and
Day, 1975).

Salicylates, Ethanol and Other Drugs

Investigation of the interaction of aspirin on acetaminophen metabolism in
experimental animals has not demonstrated any potentiation of acetaminophen-
related hepatotoxicity (Whitehouse and others, 1977). However salicylates
have been implicated in the development of papillary necrosis found in
analgesic nephropathy (Duggin, 1980).

Acetaminophen hepatotoxicity is enhanced clinically by chronic intake of
ethanol, manifested by increased hepatic necrosis or a decrease in the dose
at which severe necrosis occurs (Emby and Fraser, 1977; Goldfinger and
others, 1978). Chronic ethanol administration has been demonstrated to
increase hepatic cytochrome P450 and enhance microsomal drug metabolism.
Potentiation of acetaminophen hepatotoxicity occurs in chronic alcoholics
and patients taking other drugs such as barbiturates or imipramine (Wright
and Prescott, 1973).

Prevention of acetaminophen induced mortality and hepatotoxicity by co-
administration of phenacetin has been observed in mice (Kapetanovic and
Mieyal, 1979). Presumably this is due to inhibition of cytochrome P450
m.f.o. mediated metabolic activation of acetaminophen by phenacetin.

Compounds which Decrease Drug Metabolism.

Inhibitors of drug metabolism such as piperonyl butoxide and cobaltous
chloride inhibited protein covalent binding, partially prevented glutathione
depletion and prevented hepatic necrosis (Mitchell and others, 1973b; Potter
and others, 1974). Pretreatment of Fischer rats with cobaltous chloride
also decreased the severity of acetaminophen renal toxicity as well as
protein covalent binding in vivo and reduced in vitro activation of

acetaminophen by renal microsomes (McMurtry and others, 1978).   Cobaltous
chloride appears to act by the inhibition of cytochrome P450 synthesis
(Mitchell and others, 1973a).

Compounds which Inhibit Tissue Necrosis

Cysteine (Mitchell and others, 1973b), methionine (McLean and Day, 1975;
Prescott and others, 1976), cysteamine (Prescott and others, 1976) and
N-acetylcysteine (Prescott and others, 1977) have been found to be
effective in preventing the severe hepatotoxicity of acetaminophen and
have been successfully used for the treatment of acetaminophen overdosage.
The mechanism of action of these sulfhydryl compounds in reducing the
toxicity of acetaminophen has not been clearly defined.   D-penicillamine,
while preventing hepatotoxicity, has been suggested to potentiate nephrotoxicity (Prescott and others, 1976).   6-N-propyl-2-thiouracil has
recently been demonstrated to provide direct protection against acetaminophen
hepatotoxicity by acting as a substitute for reduced glutathione as a substrate for the GSH-S-transferases (Yamada and others, 1981).

Species and Genetic Variation

While hamsters and mice are found to be very prone to acetaminophen hepatotoxicity, rats, guinea pigs and rabbits are comparatively resistant.   The
extent of hepatic damage in different species correlated with the level of
hepatic glutathione depletion and covalent binding to hepatic microsomal
protein (Davis and others, 1974).

A study of genetic differences between C57BL/6N mice and DBA/2N mice
demonstrated that there was a correlation between aromatic hydrocarbon
(3-methylcholanthrene and β-napthoflavone) inducible N-hydroxylation of
2-acetylaminofluorene and acetaminophen hepatotoxicity (Thorgeirsson and
others, 1975).   3-methylcholanthrene pretreatment increased the incidence
and extent of acetaminophen related hepatic necrosis in the C57BL/6N mice
without showing any effect on the DBA/2N mice.   Homozygous Gunn rats,
which genetically lack glucuronidating ability, develop papillary necrosis
from a single dose of aspirin, acetaminophen or phenacetin (Axelson, 1975).

FACTORS INTERACTING TO ENHANCE OR
DECREASE CHRONIC ACETAMINOPHEN TOXICITY.

Moderate doses of acetaminophen have been reported to cause chronic hepatic
inflammation and fibrosis (Bonkowsky and others, 1978) but it is the chronic
abuse of acetaminophen in combination analgesics leading to renal papillary
necrosis which causes the most concern.   Covalent binding of acetaminophen
metabolite to kidney proteins has been studied both in vivo and in vitro
(Mudge and others, 1978; Joshi and others, 1978; McMurtry and others, 1978).
In mice, protein covalent binding of acetaminophen has been demonstrated to
be higher in renal inner medulla than in cortex and liver (Mudge and others,
1978).   In vitro studies showed that covalent binding was maximal in rabbit
kidney inner medulla, less in outer medulla and minimal in cortex (Joshi and
others, 1978).

Pretreatment with 3-methylcholanthrene induced metabolic activation of
acetaminophen in liver but not in kidney (Mudge and others, 1978; McMurtry
and others, 1978) and pointed to different mechanisms of acetaminophen

metabolism in liver and kidney.   Metabolic activation mediated by cytochrome
P450 m.f.o. requiring NADPH and O_2 has been generally regarded as the sole
pathway.   However, recently an NADPH-independent alternate pathway has been
demonstrated to activate acetaminophen in rabbit kidney inner medulla (Duggin,
1980).   No cytochrome P450 was detectable in rabbit renal inner medulla and
hence an alternate pathway which is not mediated by cytochrome P450 seemed
likely.   This pathway has now been recognized as mediated by prostaglandin
endoperoxide synthetase requiring arachidonic acid and O_2 (Mohandas and
others, 1981).

Small quantities of acetaminophen have been found to be converted to p-
aminophenol in kidney cortex when high concentrations of acetaminophen are
available as substrate (Carpenter, 1978).   Recently acetaminophen has been
demonstrated to be deacetylated by a major pathway to p-aminophenol by
urodele amphibian organ cultures, including liver and kidney (Clothier and
others, 1981).   The toxicological significance, although not yet investigated, may be in the development of renal cortical damage in overdose cases.
The differing modes of toxic metabolic activation are shown in Table 1.

TABLE 1   Hepatic and Renal Activation of Acetaminophen in Vitro.

Type of Metabolism	Tissue Prep.	Reference
Cyt. P450 m.f.o. mediated oxidation requiring NADPH, O_2	Rat, mouse, liver microsomes	Potter and others, 1973
	Rat kidney microsomes	McMurtry and others, 1978
	Rabbit renal cortex and outer medulla microsomes	Mohandas and others, 1981
PG endoperoxide synthetase mediated cooxidation requiring arachidonic acid, O_2	Rabbit renal inner medulla, outer medulla, cortex microsomes	Mohandas and others, 1981
Deacetylation	Mice kidney cortical slices	Carpenter, 1978
	Urodele amphibian liver and kidney cultured cells	Clothier and others, 1981

Oxidative metabolism of a number of organic compounds by cooxidation
mediated by prostaglandin synthetase from sheep vesicular glands in the
presence of the primary substrate arachidonic acid or the secondary substrate PGG_2 have been demonstrated (Marnett and others, 1975).   The
prostaglandin endoperoxide synthetase (PGES) mediated pathway activating
acetaminophen is predominant in renal inner medulla, less active in outer
medulla and even less in cortex (Mohandas and others, 1981).   Increase in
arachidonic acid concentration increases microsomal activation of
acetaminophen and addition of a heme compound such as methemoglobin further

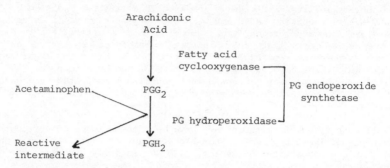

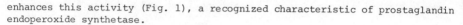

enhances this activity (Fig. 1), a recognized characteristic of prostaglandin endoperoxide synthetase.

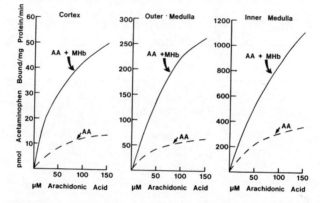

Fig. 1   Arachidonic acid (AA) mediated microsomal activation of
          acetaminophen (0.5 mM) in rabbit kidney and enhancement by 1.2
          μM methemoglobin (MHb) (0.1 M K phosphate, pH 7.8 at 37° C
          15 min).

In the rabbit kidney, cytochrome P450 mediated activation of acetaminophen requiring NADPH and O_2 was found to be highest in cortex, less in outer medulla and negligible in inner medulla (Mohandas and others, 1981). Hepatic microsomes from C57BL/6J mice and rabbit demonstrated very little activity of the prostaglandin endoperoxide synthetase mediated pathway compared to the cytochrome P450 m.f.o. mediated pathway (Mohandas and Duggin, unpublished data).

Organic hydroperoxides such as cumene hydroperoxide and t-butyl hydroperoxide have been found to initiate the cooxidative activation of acetaminophen mediated by PGES (Mohandas and Duggin, unpublished data).   Aspirin (1 mM) and indomethacin (0.2 mM) inhibit only the fatty acid cyclooxygenase activity of the enzyme PGES when the activation of acetaminophen is initiated by arachidonic acid and does not inhibit the hydroperoxide initiated cooxidation of acetaminophen.   Hence this activation of acetaminophen appears to be due to the hydroperoxidase activity of the enzyme.

The inhibition of prostaglandin biosynthesis by rabbit renal inner medullary microsomes by acetaminophen was observed previously to be dose dependant and

it was suggested that though aspirin and acetaminophen inhibited prostaglandin cyclooxygenase directly, they did so by different mechanisms
(Mattammal and others, 1979).   Aspirin has been shown to deactivate the
fatty acid cyclooxygenase activity as a result of acetylation of prostaglandin synthetase in blood platelets and ram seminal vesicles (Roth and
others, 1975).   Prostaglandin synthetase in the kidney has also been shown
to be inhibited by aspirin after transacetylation.   However, the degree of
inhibition in the medulla still leaves significant enzyme activity (Caterson
and others, 1978).   Salicylate has been demonstrated to be a potent agent
in depleting renal but not hepatic glutathione (Duggin, 1980).   The
mechanisms, in part, appear to be related to the very high concentration of
salicylate within renal cells, compared to the liver (Duggin, 1980).

Acetaminophen shows a concentration gradient within different regions of the
kidney and reaches a high concentration in the cells of renal inner medulla
compared to cortex and plasma (Duggin and Mudge, 1976).   Nevertheless even
high therapeutic doses of acetaminophen are unlikely to reach concentrations
sufficient to inhibit prostaglandin biosynthesis in the renal inner medulla.
Prostaglandin biosynthesis by rabbit renal inner medulla is stimulated by
acetaminophen at low concentrations and is inhibited by acetaminophen at
high concentrations (Fig. 2).   In this situation, it would have a
stimulatory effect on prostaglandin synthesis and hence increased
activation of acetaminophen.

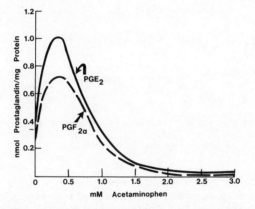

Fig. 2   Effect of acetaminophen on PG biosynthesis from 0.025 mM
          ^{14}C-arachidonic acid by rabbit renal inner medullary
          microsomes (0.1 M K phosphate, pH 7.8, 37° C, 10 min).

The apparent anomaly of synergistic toxicity between aspirin and
acetaminophen is thus explained by the stimulatory effect of acetaminophen
on prostaglandin synthetase activity in the renal medulla, the modest
inhibition by aspirin on prostaglandin synthetase activity, the lack of
effect of aspirin on the hydroperoxidase activity of the enzyme which is
the component involved in the metabolic activation of acetaminophen, the
partial exclusion of aspirin from renal medullary cells by salicylate by
competitive transport and most importantly, the glutathione depleting
effect of salicylate resulting in increased covalent binding (Duggin,
1980;   Mohandas and others, 1981).

The chemical nature of the reactive intermediate has not been definitely identified. N-hydroxyacetaminophen had been believed to be the metabolic intermediate of acetaminophen until it was shown that N-hydroxyacetaminophen was not formed in microsomal incubation mixtures with acetaminophen (Hinson and others, 1979). Recently acetaminophen has been chemically oxidized to N-acetyl-p-benzoquinoneimine which is currently considered to be the reactive intermediate (Blair and others, 1980). Whether another highly reactive intermediate is formed instead of N-acetyl-p-benzoquinoneimine, or prior to the formation of N-acetyl-p-benzoquinoneimine is still the subject of continuing research.

Although there is general agreement regarding the high reactivity of the activation product of acetaminophen, the contribution of protein covalent binding is still a subject of discussion. Covalent binding of acetamino-phen has been correlated to tissue necrosis in both liver and kidney (Jollow and others, 1973; McMurtry and others, 1978). There is certainly an inverse relationship between covalent binding, hepatotoxicity or nephro-toxicity and tissue concentration of reduced glutathione. It is quite possible that there are other factors involved in the precipitation and development of tissue necrosis in both liver and kidney and tissue covalent binding of acetaminophen is only an indication of the toxicity and not necessarily causally related. The differential relative contribution of the metabolic activation of acetaminophen by cytochrome P450 m.f.o. and prostaglandin endoperoxide synthetase is depicted in Table 2.

TABLE 2   Oxidative Activation of Acetaminophen.

Pathway 1   Liver > Renal Cortex > Renal Outer Medulla > Inner Medulla

$$\text{Acetaminophen} \xrightarrow[\text{NADPH, } O_2]{\text{Cyt. P450 m.f.o.}} \text{Reactive Intermediate.}$$

Pathway 2   Inner Medulla > Outer Medulla > Renal Cortex > Liver

$$\text{Acetaminophen} \xrightarrow[\text{Arachidonic acid, } O_2]{\text{PG endoperoxide synthetase}} \text{Reactive Intermediate.}$$

Acute toxicity of acetaminophen in the liver is mediated by cytochrome P450 m.f.o. and toxicity is increased by agents which induce the enzyme. Acute toxicity in the renal cortex is possibly mediated by three enzyme systems: cytochrome P450 m.f.o., prostaglandin endoperoxide synthetase and deacetylase. The relative importance of each remains to be determined. Chronic toxicity in the inner renal medulla is mediated exclusively by prostaglandin endoperoxide synthetase and the toxicity appears to be enhanced by salicylate.

REFERENCES

Axelson, R. A. (1975).   The induction of renal papillary necrosis in Gunn rats by analgesics and analgesic mixtures.   Br. J. Exp. Path., 56, 92-96.
Blair, I. A., A. R. Boobis, and D. S. Davies (1980).   Paracetamol oxidation: synthesis and reactivity of N-acetyl-p-benzoquinoneimine. Tetrahedron Lett., 21, 4947-4950.

Bonkowsky, H. L., G. H. Mudge, and R. J. McMurtry (1978). Chronic hepatic inflammation and fibrosis due to low doses of paracetamol. Lancet, 1, 1016-1018.

Boyer, T. D., and S. L. Rouff (1971). Acetaminophen-induced hepatic necrosis and renal failure. J. Amer. Med. Assoc., 218, 440-441.

Carpenter, H. M. (1978). Mechanisms of the nephrotoxicity of acetaminophen studied in the mouse cortex slice system. Ph.D. Thesis, University of Dartmouth, USA.

Caterson, R. J., G. G. Duggin, J. Horvath, J. Mohandas, and D. Tiller (1978). Aspirin, protein transacetylation and inhibition of prostaglandin synthetase in the kidney. Br. J. Pharmac., 64, 353-358.

Clothier, R. H., J. R. Dewar, M. A. Santos, A. D. North, S. Foster, and M. Balls (1981). A comparative study of the deacetylation of paracetamol by urodele and anuran amphibian organ cultures. Xenobiotica, 11, 149-157.

Davis, D. C., W. Z. Potter, D. J. Jollow, and J. R. Mitchell (1974). Species differences in hepatic glutathione depletion, covalent binding and hepatic necrosis after acetaminophen. Life Sci., 14, 2099-2109.

Duggin, G. G., and G. H. Mudge (1976). Analgesic nephropathy: renal distribution of acetaminophen and its conjugates. J. Pharmacol. Exp. Therap., 199, 1-9.

Duggin, G. G. (1980). Mechanisms in the development of analgesic nephropathy. Kidney Int., 18, 553-561.

Emby, D. J., and B. N. Fraser (1977). Hepatotoxicity of paracetamol enhanced by ingestion of alcohol. S. Afr. Med. J., 51, 208-209.

Goldfinger, R., K. S. Ahmed, C. S. Pitchumoni, and S. A. Weseley (1978). Concomitant alcohol and drug abuse enhancing acetaminophen toxicity. Am. J. Gastro., 70, 385-388.

Hinson, J. A., L. R. Pohl, and J. R. Gillette (1979). N-hydroxyacetaminophen: a microsomal metabolite of N-hydroxyphenacetin but apparently not of acetaminophen. Life Sci., 24, 2133-2138.

Jollow, D. J., J. R. Mitchell, W. Z. Potter, D. C. Davis, J. R. Gillette, and B. B. Brodie (1973). Acetaminophen-induced hepatic necrosis. II. Role of covalent binding in vivo. J. Pharmacol. Exp. Ther., 187, 195-202.

Jollow, D. J., S. S. Thorgeirsson, W. Z. Potter, M. Hashimoto, and J. R. Mitchell (1974). Acetaminophen-induced hepatic necrosis. VI. Metabolic disposition of toxic and nontoxic doses of acetaminophen. Pharmacology, 12, 251-271.

Joshi, S., T. V. Zenser, M. B. Mattammal, C. A. Herman, and B. B. Davis (1978). Kidney metabolism of acetaminophen and phenacetin. J. Lab. Clin. Med., 92, 924-931.

Kapetanovic, I. M., and J. J. Mieyal (1979). Inhibition of acetaminophen-induced hepatotoxicity by phenacetin and its alkoxy analogs. J. Pharmacol. Exp. Ther., 209, 25-30.

Kluwe, W. M., and J. B. Hook (1980). Effects of environmental chemicals on kidney metabolism and function. Kidney Int., 18, 648-655.

Marnett, L. J., P. Wlodawer, and B. Samuelsson (1975). Co-oxygenation of organic substrates by the prostaglandin synthetase of sheep vesicular gland. J. Biol. Chem., 250, 8510-8517.

Mattammal, M. B., T. V. Zenser, W. W. Brown, C. A. Herman, and B. B. Davis (1979). Mechanism of inhibition of renal prostaglandin production by acetaminophen. J. Pharmacol. Exp. Ther., 210, 405-409.

McLean, A. E. M., and P. A. Day (1975). The effect of diet on the toxicity of paracetamol and the safety of paracetamol-methionine mixtures. Biochem. Pharmacol., 24, 37-42.

McMurtry, R. J., W. R. Snodgrass, and J. R. Mitchell (1978). Renal necrosis, glutathione depletion and covalent binding after acetaminophen. Toxicol. Appl. Pharmacol., 46, 87-100.

Mitchell, J. R., D. J. Jollow, W. Z. Potter, D. C. Davis, J. R. Gillette, and B. B. Brodie (1973a). Acetaminophen-induced hepatic necrosis. I. Role of drug metabolism. J. Pharmacol. Exp. Ther., 187, 185-194.

Mitchell, J. R., D. J. Jollow, W. Z. Potter, J. R. Gillette, and B. B. Brodie (1973b). Acetaminophen-induced hepatic necrosis. IV. Protective role of glutathione. J. Pharmacol. Exp. Ther., 187, 211-217.

Mohandas, J., G. G. Duggin, J. S. Horvath, and D. J. Tiller (1981). Metabolic oxidation of acetaminophen (paracetamol) mediated by cytochrome P450 mixed function oxidase and prostaglandin endoperoxide synthetase in rabbit kidney. Toxicol. Appl. Pharmacol. (In press).

Mudge, G. H., M. W. Gemborys, and G. G. Duggin (1978). Covalent binding of metabolites of acetaminophen to kidney protein and depletion of renal glutathione. J. Pharmacol. Exp. Ther., 206, 218-226.

Potter, W. Z., D. C. Davis, J. R. Mitchell, D. J. Jollow, J. R. Gillette, and B. B. Brodie (1973). Acetaminophen-induced hepatic necrosis. III. Cytochrome P450 mediated covalent binding in vitro. J. Pharmacol. Exp. Therap., 187, 203-210.

Potter, W. Z., S. S. Thorgeirsson, D. J. Jollow, and J. R. Mitchell (1974). Acetaminophen-induced hepatic necrosis. V. Correlation of hepatic necrosis, covalent binding and glutathione depletion in hamsters. Pharmacology, 12, 129-143.

Prescott, L. F., J. Park, G. R. Sutherland, I. J. Smith, and A. T. Proudfoot (1976). Cysteamine, methionine and penicillamine in the treatment of paracetamol poisoning. Lancet, 2, 109-113.

Prescott, L. F., J. Park, A. Ballantyne, P. Adriaenssens, and A. T. Proudfoot (1977). Treatment of paracetamol (acetaminophen) poisoning with N-acetylcysteine. Lancet, 2, 432-434.

Roth, G. J., N. Stanford, and P. W. Majerus (1975). Acetylation of prostaglandin synthetase by aspirin. Proc. Nat. Acad. Sci., USA., 72, 3073-3076.

Thorgeirsson, S. S., J. S. Felton, and D. W. Nebert (1975). Genetic differences in the aromatic hydrocarbon-inducible N-hydroxylation of 2-acetylaminofluorene and acetaminophen-produced hepatotoxicity in mice. Mol. Pharmacol., 41, 159-165.

Whitehouse, L. W., C. J. Paul, L. T. Wong, and B. H. Thomas (1977). Effect of aspirin on a subtoxic dose of ^{14}C-acetaminophen in mice. J. Pharm. Sci., 66, 1399-1403.

Wright, N., and L. F. Prescott (1973). Potentiation by previous drug therapy of hepatotoxicity following paracetamol overdosage. Scot. Med. J., 18, 56-58.

Yamada, T., S. Ludwig, J. Kuhlenkamp, and N. Kaplowitz (1981). Direct protection against acetaminophen hepatotoxicity by propylthiouracil. J. Clin. Invest., 67, 688-695.

The Hepatotoxicity and Nephrotoxicity of Hexachlorobutadiene

E. A. Lock and J. Ishmael

Biochemical Toxicology and Pathology Sections, Imperial Chemical
Industries PLC, Central Toxicology Laboratory, Alderley Park,
Nr Macclesfield, Cheshire SK10 4TJ, UK

ABSTRACT

Hexachloro 1:3 butadiene (HCBD) is formed as a by-product during the
chlorination of hydrocarbons for the manufacture of chlorinated ethylenes
and carbon tetrachloride. Administration of HCBD (300 mg/kg, ip) to rats
produces a mild reversible hydropic swelling of the liver. This change is
associated with a swelling of mitochondria in hepatocytes located in the
periportal region of the liver. However, the major target organ for
toxicity is the kidney where HCBD produces necrosis of the pars recta of
the proximal tubule. Treatment of rats with inducers or inhibitors of
hepatic and/or renal drug metabolising enzymes followed by HCBD administration does not markedly alter HCBD-induced liver or kidney injury. In male
rats, HCBD causes a depletion of hepatic but not renal non-protein
sulphydryl content (NP-SH) and pretreatment of animals with diethylmaleate,
which reduces tissue glutathione content, markedly enhances the nephrotoxicity of HCBD. Our findings to date indicate that glutathione plays a
protective role against HCBD-induced renal tubular necrosis which suggests
a metabolic activation reaction may be involved in the nephrotoxicity.

KEYWORDS

Hexachloro 1:3 butadiene; renal tubular necrosis; liver damage; glutathione
depletion; P-450 inducers; P-450 inhibitors.

INTRODUCTION

Hexachloro 1:3 butadiene (HCBD) is formed as a by-product during the
manufacture of chlorinated ethylenes and carbon tetrachloride. Gradiski
and Magadur (1974) showed HCBD was the most toxic of a series of chlorinated
solvents to the mouse. The oral LD50 in the mouse is about 80 mg/kg,
whereas in the rat it is less toxic, the LD50 being about 350 mg/kg
(Gradiski and co-workers, 1975; Kociba and co-workers, 1977). HCBD does
not produce necrosis in the liver but has been reported to increase the
liver to body weight ratio following a single injection (Lock and Ishmael,
1981) or feeding in the diet (Harleman and Seinen, 1979). The kidney is
the major target organ, where HCBD produces necrosis of the proximal
tubules in the rat following several routes of administration (Gradiski and
co-workers, 1975; Kociba and co-workers, 1977; Berndt and Mehendale, 1979;
Harleman and Seinen, 1979; Lock and Ishmael, 1979). The toxic mechanism by

which this compound damages the kidney is not understood. In this paper we describe (1) the toxicity of HCBD to rat liver and kidney, (2) the effect of modifiers of drug metabolising enzymes on HCBD-induced liver and kidney injury, (3) the role of glutathione in the toxicity.

RESULTS AND DISCUSSION

HCBD-Induced Liver Injury

A single administration of HCBD (300 mg/kg, ip) produced within 24 h a significant increase in liver to body weight ratio which was associated with a significant increase in liver water and K^+ concentration and a small but non-significant increase in Na^+ (Table 1). However, the concentration of Na^+ plus K^+ in total liver water did not change (Table 1). No change was seen in cytochrome P-450 content (Table 1) or increase in plasma markers of liver dysfunction. The increase in liver water was rapid, reaching a peak 16-24 h after dosing and then returning to control levels over the following three days.

TABLE 1   Water, sodium, potassium and cytochrome P-450 content of rat liver 24 h after HCBD (300 mg/kg, ip)

Parameter	Control	HCBD
Liver/body wt x 100	3.19±0.04	4.37*±0.06
Water (gH_2O/g dry wt)	2.26±0.02	2.73*±0.04
Sodium (μeq/g dry wt)	99± 5	113 ± 8
Potassium (μeq/g dry wt)	318± 3	369*± 7
Concentration $Na^+ + K^+$ in cell water (mM)	185± 2	177 ± 4
Cytochrome P-450 (nmol/total liver)	293±19	300 ±23

Results are means ± SE with five animals per group. *Significantly different from control P<0.05. Water content was determined as weight loss on drying at 105°. The dried liver tissue was extracted with 5% trichloro-acetic acid and the Na^+ and K^+ determined by flame photometry. Cytochrome P-450 was determined on whole liver homogenate by the method where both cuvettes are gassed with CO and one is reduced with dithionite.

Detailed morphological studies showed that HCBD produced no consistent alteration in the liver at the light microscopic level, although some animals showed slight vacuolation of periportal hepatocytes 16 and 24 h after dosing. Ultrastructural changes showed that by 8 h when there was a significant increase in liver water the mitochondria of the periportal hepatocytes were swollen and this was very marked by 24 h (Fig. 1). In addition to mitochondrial swelling some proliferation of smooth endoplasmic reticulum in periportal cells was seen at 24 h.

An interesting observation is the maintenance of the normal concentration of Na^+ and K^+ during the time of maximum increased water. These cation and water changes induced by HCBD in rat liver are identical to those produced by carbon disulphide (CS_2) (Butler, Hempsall and Magos, 1974). However, CS_2 when given to rats pretreated with phenobarbitone produces centrilobular hydropic degeneration (Bond and co-workers, 1969; Magos and Butler, 1972). Following CS_2 the additional water has been shown to be located predominantly within the cisternae of the rough endoplasmic reticulum (Butler, Chandra and Magos, 1974), which may be related to the reduction of cytochrome P-450 reported by Bond and DeMatteis (1969). Thus,

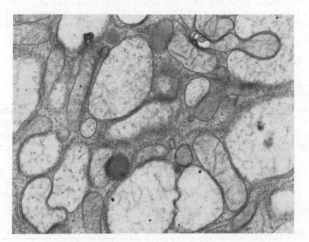

Fig. 1.   Marked mitochondrial swelling in a periportal
          hepatocyte 24 h after administration of HCBD (300
          mg/kg, ip) x 19,500.

although the cation changes are similar with HCBD and CS_2 the ultrastructural changes are seen to occur in different parts of the liver lobule
and in different intracellular compartments. Additionally HCBD does not
appear to cause a loss of cytochrome P-450 (Table 1).

HCBD-Induced Renal Injury

Administration of HCBD (200 mg/kg, ip) causes necrosis of the pars recta of
the proximal tubule situated in the outer stripe of the outer medulla of
the rat kidney. The earliest morphological changes detectable by light
microscopy were observed after 8 h, with several proximal tubules showing
necrosis. By 16 h, a distinct band of tubular necrosis was seen in the
outer stripe of the outer medulla (Fig. 2).

Ultrastructural changes were seen as early as 1 h after HCBD (300 mg/kg,
ip) although necrosis was not marked until 8 h. Mitochondrial swelling was
seen 1-4 h after dosing in the S_1 and S_2 segments of the proximal tubule.
By 8 h the major pathological changes were largely confined to the S_3
segment and consisted of loss of brush border, mitochondrial swelling and
cellular necrosis. Thus in the rat HCBD produces a site-specific nephrotoxic
effect on the S_3 segment of the proximal tubule, located in the outer
stripe of the outer medulla.

The Effect of Modifiers of Drug Metabolising Enzymes on HCBD-Induced Liver and Kidney Injury

A body of evidence is developing which suggests that certain halogenated
ethylenes can be transformed into highly reactive intermediates in vivo.
For example, vinyl chloride and dichloroethylene are thought to be metabolically activated to an epoxide which is the ultimate reactive and
carcinogenic metabolite of these compounds (IARC Monograph, 1979). We
speculated that the toxicity of HCBD requires metabolic activation in vivo
of one of the double bonds, the reactive intermediate may be an epoxide,

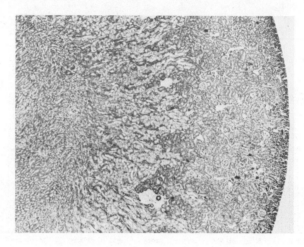

Fig. 2. Kidney of rat 16 h after injection of HCBD (200
mg/kg, ip) showing a distinct band of tubular necrosis
in the outer stripe of the outer medulla. Haematoxylin
and eosin x 30.

which would be expected to be a strongly electrophilic species capable of
alkylating nucleophilic sites on tissue macromolecules. Drug metabolising
enzymes are capable of catalysing the above reaction (i.e. cytochrome(s)
P-450). In an attempt to determine the role of metabolic activation in
HCBD-induced toxicity we looked at the effect of modifying hepatic and
renal cytochrome P-450's on the extent of liver and kidney injury. Renal
injury was assessed by plasma urea, light microscopy and p-aminohippurate
transport (PAH) into thin slices of renal cortex whilst liver injury was
determined by plasma alanine aminotransferase (ALT) activity and light
microscopy. Administration of HCBD to rats treated with the hepatic P-450
inhibitors SKF525A or piperonyl butoxide did not alter the response of the
liver or kidney to injury (Fig. 3). Treatment of animals with inducers of
P-450's, phenobarbitone, β-naphthoflavone, A-1254 or Isosafrole, followed
by HCBD also did not appear to alter either liver or kidney injury (Fig. 4
and Fig. 5), although Isosafrole treatment did produce a less marked rise
in plasma urea and no decrease in PAH accumulation. Previous studies (Lock
and Ishmael, 1981) had shown a small enhancement of nephrotoxicity by
pretreatment with A-1254, however this has not proved repeatable (Fig. 4).
These studies indicate that altering drug metabolising enzyme activity does
not appear to alter liver or kidney injury produced by HCBD. These findings
are in contrast to those reported for vinyl chloride or dichloroethylene
toxicities where the degree of organ toxicity can be altered by treatment
with modifiers of drug metabolising enzymes (Jaeger and co-workers, 1976;
Reynolds and co-workers, 1975). Our studies indicate that either metabolic
activation is not a prerequisite for toxicity or that the P-450 modifiers
used do not inhibit or induce those enzymes responsible for HCBD-induced
toxicity.

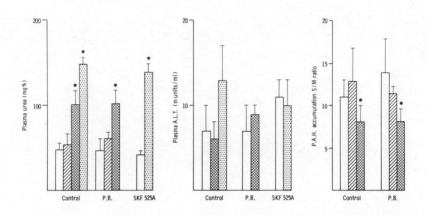

Fig. 3. Plasma urea and alanine aminotransferase and PAH
accumulation in renal slices from rats treated with
SKF525A or piperonyl butoxide and then HCBD or corn
oil for 24 h. Animals were dosed with corn oil (☐) or
HCBD ip at 100 mg/kg (▨), 200 mg/kg (▩) or 300 mg/kg
(⬚). Results are mean ± SE with 5 animals per
treatment. *Significantly different from no HCBD
P<0.05. SKF525A was given at 75 mg/kg, sc in saline
1 h before and 6.5 h after HCBD, piperonyl butoxide
(PB) was given at 400 mg/kg sc, 1 h before HCBD. PAH
accumulation was measured as described by Berndt and
Mehendale (1979).

The Effect of HCBD on Renal and Hepatic Non-Protein Sulphydryl Content and the Effect of Diethylmaleate Treatment

Glutathione is used in the conjugation of foreign compounds that are
excreted as mercapturic acid (Boyland and Chasseaud, 1969). In addition an
important role of glutathione in the body is to protect vital nucleophilic
sites in hepatocytes, renal tubular cells (and presumably other tissues)
from electrophilic attack by alkylating metabolites of drugs e.g. acetaminophen (Mitchell and co-workers, 1973), bromobenzene (Jollow and co-workers,
1974). If HCBD is metabolically activated at one of the double bonds then
the electrophilic species generated would be capable of reacting with
glutathione. We therefore decided to look at the effect of HCBD on liver
and kidney NP-SH content (mainly glutathione). Increasing concentrations
of HCBD up to 900 mg/kg ip produced in 4 h a dose related decrease in liver
NP-SH in male rats, the maximum effect occurring at about 750 mg/kg; no
effect being seen at 150 mg/kg (Fig. 6). However no decrease in renal
NP-SH was seen (Fig. 6).

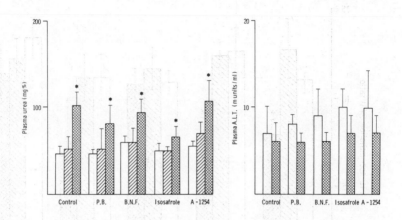

Fig. 4.   Plasma urea and alanine aminotransferase in rats
          treated with various inducers and then HCBD or corn
          oil for 24 h. Animals were dosed with corn oil (☐)
          or HCBD ip at 100 mg/kg (▨) or 200 mg/kg (▨).
          Results are mean ± SE with 5 animals per treatment.
          * Significantly different from no HCBD P<0.05.
          Phenobarbitone (PB) was given at 75 mg/kg/day ip for 3
          days in saline, Aroclor 1254 (A-1254) at 300 mg/kg ip
          in corn oil, β-naphthoflavone (BNF) at 100 mg/kg/day
          or isosafrole at 200 mg/kg/day ip for 4 days in corn
          oil. HCBD was administered on day 4 for phenobarbitone
          treated rats and day 5 for other inducers.

Female rats are more sensitive to HCBD-induced renal damage, a dose of 50
mg/kg, ip producing a rise in plasma urea (Table 2) and tubular necrosis to
a similar extent to that seen at 200 mg/kg in males. Increasing concentration of HCBD up to 600 mg/kg ip in female rats produced a decrease in
liver NP-SH at 600 mg/kg by 4 h, and a dose-related decrease in renal
NP-SH, the maximum effect occurring at about 450 mg/kg (Fig. 6). Thus the
female rat appears to be more susceptible to renal injury produced by HCBD
than the male and this increased sensitivity may be related to a marked
depletion in renal NP-SH in the female but not male rat. Treatment of male
rats with diethylmaleate, a compound which is known to deplete tissue NP-SH
content markedly enhanced the nephrotoxicity of HCBD, without affecting the
liver. Fig. 7 shows that as early as 4-8 h after HCBD administration there
is a marked increase in plasma urea, which is not observed at that time
following HCBD administration alone. These studies indicate (i) that HCBD
or a metabolite may react with NP-SH, if so (ii) this reaction occurs at a
different rate in female compared to male rat kidney, (iii) that tissue
NP-SH appears to play a protective role against HCBD-induced renal damage.

In summary, our data at present are not entirely consistent. We have no
good evidence for metabolic activation of HCBD via P-450, although formation
of a glutathione conjugate in the liver, which is transported to the kidney

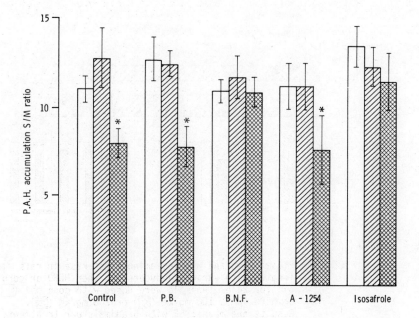

Fig. 5. PAH accumulation by slices of renal cortex from rats
treated with various inducers and then HCBD or corn
oil for 24 h. Animals were dosed with corn oil (☐)
or HCBD ip at 100 mg/kg (▨) or 200 mg/kg (▨).
Results are mean ± SE with 5 animals per treatment.
*Significantly different from no HCBD P<0.05. For
dosing regimen see legend to Fig. 4. PAH accumulation
was measured as described by Berndt and Mehendale
(1979).

TABLE 2 Plasma urea in male and female rats, 24 h after HCBD administration

Parameter	Sex	\multicolumn{4}{c}{HCBD (mg/kg)}
		0	50	100	200
Plasma urea (mg%)	Male	39±3	40± 3	51±4	80±4
Plasma urea (mg%)	Female	40±2	145±20	156±8	189±7

Results are mean ± SE with 4 animals per group.

and activated is possible but not consistent with the enhanced renal damage
produced by NP-SH depletion. Only by understanding the metabolism of HCBD
in both the liver and kidney and exploiting the male, female differences
will we be able to postulate a mechanism of toxicity. The reactions
responsible for the depletion of NP-SH are currently being studied.

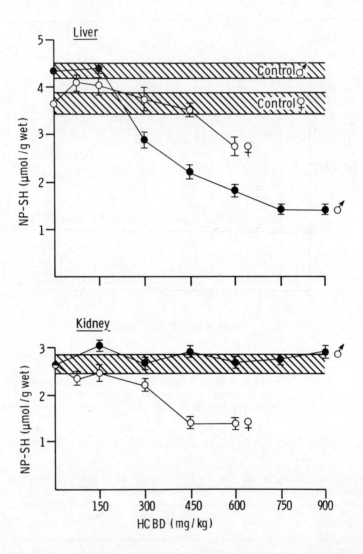

Fig. 6. The effect of varying doses of HCBD on NP-SH content
in male and female rat liver and kidney. Results are
mean ± SE with at least 3 animals per HCBD concentration. NP-SH was determined on tissue extracts
prepared in buffered ethanol as described by Johnson
(1966) by the method of Beutler, Duron and Kelly
(1963).

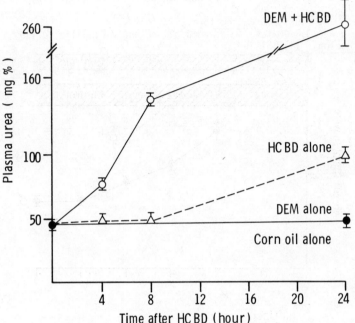

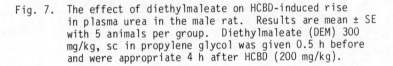

Fig. 7. The effect of diethylmaleate on HCBD-induced rise
in plasma urea in the male rat. Results are mean ± SE
with 5 animals per group. Diethylmaleate (DEM) 300
mg/kg, sc in propylene glycol was given 0.5 h before
and were appropriate 4 h after HCBD (200 mg/kg).

Acknowledgements

The authors would like to thank Dr I S Pratt for the electron microscopy,
Dr J B Hook for his contribution to some of the work and Mr E Howard and
Mrs P Berry for valuable technical assistance.

References

Berndt, W.O. and H.M. Mehendale (1979) Toxicology, 14, 55-65
Beutler, E., O. Duron and B.M. Kelly (1963) J. Lab. Clin. Chem., 61 882-888
Bond, E.J. and F. DeMatteis (1969) Biochem. Pharmacol., 18, 2531-2549
Bond, E.J., W.H. Butler, F. DeMatteis and J.M. Barnes (1969) Brit. J. Ind.
  Med., 26, 335-337
Boyland, E., and L.F. Chasseaud (1969) Advan. Enzymol., 32, 173-219
Butler, W.H., S.V. Chandra and L. Magos (1974) J. Path., 112, 147-152
Butler, W.H., V. Hempsall and L. Magos (1974) J. Path., 113, 53-59
Gradiski, D., J.L. Magadur (1974) Eur. J. Toxicol., 7, 247-254
Gradiski, D., P. Duprat, J.L. Magadur, and E. Fayein (1975) Eur.J. Toxicol.,
  8, 180-187

Harleman, J.M. and W. Seinen (1979) Toxicol. Appl. Pharmacol, 47, 1-14
IARC Monographs on the evaluation of the carcinogenic risk of chemicals to
    humans (1979) 19, 377-459
Jaeger, R.J., F.E. Mullen., L.J. Coffman and S.D. Murphy (1976) Proc. Eur.
    Soc. Toxicol., 17, 301-308
Johnson, M.K. (1966) J. Chromatogr., 23, 474-475
Jollow, D.J., J.R. Mitchell, N. Zampaglione and J.R. Gillette (1974)
    Pharmacology, 11, 151-169
Kociba, R.J., D.G., Keyes, G.C. Jersey, J.J. Ballard., D.A. Dittenber.,
    J.F. Quast, C.E. Wade, C.G. Humiston and B.A. Schwetz (1977) Am. Ind.
    Hyg. Assoc. J., 38, 589-602
Lock, E.A. and J. Ishmael (1979) Arch. Toxicol., 43, 47-57
Lock, E.A. and J. Ishmael (1981) Toxicol. Appl. Pharmacol., 57, 79-87
Magos, L., and W.H. Butler (1972) Brit. J. Ind. Med., 29, 95-98
Mitchell, J.R., D.J. Jollow, W.Z. Potter, J.R. Gillette and B.B. Brodie
    (1973) J. Pharmacol Exp. Ther., 187, 185-194
Reynolds, E.S., M.T. Moslen, S. Szabo, R.J. Jaeger and S.D. Murphy (1975)
    Am. J. Path., 81, 219-231

Modulation of Nephrotoxicity by Environmental Chemicals

G. Rush, J. Newton and J. B. Hook

Department of Pharmacology and Toxicology, and Center for
Environmental Toxicology, Michigan State University, East Lansing,
Michigan 48824, USA

ABSTRACT

Environmental contaminants such as polybrominated biphenyls (PBBs) and polychlorinated biphenyls (PCBs) produce no detectable alteration in normal renal function.
There is a growing body of evidence however, that these contaminants alter the
biochemical pathways responsible for the metabolic activation of other chemicals
which may be nephrotoxic. Chloroform nephrotoxicity was markedly enhanced by PBB
ingestion in mice and the degree of enhancement was proportional to the concentration of PBBs in the diet. The nephrotoxicity of carbon tetrachloride, trichloroethylene
and 1,1,2-trichloroethane was also markedly enhanced in PBB treated mice. Similarly,
the nephrotoxicity of acetaminophen was enhanced in rats treated with PBBs. On the
other hand, PCBs reduced the nephrotoxicity of chloroform in mice. The
nephrotoxicity of chloroform was also reduced by exposure to TCDD. Thus, a variety
of environmental chemicals may influence metabolism within the kidney and
subsequently alter the toxicity of certain compounds that require metabolic activation
to a nephrotoxic product.

KEY WORDS

polybrominated biphenyls; polychlorinated biphenyls; dioxins; nephrotoxicity; kidney;
chloroform; acetaminophen; environmental contamination

INTRODUCTION

The mammalian kidney, because of its high rate of perfusion, active transport
capabilities and concentrating functions, is often exposed to much higher concentrations of chemicals than are other organs. Consequently, the kidney is highly
susceptible to the toxic effects of a variety of chemicals.

A chemical may act directly or indirectly on the kidney to produce a toxic response.
For instance, agents like heavy metals and antibiotics like gentamicin probably act
directly to interfere with some biochemical mechanism required for cellular integrity.
On the other hand, an ingested chemical may require metabolic activation prior to
becoming toxic. Alternatively, chemicals may produce more subtle effects manifest
primarily as biochemical changes that alter the response of the kidney to the toxic
effects of other compounds. Exposure to these chemicals, be it in the workplace or

through environmental contamination, may produce no detectable correlating functional nephropathy.

Recently, the metabolism of chemicals to toxic, reactive intermediates has been implicated in chemically induced mutagenesis, teratogenesis, necrogenesis and other disorders (Ames, 1973; Gillette, 1974). Relationships between the formation of reactive metabolites and the development of acute cellular injury have been studied most extensively in the rodent liver. Toxic intermediates of xenobiotic metabolism may alter normal cell function by a number of different mechanisms such as covalent binding with essential cellular macromolecules and/or by stimulating the peroxidation of membrane lipids (Boyd, 1980).

Chemicals that influence the pathways involved in the production of reactive intermediates may alter the toxicity of other agents. The purpose of this paper is to review the interactions between environmental agents that influence these pathways in the kidney and their influence on other potentially toxic agents.

Drug Metabolism

With the exception of fatty acid hydroxylation, mixed function oxidase (MFO) activity in the kidney is generally very low in comparison to that of the liver. However, unlike the liver, renal MFOs may be confined to a specific population of renal cells. In the kidney, there is a cortical-papillary gradient (highest in the cortex lowest in the papilla) for MFOs and P-450 concentrations (Zenser, 1978). In addition, rats treated with 2,3,7,8- tetrachlorodibenzo-p-dioxin (TCDD), an inducer of microsomal enzymes, have increased renal MFO activities and proliferation of the smooth endoplasmic reticulum in the S_3 cells of the proximal tubule while the anatomically-adjacent S_2 cells and cells of the distal tubule are unaffected (Fowler, 1977). Thus, microsomes prepared from whole kidney cortex, which contain many different types, may greatly dilute out the MFOs.

ENVIRONMENTAL CONTAMINANTS

A list of common chemical pollutants that increase renal enzyme activities is shown in Table 1.

TABLE 1   Environmental Pollutants that Increase Renal Xenobiotic Metabolizing Enzyme Activities

3,4-Benzo(a)pyrene
Chlorinated dibenzodioxins (TCDD)
Dichlorodiphenyltrichloroethane (DDT)
Polybrominated biphenyls (PBBs)
Polychlorinated biphenyls (PCBs)
Hexachlorobenzene

(From Kluwe, 1980.)

There has been much interest recently in the toxicological potential of PBBs since the commercial fire retardant, Firemaster BP6 (Michigan Chemical Co., St. Louis, MI), primarily hexabromobiphenyl, was inadvertently mixed into domestic animal feed in south central Michigan, resulting in exposure of commercial livestock to high concentrations of dietary PBBs (Mercer, 1976). Secondary exposure of the human population occurred through consumption of meat and dairy products derived from contaminated livestock (Chen, 1977). PBBs are nonpolar, lipophylic and for the most part, chemically unreactive compounds. Because of these physical properties PBBs have an extremely long environmental and biological half-life.

The forced feeding of large amounts of PBB (25 g/day) to cows produced dilatation of renal tubules and collecting ducts and elevations of serum urea nitrogen and urine protein concentrations (Moorhead, 1977). However, the cows also appeared emaciated and the relative contributions of PBBs treatment and body wasting to the reported symptoms are difficult to distinguish. Lower doses (0.25 g/day) produced no kidney abnormalities. Rats ingesting 5 mg/kg/day of PBBs for up to 3 months exhibited normal renal function. No changes were detected in such functional parameters as clearance of inulin (glomerular filtration), clearance of para-aminohippurate (effective renal plasma flow) or fractional excretion of sodium (Table 2).

Similarly, renal morphology was also normal following 3 months dietary exposure to PBBs. In contrast to physiological function, renal microsomal MFO activities were markedly altered by PBBs (Table 3). Renal aryl hydrocarbon hydroxylase (AHH), biphenyl-4-hydroxylase and biphenyl-2-hydroxylase were selectively induced by PBB while epoxide hydrolase was reduced (Table 3) (McCormack, 1978).

TABLE 2   Effect of Feeding PBBs on Glomerular Filtration Rate (GFR), Effective Renal Plasma Flow (ERPF), and Fractional Sodium Excretion (FE_{Na})

Treatment	GFR (ml/min)	ERPF (ml/min)	FE_{na}(%)
Control	2.46+0.16*	10.78+0.63	0.17+0.04
PBB	2.34+0.21	8.77+0.97	0.12+0.03

*Values are means + S.E.M. for four animals.
(From McCormack, 1978.)

TABLE 3   Effect of PBB-feeding on Renal Arylhydrocarbon Hydroxylase (AHH), Epoxide Hydrolase (EH), Biphenyl-2-Hydroxylase (BP-2-OH) and Biphenyl-4-hydroxylase (BP-4-OH) Activities*

Treatment	AHH	EH	BP-2-OH	BP-4-OH
Control	2.94+1.35*	0.14+0.06	0.01+0.01	0.04+0.01
PBB	32.82+1.73	0.02+0.01	0.11+0.01	0.22+0.02

*Values are mean + S.E.M. for three animals.
Fluorescence units/mg protein/min.
Nanomoles of product/mg protein/min.
(From McCormack, 1978.)

PCBs are similar to PBBs in many respects. They are complex mixtures of halogen-substituted biphenyls and related compounds, they are lipid soluble, resistant to metabolic degradation and are accumulated in fatty tissues. PCBs have been used as flame retardants, plasticisers, and heat dispersing agents in electrical transformers. Because of their many uses, PCBs are global contaminants, though their current manufacture and use is restricted. Many different formulations of PCBs have been marketed (for example, various Aroclors and Kanneclors), and some have been reported to contain small amounts of highly toxic chlorinated dibenzofurans and dibenzodioxins as contaminants. The contributions of these contaminants to the effects of commercial PCB mixtures in mammals is unknown (Dustman, 1971; Kluwe, 1980).

The acute toxicity of PCBs, like that of PBBs, is relatively low. Ingestion of subtoxic amounts, however, stimulates the activities of many xenobiotic metabolizing enzymes. Occupational exposure to PCBs has been reported to affect drug disposition in man (Alvares, 1977) indicating that the response to metabolically activated toxicants may be altered by exposure to PCBs. PCBs are structurally similar to PBBs, and the effects of PCBs on MFO activities are qualitatively similar to PBBs. PCBs induce renal P-450 and microsomal enzyme activities in rodent kidney but are less potent in this respect than PBBs.

TCDD which has extremely low LD50 values in mammals (0.0006 to 0.115 mg/kg) (Schwetz, 1973) has been found in commercial products such as the wood preservative pentachlorophenol, the herbicide 2,4,5-trichlorophenoxyacetic acid and other products synthesized from chlorinated phenols (Langer, 1973). Administration of relatively large amounts of TCDD to rodents produced direct renal injury; hydronephrosis in male and female offspring of TCDD-treated dams and degenerative changes in kidneys of adult animals have been reported (Moore, 1973; McConnell, 1978). Higher species, such as nonhuman primates, appear to be more susceptible to the nephrotoxic effects of TCDD than are lower species, such as rodents. The opposite is true for the hepatotoxic effects of TCDD (Moore, 1979). These differences may be a consequence of species differences in TCDD distribution and disposition.

TABLE 4   Effects of Polybrominated Biphenyls (PBBs) on Chloroform-induced Nephrotoxicity in Mice*

Function	Chloroform		
	0.000 ml/kg	0.005 ml/kg	0.025 ml/kg
BUN, mg/dl			
At 0 ppm PBBs	21+4	27+4	26+3
At 1 ppm PBBs	22∓4	23∓4	35∓4
At 25 ppm PBBs	22∓2	22∓2	47∓5†
At 100 ppm PBBs	21∓2	28∓2	81∓9†
PAH, S/M*			
At 0 ppm PBBs	7.8+0.4	7.6+0.5	6.2+0.5
At 1 ppm PBBs	7.5∓0.3	5.8∓0.6	4.4∓0.5†
At 25 ppm PBBs	8.1∓0.5	5.5∓0.8	4.1∓0.6†
At 100 ppm PBBs	8.4∓0.4	5.4∓0.6	3.7∓0.4†

*Elevations of BUN and reductions of PAH S/M are signs of kidney injury 48 hr after i.p. chloroform (S/M is slice-to-medium concentration ratio). Each value is the mean + SEM from six mice.
†Significantly different from control (same dietary concentration of PBBs, 0.000 ml/kg chloroform), P<0.05.
(Data modified from Kluwe and Hook, 1980.)

Administration of TCDD increases enzyme activities in both kidney and liver. The magnitudes of increase, however, are generally greater in kidney than in liver (Aitio, 1978; Hook, 1975). Like PBBs, TCDD is a potent inducer of renal AHH but not renal EH or glutathione-S-transferase [generally regarded as detoxification enzymes (Aitio, 1978)].

Interactions with Other Nephrotoxic Agents

Environmental contaminants like PBBs, PCBs and TCDD, by altering the pathways responsible for both detoxification and bioactivation, are of toxicological importance. With the exception of TCDD, these chemicals (PBBs, PCBs) in general, have no nephrotoxic effects when administered alone. However, they can alter the toxic response to other known nephrotoxicants. Halogenated aliphatic hydrocarbons, like chloroform and carbon tetrachloride, are hepato- and nephrotoxic chemicals that are thought to be converted to toxic products via microsomal metabolism (Butler, 1961; Pohl, 1979). Chloroform nephrotoxicity is potentiated by PBBs. Administration of PBBs alone or subtoxic doses of chloroform has no effect on renal toxicity. However, in animals treated with chloroform subsequent to PBBs exposure, nephrotoxicity is evident (Table 4).

Ingestion of PBBs was also shown to enhance the nephrotoxicity of other halogenated hydrocarbons. Carbon tetrachloride, trichloroethylene, and 1,1,2-trichloroethane produced more renal injury in PBBs-treated mice than they did in control mice (Kluwe, 1979). Thus, PBBs exposure may enhance the susceptibility of the kidney to the nephrotoxic effects of chlorinated aliphatic hydrocarbons.

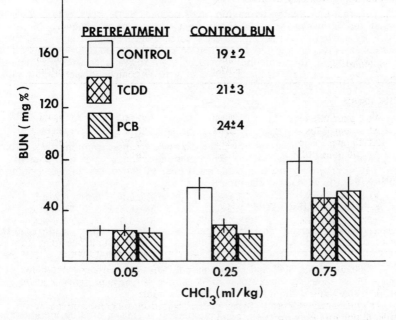

FIG. 1. Effects of PCBs and TCDD on chloroform induced changes in blood urea nitrogen (BUN). Control mice pretreated with TCDD or PCBs for varying periods of time were challenged with single i.p. injections of $CHCl_3$. (From Kluwe, 1978.)

The nephrotoxicity of acetaminophen (APAP) is considered to be associated with the production of a reactive metabolite, which may also be responsible for reducing renal concentration of nonprotein sulphydryl groups (primarily glutathione). Fischer 344 rats pretreated with PBBs exhibited marked renal functional impairment after a dose of APAP that produced no changes in naive animals (Kuo, 1981). The ability of APAP to deplete nonprotein sulphydryls in the isolated perfused rat kidney was enhanced by prior treatment of the donor rats with PBBs and was reduced by piperonyl butoxide. More recently, excretion of the mercapturic acid conjugate of APAP (presumed to be indicative of the conjugation of a reactive intermediate with glutathione) by the isolated perfused rat kidney was enhanced three-fold to four-fold by PBBs, whereas formation of the nontoxic glucuronide and sulfate conjugates were decreased by 20% (Newton, 1979).

Although PBBs and PCBs are very similar in their patterns of microsomal enzyme induction, their effects on the pathways leading to metabolic activation appear to be different. PBBs potentiate the nephrotoxic effects of chloroform (Table 4), while both PCBs and TCDD markedly reduced the nephrotoxic effects of chloroform (Fig. 1). Similarly, CCl_4-induced renal damage was increased by PBBs but not by PCBs (Kluwe, 1979). Thus, in addition to being more potent as modifiers of drug metabolism than PCBs, PBBs also affect enzymatic toxification pathways in a qualitatively different manner. In addition, the PBBs and PCBs preparations used in all of the studies mentioned above were commercially available products (Firemaster BP6, Aroclor 1254) and consist of mixtures of many different polyhalogenated biphenyls and small quantities of other halogenated chemicals. Quantitative or qualitative differences in the manner in which PBBs and PCBs affect the biotransformation of certain chemicals to toxicants could result from different congeners present or from contaminants in the mixtures rather than from a difference in the type of halogen (Br, Cl) attached to the biphenyl rings.

The fact that these polyhalogenated biphenyls induce MFOs does not necessarily indicate that the pathways for metabolic activation have been induced. There are alternative explanations. For example, these agents (PCBs, PBBs) may selectively alter renal enzymes responsible for detoxification of halogenated hydrocarbons either prior to or subsequent to metabolic activation. In addition, these environmental contaminants may alter the pharmacokinetics of a toxic compound such that smaller or greater quantitites are delivered to the kidney.

SUMMARY

In laboratory animals the nephrotoxic effects of agents such as chloroform and acetaminophen are markedly altered by prior exposure to these contaminants. Thus, the detrimental effect on the kidney from contamination of the environment by chemicals that alter mixed function oxidases (PBBs, PCBs) resides in that potential interaction that exists with other chemicals.

ACKNOWLEDGEMENTS

This research was supported by USPHS grant No. ES00560 and a grant from the Michigan Department of Agriculture. Michigan Agricultural Experiment Station Journal article No. 10014. We wish to thank D. Hummel and M. Whiting for their help in preparing the manuscript.

REFERENCES

Aitio, A., and Parkki, M.G. (1978). Organ specific induction of drug metabolizing enzymes by 2,3,7,8-tetrachorodibenzo-p-dioxin in the rat. Toxicol. Appl. Pharmacol., 44, 107-114.

Alvares, A.P., Fischbein, A., Anderson, K.E., and Kappas, A. (1977).   Alterations in
drug metabolism in workers exposed to polychlorinated biphenyls.   Clin.   Pharmacol. Ther., 22, 140-146.
Ames, B.N., Durston, W.E., Yamasaki, E., and Lee, F.D. (1973).   Carcinogens as
mutagens: A simple test system combining liver homogenates for activation and
bacteria for detection. Proc. Natl. Acad. Sci. USA, 78, 2282-2285.
Boyd, M.R. (19??).   Biochemical mechanisms in chemical induced lung injury,   Roles
of metabolic activation. CRC Crit. Rev. Toxicol., 103-176.
Butler, T.C. (1961).   Reduction of carbon tetrachloride in vivo and reduction of carbon
tetrachloride and chloroform in vitro by tissues and tissue homogenates.   J.
Pharmacol. Exp. Ther., 143, 311-319.
Chen, E. (1977).   Michigan: If something odd happens.... Atlantic Michigan, 240, 2-20.
Dustman, E.H., Stickel, L.F., Blus, L.J., Reichel, W.L., and Wiemeyer, S.N. (1971).
The occurrence and significance of polychlorinated biphenyls in the environment.
Trans. 36th North Amer. Wildlife and Nat. Res. Conf., Wildlife Management
Institute, Washington, D.C., p. 118.
Fowler, B.A., Hook, G.E.R., and Lucier, G.W. (1977).   Tetrachlorodibenzo-p-dioxin
induction of renal microsomal enzyme systems: Ultrastructural effects on pars
recta (S_3) proximal tubule cells of the rat kidney.   J. Pharmacol. Exp. Ther.,
203, 712-721.
Gillette, J.R., Mitchell, J.R., and Brodie, B.B. (1974).   Biochemical mechanisms of
drug toxicity. Ann. Rev. Pharmacol., 14, 271-289.
Hook, G.E.R., Haseman, K., and Lucier, G.W. (1975).   Induction and suppression of
hepatic and extrahepatic microsomal foreign compound metabolizing enzymes
systems by 2,3,7,8-tetrachlorodibenzo-p-dioxin. Chem. Biol. Interactions, 10,
199-214.
Kluwe, W.M., and Hook, J.B. (1978).   Polybrominated biphenyl-induced potentiation of
chloroform toxicity. Toxicol. Appl. Pharmacol., 45, 861-869.
Kluwe, W.M., Herrmann, C.L., and Hook, J.B. (1979).   Effects of dietary
polychlorinated biphenyls and polybrominated biphenyls on the renal and hepatic
toxicities of several chlorinated hydrocarbon solvents in mice.   J. Toxicol.
Environ. Hlth., 5, 605-615.
Kluwe, W.M., and Hook, J.B. (1980).   Effects of environmental chemicals on kidney
metabolism and function. Kidney Int., 18, 648-655.
Kuo, C-H., McNish, R.W., Mehl, S.L. and Hook, J.B. (1981).   Effect of enzyme indcers
on acetaminophen (APAP)-induced nephrotoxicity and hepatotoxicity.   Toxicologist 1, 10.
Langer, H.G., Brody, T.P., and Briggs, P.R. (1973).   Formation of dibenzodioxins and
other condensation products from chlorinated phenols and derivatives. Environ.
Hlth. Perspec., 5: 3-7.
McConnell, E.E., Moore, J.A., and Dalgard, D.W. (1978).   Toxicity of
2,3,7,8-tetrachlorodibenzo-p-dioxin in rhesus monkeys (macaca mulatta) follow-
ing a single oral dose. Toxicol. Appl. Pharmacol., 43, 175-187.
McCormack, K.M., Kluwe, W.M., Rickert, D.W., Sanger, V.L., and Hook, J.B. (1978).
Renal and hepatic microsomal enzyme stimulation and renal function following
three months of dietary exposure to polybrominated biphenyls. Toxicol. Appl.
Pharmacol., 44, 539-553.
Mercer, H.D., Teske, R.H., Condon, R.J., Furr, A., Meerdink, G., Buck, W., and Fries,
G. (1976).   Herd health status of animals exposed to polybrominated biphenyls.
J. Toxicol. Environ. Hlth., 2, 335-349.
Moore, J.A., Gupta, B.N., Zinkl, J.G., and Vos, J.G. (1973).   Postnatal effects of
maternal exposure to 2,3,7,8-tetrachlorodibenzo-p-dioxin (TCDD).   Environ.
Hlth. Perspec., 5, 81-85.
Moore, J.A., McConnell, E.E., Dalgard, D.W., and Harris, M.W. (1979).   Comparative
toxicity of halogenated dibenzofurans of guinea pigs, mice and rhesus monkeys.
Ann. N.Y. Acad. Sci., 320, 151-163.

Moorhead, P.D., Willett, L.B., Brumm, C.J. and Mercer, H.D. (1977).   Pathology of experimentally-induced polybrominated biphenyl toxicosis in pregnant heifers. J. Am. Vet. Med. Assoc., 170, 307-313.

Newton, J.F., Kluwe, W.M., and Hook, J.B. (1979).   Acetaminophen (APAP)-induced glutathione depletion in the isolated perfused kidney (IPK).   Toxicol. Appl. Pharmacol., 48, A19.

Pohl, L.R. (1979).   in Reviews of Biochemical Toxicology (Eds. E. Hodgson, J. Bend and R.M. Philpot), p. 79, Elsevier-North Holland, New York.

Schwetz, B.A., Norris, J.M., Sparshu, G.L., Rose, W.K., Gehring, P.J., Emerson, J.L., and Gerbig, G.C. (1973).   Toxicity of chlorinated dibenzo-p-dioxins.   Environ. Hlth. Perspec., 5, 87-99.

Zenser, T.V., Mattammal, M.B., and Davis, B.B. (1978).   Differential distribution of the mixed-function oxidase activities in rabbit kidney.   J. Pharmacol. Exp. Ther., 207, 719-725.

SYMPOSIUM

Heme Synthesis and Degradation: Its Role in Predicting Drug Toxicity

Chairmen: U. A. Meyer, G. D. Sweeney

Heme Synthesis and Degradation:
Its Role in Predicting Drug Toxicity —
Opening Remarks

U. A. Meyer* and G. D. Sweeney**

*Div. of Clin. Pharmacol., Univ. Hospital, Zurich, Switzerland
**Dept. of Medicine, McMaster Univ., Hamilton, Ont. L8N 3Z5,
Canada

INTRODUCTORY REMARKS

The pathways of heme metabolism have long been recognized as targets for
toxic processes and the purpose of this symposium is to explore the reasons
for this.   These introductory remarks will define essential terms, describe
some functions of heme, examine the properties of the heme biosynthetic and
degradative pathways which have accorded these a special place in toxicology; and review briefly the history of the involvement of heme metabolism
in human toxicity.

All aerobic cells possess the machinery to both make and degrade heme, which
is the prosthetic group of a large number of hemoproteins.   Hemoproteins
transport oxygen (hemoglobin and myoglobin), transport electrons (mitochondrial cytochromes), activate oxygen (tryptophan oxygenase, P-450 cytochromes), activate hydrogen peroxide (peroxidases) or decompose hydrogen
peroxide (catalases).   The quantities of intermediates (δ-aminolevulinic
acid, porphobilinogen, porphyrinogens) accumulating and being lost by
irreversible oxidation is very small, totaling approximately 1% of daily
heme synthesis.   Small changes in the efficiency of precursor conversion
to heme are thus readily detected.

In the human, the bone marrow synthesizes roughly 300 mg of heme per day to
serve the needs for hemoglobin synthesis; the liver manufactures approximately 100 mg per day, most of which is utilized to maintain microsomal
cytochrome systems.   Kidney, gut, lung and spleen make smaller amounts of
heme and even smaller quantities are made in the remaining tissues.   Half-
lives for the hemoproteins in rats range from 30 days for red cell hemoglobin to about 8 to 48 hours for microsomal cytochrome P-450 and even
shorter half-lives for tryptophan oxygenase.

The terms heme, hemin and hematin are used as if they were interchangeable.
Heme is the complex of iron (II) and protoporphyrin IX; the oxidized (iron -
III) state of hemin usually refers to hemin chloride prepared from blood and
to hematin for the compound in which the chloride ion of hemin is replaced

by an hydroxyl ion.

What are the features of heme metabolism which justify devoting a symposium
on toxicology to the disorders of this particular pathway?   First, heme
synthesis is essential to maintain the integrity of processes already
listed.   Second, the pathways of synthesis (via porphyrins) and degradation
(to bile pigments) are separate pathways and are concerned only with heme
metabolism.   Third - and perhaps most important - the synthesis of heme in
the liver is under high gain feedback control;   failure of heme synthesis to
satisfy requirements can result in increases in precursor formation.   Finally, accurate methods to measure the precursors, aminolevulinic
acid and porphobilinogen are available and porphyrins can be measured in
circulating fluids or excreta by extremely sensitive fluorimetric methods
in concentrations down to 10^{-14}M.   Only heme has defied determined attempts
to measure accurately its free concentration in biological systems.   The
bile pigments, familiar products of heme degradation similarly are easily
detected although once exposed to bacterial activity their chemistry tends
to become inconveniently complex.

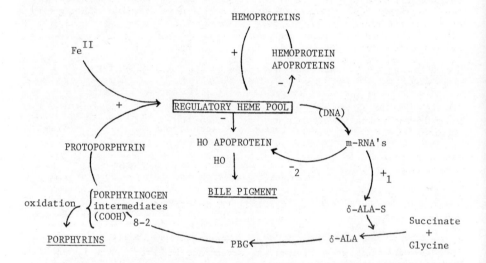

Fig. 1. Postulated control of the regulatory heme pool
        in liver. + and - signs indicate formation and
        depletion of available unbound heme and also 2
        important regulatory pathways which possibly
        involve transcriptional and translational events
        (1) δ-aminolevulinate synthase (δ-ALA-S)
        controlling heme biosynthesis, and (2) synthesis
        of heme oxygenase (HO) apoprotein which will
        bind heme and degrade it to bile pigment.
        (PBG - porphobilinogen).

In the liver, many aspects of the regulation of heme biosynthesis and breakdown can be explained if the pool of "uncommitted", "free" or "regulatory"
heme is assumed to also supply heme for degradation by heme oxygenase and

for hemoprotein synthesis. The sensitivity of heme synthesis and breakdown to changes in the "regulatory heme pool" is a prime determinant of the value of studies on this pathway as indicator of toxicity.

Biosynthesis of heme involves at least 8 enzymes which carry the reactions from simple precursors to heme, the principal end-product of this irreversible sequence. The process is initiated in the mitochondrion where succinyl CoA and glycine condense to form the aminoketone δaminolevulinic acid (ALA). In the cytoplasm, two moles of ALA form the monopyrrole, porphobilinogen, which cyclizes to form uroporphyrinogen, the first of the tetrapyrroles. Of four possible isomeric uroporphyrinogens, only III is a precursor for protoporphyrin (Type IX of XV possible isomers). Biosynthesis continues with the porphyrinogens (hexahydroporphyrins) as intermediates until the re-entry of coproporphyrinogen into mitochondria and the oxidation of protoporphyrinogen and the insertion of iron (as iron II) into protoporphyrin to form heme. Much evidence points to the regulation of this pathway by heme with one exception, if iron is deficient, ALA-S is not de-repressed.

While bone marrow and liver are the principal sites of heme production, and the spleen the principal site of heme degradation, permeability barriers tend to protect bone marrow cells from a number of compounds which might otherwise interfere with normal heme biosynthesis. On the other hand, the liver, the second most important site of heme synthesis, is remarkably unprotected by permeability barriers from a wide range of materials delivered directly from the gut or the systemic circulation. This organ therefore is a frequent target of toxic effects manifesting as abnormal heme biosynthesis or degradation.

The sedative drugs sulfonal and trional, now obsolete, were used in Europe prior to the advent of barbiturates and were recognized as causing a chemical porphyria. A similar porphyria caused by "Sedormid" was reported in the late 1940's and studies of structure activity relationships led to discovery of similar but more potent effects of its congener, 2-ally-2-isopropylacetamide (AIA) which will be referred to repeatedly in this symposium. AIA induces hepatic microsomal cytochrome P-450, is metabolised by this hemoprotein which may be destroyed in the process and AIA massively induces ALA synthase. Dr. Meyer will be exploring aspects of this complex toxic interaction in the first paper of this Symposium.

It is over 25 years since Schwartz and Ikeda (1955) reported that compounds like Sedormid cause green pigments to accumulate in liver. Much is now known of these abnormal heme degradation products as we shall learn from Dr. de Matteis in the third paper. Preceding this, Dr. Kikuchi will present his important studies on the normal pathways of heme degradation via heme oxygenase.

Both Drs. de Matteis and Tephly will speak of 3,5-dicarbethoxycarbonyl-1-1,4-dihydrocollidine (DDC). In some systems this toxin inhibits the incorporation of iron into protoporphyrin. Historically, however, it should be remembered as the agent used by Granick and Urata (1963) to demonstrate the inducibility of δ-ALA-S, the crucial regulator of heme synthesis.

Various metals apart from iron modulate heme synthesis and degradation. Inhibition of heme synthesis in the liver, transient increase in the activity of δ-ALA-S and marked stimulation of heme oxygenase, e.g. by cobalt, suggests a complicated situation which Dr. Tephly will examine in our fourth paper.

The final presentation by Dr. Sweeney will consider effects on heme

biosynthesis of toxic haloaromatic hydrocarbons including hexachlorobenzene
and 2,3,7,8-tetrachlorodibenzo(p)dioxin (TCDD). Toxicity of these compounds
may be different in that they appear not to affect heme synthesis or degradation directly, or through metabolites, but rather to decrease the activity
of uroporphyrinogen decarboxylase (UD) through processes which first require
induction of drug metabolism in the liver, and the presence of excess iron.

This Symposium has emphasised toxicity mediated through effects upon the
liver. Apart from differences in the regulation of heme synthesis in the
bone marrow, permeability barriers protect this site from direct toxins
and the effect of microsomal cytochromes activating compounds such as AIA
is absent. However, it must not be forgotten how valuable monitoring
various aspects of heme biosynthesis has been in assessing lead poisoning.
Lead influences various steps in heme biosynthesis in both liver and bone
marrow and a most valuable screen to detect lead poisoning in human populations is the measurement of zinc protoporphyrin in red cells from finger-
pricked blood. Finally, we should not overlook the interaction between
genetically abnormal individuals and a wide range of drugs which manifests
as a disturbance of heme biosynthesis. The porphyrias are referred to
here and in this interesting group of inborn errors of metabolism consideration of which is beyond the scope of this Symposium, we find greatly
increased sensitivity to a wide range of medicinal drugs, alcohol, possibly
cigarette smoke and environmental contaminants.

REFERENCES

DeMatteis, F. and W. N. Aldridge (Eds., 1978). Heme and Hemoproteins.
    Handbook of Experimental Pharmacology, Vol. 44, Springer-Verlag, Berlin-
    Heidelberg.
Elder, G. H. (1980). In A. Jacobs, M. Norwood (Eds.), Iron in Biochemistry
    and Medicine. 2nd ed. Academic Press, London, pp.245-292.
Granick, S., and G. Urata (1963). Increase in activity of δ-aminolevulinic
    acid synthetase in liver mitochondria induced by feeding of 3,5-
    dicarbethoxy-1,4-dihydrocollidine. J. Biol. Chem., 238, 821-827.
Meyer, U. A. and R. Schmid (1978). In J. B. Stanbury, J. B. Wyngaarden and
    D. S. Fredrickson (Eds.), The Metabolic Basis of Inherited Disease. 4th
    ed. McGraw Hill Book Co., New York, Chap. 50, pp.1166-1220.
Schwartz, S., and K. Ikeda (1955). In G. Wolstenholme and A. Millar (Eds.),
    CIBA Foundation Symposium on Porphyrin Biosynthesis and Metabolism.
    J. & A. Churchill Ltd., London, pp. 209-226.

Effect of Drugs and Chemicals on δ-Aminolevulinic Acid Synthase, the Rate-limiting Enzyme of Heme Synthesis

U. A. Meyer

Division of Clinical Pharmacology, Department of Medicine,
University Hospital, University of Zurich, 8091 Zurich, Switzerland

ABSTRACT

δ-Aminolevulinic acid synthase (ALA synthase) is the first and rate-limiting enzyme in heme biosynthesis. This review focuses upon the effects of drugs and chemicals on its activity. In the liver, in differentiated erythroid cells and presumably in other tissues ALA synthase is regulated by feedback repression by heme, the endproduct of the pathway. Indirect evidence suggests that a small, readily exchangeable and rapidly turning over heme pool controls ALA synthase by changing its rate of synthesis. After exposure of the liver to a large number of drugs and chemicals, ALA synthase is induced; induction of ALA synthase may reflect either a physiological adaptive response or drug toxicity. Most if not all of the drugs and chemicals that cause increased ALA synthase activity do so by primarily or secondarily affecting the postulated regulatory heme pool. The following mechanisms have been considered: 1. Inhibition of heme synthesis. 2. Increased heme breakdown. 3. Induction of apoproteins. 4. Combined effects.

Common to all compounds or treatments which cause excessive or prolonged induction of ALA synthase and consequently lead to experimental porphyria with increased formation, accumulation and excretion of heme precursors, is that they affect the regulatory heme pool, by more than one mechanism. Thus, drugs and chemicals which induce cytochrome P450 apoproteins and at the same time inhibit enzymes of heme synthesis and/or accelerate heme breakdown cause the highest increases in ALA synthase activity.

KEYWORDS

δ-aminolevulinic acid, heme biosynthesis, hemoproteins, cytochromes P450, induction, repression, experimental porphyria, hepatic porphyria.

INTRODUCTION

The sequence of 8 enzymatic reactions leading to heme starts with the formation of δ-aminolevulinic acid (ALA;). The substrates involved in this reaction are succinyl CoA, which is generated predominantly by the tricarboxylic acid cycle, and glycine. ALA synthase, an enzyme functional in mitochondria which requires pyridoxal phosphate as a cofactor, catalyzes the reaction (Meyer and Schmid, 1978; Elder, 1980). Although mammalian tissues contain transaminases potentially capable of catalyzing the conversion of ALA to or the generation of ALA from γ, δ-dioxovaleric acid (Varticovsky, Kushner and Burnham, 1980), most of the ALA formed in liver and bone marrow undoubtedly is synthesized by ALA synthase.

In the liver and probably in most other tissues the step of ALA formation is decisive for heme biosynthesis, since ALA synthase is the rate-limiting enzyme for the entire sequence of reactions. Thus, the normal Vmax of ALA synthase is as low or lower than that of the other enzymes and is proportional to the rate of heme synthesis in any particular tissue. Moreover, under normal circumstances, the substrate concentration of each enzyme beyond ALA apparently is well below its Michaelis constant. This ensures that accumulation of intermediates is minimal. However, if activity of ALA synthase and thereby ALA formation is markedly increased, other enzymes, e.g. uroporphyrinogen I synthase (porphobilinogen deaminase) may become rate-limiting and this may cause accumulation of intermediates. Alternatively, inherited or acquired partial deficiencies of enzymes beyond ALA, as occurs in certain types of inherited or acquired (toxic) human porphyrias, in lead poisoning or in chemically induced experimental porphyrias in animals, may make this enzymatic step rate limiting and cause accumulation of heme precursors. The pattern of precursor accumulation will depend upon the kinetic para meters of the affected enzymes and their substrate concentrations (Tschudy and Bonkowsky, 1973). Increased accumulation and excretion of heme precursors thus indicates either massively increased activity of ALA synthase or partial defects in more distal enzymes or, as discussed below, combination of the two processes.

The role of ALA synthase during erythropoiesis in the bone marrow is complex. During erythroid differentiation ALA-synthase does not appear to become rate-limiting for heme synthesis until all the enzymes of the pathway have been expressed by sequential activation of the appropriate genes. ALA synthase probably is the rate-limiting enzyme in erythroid cells actively synthesizing heme, but the regulation of its activity markedly differs from that of hepatic ALA synthase (Meyer and Schmid, 1978; Elder, 1980). In fact, recent studies suggest that molecular differencies may exist between erythroid and non-erythroid forms of ALA synthase (Bishop, Kitchen and Wood, 1981).

REGULATION OF ALA SYNTHASE ACTIVITY

There is little doubt that at least in the liver the primary
regulatory control of heme formation is exercised at the level
of ALA synthase activity (Meyer and Schmid, 1978). Under
certain conditions, the rate of ALA formation may be limited
by lack of substrate or cofactor. Thus because of the high Km
of ALA synthase for glycine experimental depletion of glycine
may inhibit ALA formation (Tephly, Condie and Piper, 1973) and
drug induced changes in vitamin B6 metabolism have caused
decreases in enzyme activity (Bottomley, 1980). More recently,
we have been able to further characterize the inhibition of
ALA formation by acetate (Piper and Tephly, 1974) as being
caused by competion of acetate with succinate for Coenzyme A
(Giger and Meyer, 1981).

Numerous studies in mammalian and avian liver provide convincing evidence that ALA synthase is under negative feedback
regulation by heme, the end product of the pathway. Three
different modes of feedback regulation have been proposed: 1)
feedback repression of the synthesis of ALA synthase by
heme, 2) feedback inhibition of ALA synthase activity by heme,
and 3) heme inhibition of the transfer of soluble cytosolic
ALA synthase into mitochondria (Meyer and Schmid, 1978). Heme
inhibition of enzyme synthesis by repressing translation or by
decreasing the amount of mRNA available for translation
(Whiting 1976) appears to be the most important mechanism,
since ALA synthase in intact rat liver mitochondria is not
inhibited at rates of heme formation 75 times higher than
those in vivo (Wolfson, Bartczak and Bloomer, 1979) and the
role of heme inhibition of translocation of ALA synthase from
the ribosomal site of synthesis to the mitochondrial matrix
under physiological conditions is still unclear (Yamauchi,
Hayashi and Kikuchi, 1980). Repression of ALA synthase by heme
may occur at concentrations of heme of 10^{-7} to 10^{-8}M
(Granick, Sinclair, Sassa, Grieninger 1975).

A large number of compounds of diverse structure including
drugs, carcinogens, insecticides and other chemicals as well
as synthetic and natural steroids and other endogenous substances induce ALA synthase in avian and mammalian liver. The
increase in enzyme activity has been shown to involve an
increase in the level of ALA synthase mRNA (Brooker, May and
Elliott, 1980) and an increase in immunologically identified
enzyme protein (Whiting 1976). The exact mechanism of the
induction of ALA synthase by drugs and chemicals is still
unclear. Several alternative possibilities will be discussed
below.

A variety of exogenous and endogenous factors modify the
induction of ALA synthase by chemicals in the liver. Of
particular relevance are the effects of carbohydrates and
fasting, of iron and of steroid hormones (Meyer and Schmid,
1978; Elder, 1980). A detailed consideration of these factors
is beyond the scope of this review.

Regulation of ALA synthase by heme in erythroid cells is more
complex and the effects of heme may alter as erythroid differentiation proceeds. Initially, heme may induce ALA synthase

by provoking erythroid differentiation. Later on, as the
pathway of heme and hemoglobin synthesis is established,
endproduct repression or inhibition of heme synthesis and
translational control of globin synthesis by heme ensure
coordination of heme and globin synthesis. Only a few factors
which alter ALA synthase activity in erythroid cells have been
identified. Erythropoietin and hypoxia as well as certain
steroids increase ALA synthase in this tissue (Meyer and
Schmid, 1978).

> MECHANISMS BY WHICH DRUGS AND CHEMICALS
> INDUCE ALA SYNTHASE.
> Role of a regulatory heme pool.

The principal control of hepatic ALA synthase activity by
heme repression requires the existence of a regulatory heme
pool (Fig. 1). Most aspects of the regulation of hepatic heme
and hemoprotein synthesis and breakdown can be explained if a
small, readily exchangeable and rapidly turning over pool with
an approximate concentration of 0.05 to 0.1 uM (Granick,
Sinclair, Sassa and Grieninger, 1975; Badawy, 1978) is postulated. This hypothetical pool would influence the synthesis of
ALA synthase, supply heme for hemoprotein assembly and act as
a substrate for heme oxygenase. Among other observations, this
concept is based on the findings that certain chemicals
which enhance the activity of ALA synthase cause a rapid
depletion of hepatic heme and that the exogenous heme decreases ALA synthase activity and is effective in the treatment of inducible acute hepatic porphyrias (Meyer and Schmid,
1978; Elder, 1980; Giger and Meyer, 1981).On the basis
of these considerations, it is postulated that most if not all
of the drugs and chemicals which cause increased ALA synthase
may do so by primarily or secondarily decreasing the regulatory heme pool (Table 1).

> TABLE 1. MECHANISMS BY WHICH DRUGS INDUCE
>   HEPATIC ALA-SYNTHASE
>
> 1 FEEDBACK REPRESSION BY HEME
>
> a) Inhibition of heme synthesis
> b) Increase of heme breakdown
> c) Induction of apoproteins e.g.
>   apocytochromes P450
> d) Combinations of a), b) and c)
>   (experimental porphyria)
>
> 2 DIRECT ACTION ON NUCLEUS WITH
>   INCREASE IN INDUCTION-SPECIFIC RNA
>
> 3 EFFECT ON $T_{1/2}$ ALA-SYNTHASE

Inhibition of heme synthesis

The scheme shown in Fig. 1 would predict that inhibition of heme synthesis will deplete the regulatory heme pool and induce ALA synthase. Evidence that this mechanism may occur is derived from our studies on the effects of lead chloride, which inhibits several enzymes of heme synthesis in rats (Maxwell and Meyer, 1976) and of levulinic acid, a competitive inhibitor of porphobilinogen synthase (ALA dehydrase) which resulted in increased hepatic activity of ALA in synthase in rats (J. Reubi and U.A. Meyer, unpublished observation). Similarly, succinylacetone, a potent inhibitor of porphobilinogen synthase endogenously formed in certain patients with tyrosinemia (Lindblad, Lindstedt and Steen, 1977), when added to cultured chick embryo hepatocytes caused induction of ALA synthase at a concentration of 3×10^{-4}M (U.Giger and U.A. Meyer, unpublished observation). In spite of these initial observations, experimental evidence for a quantitative relationship between inhibition of total cellular heme synthesis and ALA synthase induction is still lacking. This may be so because at the level of inhibition of total cellular heme synthesis at which ALA synthase induction may occur most chemicals used were prohibitively toxic. The induction caused by the mentioned chemicals (lead chloride, levulinic acid, succinylacetone) was relatively weak, in the order of 200% of controls. A number of other chemicals, e.g. iron chelators (Sinclair and Granick, 1975) and acetate (U. Giger and U.A. Meyer, 1981) which inhibits ALA formation and thereby heme synthesis, do not induce ALA synthase when given alone in nontoxic doses but lead to a marked potentiation of ALA synthase induction by lipophilic compounds. At least part of the effect of 3,5-diethoxy carbonyl-1,4-dihydrocollidine (DDC), which causes massive induction of hepatic ALA synthase with consequent accumulation of heme precursors is due to inhibition of hepatic heme synthesis at the stage of ferrochelatase, as will be discussed in other contributions to this Symposium (Tephly, Gibbs and De Matteis, 1979).

Increase of heme breakdown

The effects of certain chemicals which cause massive induction of hepatic ALA synthase and cause experimental porphyria is related to their property of destroying the heme of cytochrome P450 and possibly other hemoproteins, as exemplified by 2-allyl-2 isopropylacetamide (Meyer and Marver, 1971). These compounds and their mechanism of action will be discussed separately in the paper on "Liver Heme as Target of Drug Toxicity" of this Symposium.

Induction of apoproteins

Among the reactions that compete for heme in the cell are the syntheses of microsomal, mitochondrial and cytosolic hemoproteins (Fig.1). From their respective concentrations and turnover rates, the amount of heme needed to maintain their steady state concentrations have been calculated (Meyer and Schmid, 1978). It is apparent from these calculations that the group of cytochrome P450 hemoproteins which function as terminal oxidases in drug metabolism account for the major

part of the total hepatic heme synthesized. The concentration
of cytochrome P450 increases in response to numerous lipophilic drugs, classically represented by phenobarbital, and
expectedly, induction of cytochrome P450 regularly is accompanied by an increase in ALA synthase. Using sensitive assays
for ALA synthase activity we have not encountered an experimental situation in which marked induction of cytochrome P450
was not accompanied by increased ALA synthase activity. This
and other laboratories also have presented experimental
evidence indicating that lipophilic drugs such as phenobarbital and other chemicals primarily induce the synthesis of
apocytochromes P450 (De Matteis and Gibbs, 1972; Correia and
Meyer, 1975); Rajamanickam, Satyanarayaha Rao and Padmanaban,
1975; Meier, Spycher and Meyer, 1978) which through their
heme-binding capacity divert heme from the intracellular pool
regulating ALA synthase. The secondary rise of hepatic
ALA synthase following apocytochrome P450 induction by these
compounds may be envisioned as a coordinated adaptive response
providing the additional heme for hemoprotein synthesis,
although the exact manner by which induction of apocytochrome
and heme synthesis are coordinated, remains to be elucidated.

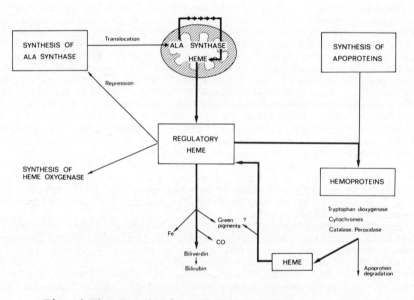

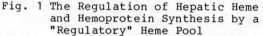

Fig. 1 The Regulation of Hepatic Heme
and Hemoprotein Synthesis by a
"Regulatory" Heme Pool

Combined mechanisms

In marked contrast to the large number of drugs and chemicals
that induce cytochrome P450 and secondarily lead to a controlled and coordinated induction of ALA synthase, a small number
of chemicals affect heme synthesis in such a way as to produce
so-called experimental or toxic porphyria characterized by a
massive increase in ALA synthase and marked hepatic overproduction, accumulation and excretion of heme precursors.
There is evidence that these compounds affect the postulated
regulatory heme pool by at least two different mechanisms:
Depletion of hepatic heme by inhibition of heme synthesis or
heme destruction and induction of apocytochromes P450 (Maxwell
and Meyer, 1976; De Matteis, 1978). Two of the best known
chemicals causing experimental porphyria may again serve to
illustrate this point. 2-Allyl-2-isopropylacetamide enhances
heme catabolism by covalently binding to the heme of P450 and
at the same time 2-allyl-2-isopropylacetamide is a substrate
and an inducer of cytochrome P450. DDC inhibits the last step
of heme synthesis and also is an inducer of apocytochrome
P450. Moreover, lipophilic drugs such as phenobarbital,
when given alone cause only moderate increases in ALA synthase
activity but lead to marked ALA synthase induction in rats
which have been given large doses of lead chloride (Maxwell
and Meyer, 1976). Similarly, acetate, succinylacetone and
levulinate, when added to cultured chick embryo hepatocytes potentiated the induction of ALA synthase by phenobarbital (Giger and Meyer, 1981; U.Giger and U.A. Meyer, unpublished observation). These observations suggest that depletion
of the regulatory heme pool by partial inhibition of heme
synthesis or increased heme breakdown sensitizes ALA synthase
to massive induction by compounds, which in the absence of
such interference would only moderately affect ALA synthase.
Obviously, the excessive induction of ALA synthase and
accumulation of heme precursors after porphyrogenic chemicals
reflects toxicity, while the moderate increase of ALA synthase
after drugs like phenobarbital reflects "physiological"
adaptation of the cell to increased needs. Sensitive assays
for ALA synthase and heme precursors, particularly easy
detection of minute of fluorescent porphyrins in tissues and
cells frequently allow early differentiation of the "adaptive
response" from "toxicity".
Alternative mechanisms of induction of ALA synthase by drugs
unrelated to heme repression such as direct action in the
nucleus to increase induction-specific RNA or a direct effect
of certain drugs on translation of ALA synthase or on the
halflife of the enzyme have been proposed on the basis of
indirect studies. (Granick and Sassa, 1971; Tyrell and Marks,
1972)

INDUCTION OF HEPATIC ALA SYNTHASE
BY DRUGS IN HUMAN HEPATIC PORPHYRIA

The concept of "combined effects" on a regulatory heme pool
controlling ALA synthase may also explain the unique sensitivity of patients with intermittent acute porphyria, hereditary
coproporphyria and variegate porphyria. In these disorders
genetic partial deficiencies of enzymes of heme synthesis

cause increased inducibility of hepatic ALA synthase in
response to induces of apocytochromes P450, e.g. phenobarbital. The result is massive accumulation and excretion of
potentially neurotoxic ALA and other heme precursors and
apparently decreased induction of cytochrome(s) P450 and
its monooxygenase function (for review see Maxwell and Meyer,
1978). When considering drugs for use in the patient with
hepatic porphyria one should therefore select drugs with a
weak potential for induction of cytochromes P450. When testing
drugs for safe use in patients with porphyria, the normal
laboratory animal may not be the appropriate model, but ALA
synthase induction should be tested under the condition of an
experiemntal partial block in heme biosynthesis. Chick embryo
liver or cultured chick embryo hepatocytes appear to be the
best model with "predictive value". In addition to the unique
pharmacokinetics in a cell culture system, chick embryo liver
is characterized by a low activity of ferrochelatase, the last
enzyme of heme synthesis, thus imitating a "partial defect"
in heme synthesis (for review, see Marks, 1981).

ACKNOWLEDGMENT

The reported studies were supported by grant 3.964.78 from
the Swiss National Foundation for Scientific Research. The
skilful secretarial assistance of Ms. M. Bucher in the preparation of this manuscript is gratefully acknowledged.

REFERENCES

Badawy, A.A.-B. (1978). Biochem.J.,172, 487-494.
Bishop, D.F., H. Kitchen, and W.A.Wood (1981). Arch.Biochem.
    Biophys.206, 380-391.
Bottomley, S.S. (1980). In A. Jacobs and M. Worwood (Eds.),
    Iron in Biochemistry and Medicine, II, Academic Press,
    London and New York. pp. 363-392.
Brooker, J.D., B.K. May, and W.H. Elliott (1980). Europ.J.
    Biochem.106, 17-24.
Correia, M.A., and U.A.Meyer (1975). Proc.Natl.Acad.Sci.USA
    72, 400-404.
De Matteis, F., and A. Gibbs (1972). Biochem.J.126,1149-1160.
De Matteis, F. (1978). In F.De Matteis and W.N. Aldridge
    (Eds.),Heme and Hemoproteins,Handbook of Exp.Pharmacology,
    vol. 44, Springer Verlag, Berlin, Heidelberg and New York,
    pp. 129-156.
De Matteis, F., A.Gibbs, and T.R. Tephly (1980). Biochem.J.
    188, 145-152.
Elder, G.H. (1980). In A. Jacobs and M. Worwood (Eds.) Iron in
    Biochemistry and Medicine II, Academic Press, London and
    New York, pp. 245-292.
Giger, U., and U.A. Meyer (1981). Biochem. J. 198,(in press).
Granick, S. and S.Sassa (1971). In H.J. Vogel (Ed.) Metabolic
    Regulation (vol.5 of Metabolic Pathways) Academic Press,
    New York and London, pp.77-141.
Granick, S., P. Sinclair, S. Sassa, and G.Grieninger (1975).
    J.Biol.Chem.250, 9215-9225.

Lindblad B., S. Lindstedt,and G.Steen (1977). Proc.Natl.Acad.
Sci.USA 74, 4641-4645.
Marks, G.S.(1981). Trends in Pharmacol. Sci.2, 59-61.
Maxwell, D.J.,and U.A. Meyer (1976). Eur.J.Clin.Invest.6,
373-380.
Maxwell, D.J., and U.A. Meyer (1978). In F. De Matteis and
W.N. Aldridge (Eds.) Heme and Hemoproteins, Handbook of
Exp.Pharmacology vol. 44, Springer Verlag, Berlin, Heidel-
berg and New York, pp. 239-254.
Meier, P.J., M.A. Spycher, and U.A. Meyer (1978). Exp.Cell.
Res. 111, 479-483.
Meyer, U.A., and H.S. Marver (1977). Science 171, 64-66.
Meyer, U.A., and R. Schmid (1978). In J.B. Stanbury, J.B.
Wyngaarden and D.S. Fredrickson (Eds.) The Metabolic Basis
of Inherited Disease, McGraw-Hill, New York, pp. 1066-1220.
Piper, W.N., and T.R. Tephly (1974). Arch.Biochem.Biophys.154,
351-356.
Rajamanickam, C., M.R. Satyanarayana Rao, and G.Padmanaban.
J.Biol.Chem. 250, 2305-2310.
Sinclair, P.R., and S.Granick (1975). In A.D. Adler (Ed.) The
Biological Role of Porphyrins and Related Structures. Ann.
New York Acad.Sci. 244, pp 509-518.
Tephly, T.R., L.W. Condie, and W.N. Piper (1973). Enzyme 16,
187-195.
Tephly, T.R., A.H. Gibbs and F. De Matteis (1979). Biochem. J.
180, 241-244.
Tschudy, D.P., and H.L. Bonkowsky (1973). Mol.Cell.Biochem.2,
55-62.
Tyrrell, D.L.J., and G.S. Marks (1972). Biochem.Pharmacol.21,
2077-2093.
Varticovski, L., J.P. Kushner, and B.F. Burnham (1980).
J.Biol.Chem. 255, 3724-3747.
Whiting, M.J. (1976). Biochem.J. 158, 391-400.
Wolfson, S.J., A. Bartczak, and J.R. Bloomer (1979). J.Biol.
Chem.254, 3543-3546.
Yamauchi, K., N.Hayashi, and G. Kikuchi (1980). J.Biol.
Chem.255, 1746-1751.

Effects of Drugs and Metals on Heme Degradation by the Heme Oxygenase System

G. Kikuchi, T. Yoshida and S. Ishizawa

Department of Biochemistry, Tohoku University School of Medicine,
Sendai, Japan

ABSTRACT

Rat hepatic heme oxygenase can be induced by treatment with various substances, including hemin and non-heme substances. The heme oxygenase induction seemed to involve two apparently different mechanisms; the one, heme-mediated and the other, independent of mediation by heme. Far more extensive induction occurred in the heme-independent system than in the heme-mediated system. Polysome-directed cell-free synthesis of heme oxygenase revealed that the functional mRNA for heme oxygenase was actually increased in the liver of rats treated with either hemin or non-heme inducers apparently in proportion to the activities of heme oxygenase in respective livers.

KEYWORDS

Heme oxygenase; induction of heme oxygenase; Cd^{2+}; Co^{2+}; bromobenzene; carbon disulfide; substrate-mediated induction; cell-free synthesis of heme oxygenase.

INTRODUCTION

The microsomal heme oxygenase system plays an essential role in the physiological heme catabolism. The heme oxygenase system is composed of two proteins, heme oxygenase and NADPH-cytochrome P-450 reductase, and catalyzes the oxidation of heme at α-methene bridge to form biliverdin IXα at the expense of NADPH and molecular oxygen. Recently we purified heme oxygenase to apparent homogeneity from pig spleen and rat liver, and studies with the purified heme oxygenase preparations revealed that the mechanism of heme degradation catalyzed by this enzyme system is essentially similar to that of heme decomposition by the so-called coupled oxidation of myoglobin or hemoglobin and ascorbic acid. The possible sequence of heme degradation in the heme oxygenase reaction is shown in Fig. 1. Heme degradation starts from the oxygenated form of the heme·heme oxygenase complex, and for the onset of heme degradation, the second electron is indispensable. Chemical nature of the 688 nm substance in Fig. 1 remains to be elucidated. Also it is unclear whether carbon monoxide is liberated before or after the formation of

this intermediate.   Release of iron from the biliverdin-iron chelate is
facilitated by reduction of iron.   The whole process of heme degradation is
catalyzed by a single enzyme, heme oxygenase, and in microsomes the reducing
equivalents are supplied solely from the NADPH-cytochrome P-450 system.   In
the heme oxygenase reaction heme acts as both the substrate and coenzyme
which activates molecular oxygen, and the heme oxygenase protein provides a
suitable site for the rapid autocatalytic oxidation of the bound heme (Kikuchi and Yoshida, 1980).

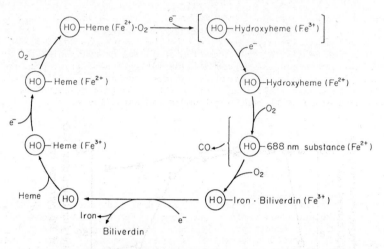

Fig. 1.   Possible mechanism of heme degradation in the
heme oxygenase reaction.

The activity of heme oxygenase is higher in those tissues normally involved in the sequestration and breakdown of red cells such as spleen, liver
and bone marrow.   Heme oxygenase, however, can be induced in liver (Tenhunen
and others, 1970),   kidney (Pimstone and others, 1971a)   and macrophages
(Pimstone and others, 1971b; Shibahara and others, 1978) by the administration of heme or hemoglobin, possibly in a substrate-mediated induction.   By
the combined use of [^{3}H]leucine and a rabbit antibody(IgG) prepared against
a purified pig spleen heme oxygenase,   we demonstrated that the functional
mRNA for heme oxygenase was actually increased in the cultured hemin-induced
pig alveolar macrophages (Shibahara and others, 1979).   The polysome-directed, cell-free synthesis of heme oxygenase also revealed that free polysomes
were the major site of synthesis of heme oxygenase.
However, since 1974 a number of non-heme substances such as metal ions
(Maines and Kappas, 1975, 1976, 1977) and some organic compounds (Järvisalo
and others, 1978; Guzelian and Elshourbagy, 1979) were reported to greatly
increase the heme oxygenase activity in rat hepatic and renal microsomes.
Induction of heme oxygenase by these substances was accompanied by various
perturbations of heme metabolism such as alteration in the activity of δ-
aminolevulinate (abbreviated as ALA) synthase and decrease in microsomal
contents of heme and hemoproteins.   It is very important and interesting to
clarify the mechanisms as to how these substances induce de novo synthesis
of heme oxygenase protein and how these substances perturb the heme metabolism.   In the present paper we will report the results of our study on
the effects of various inducing agents on the heme oxygenase activity as
well as other parameters related to heme metabolism.

EXPERIMENTAL OBSERVATIONS

Induction by Administration of Hemin

Effects of intraperitoneal injection of hemin (20 mg or 30 μmol/kg body
weight) on the heme oxygenase activity, the ALA synthase activity, the content of cytochrome P-450 and the degree of heme saturation of tryptophan
pyrrolase in the liver are shown in Fig. 2. The degree of heme saturation
of tryptophan pyrrolase has been considered to be a sensitive and reliable
index of the "regulatory heme" pool in the liver (Welch and Badawy, 1980;
Yamamoto and others, 1981).   Heme oxygenase was assayed by the method of
Yoshida and Kikuchi (1978a) and one unit of the enzyme was defined as the
amount of enzyme catalyzing the formation of 1 nmol of bilirubin/hr. Activity of ALA synthase and the degree of heme saturation of tryptophan pyrrolase were determined as described by Yamamoto and others (1981); 1 unit
of ALA synthase should yield 1 nmol of ALA/hr.   Content of cytochrome
P-450 was determined by the method of Omura and Sato (1964).

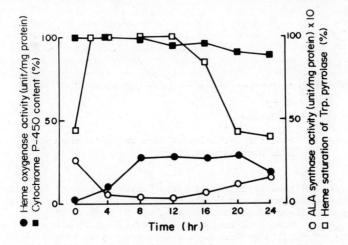

Fig. 2. Time courses of effects of hemin.

Injection of hemin brought about a full saturation of tryptophan pyrrolase
with heme, and the full saturation was maintained for at least 12 hr.   Injection of hemin also caused an extensive reduction of the level of ALA synthase
which also continued for about 12 hr.   It is apparent that the regulatory
heme pool in the liver cell was greatly increased by the hemin injection.
In concomitance with the increase of the degree of heme saturation of
tryptophan pyrrolase, the heme oxygenase activity began to increase, supporting the view of the substrate-mediated induction.   A maximum activity was
attained 8 hr after the hemin injection and this level was maintained for
the subsequent 12 hr.   The maximum activity attained was 30 units/mg protein which was about 15 fold of the activity in the control rat.   Injection
of hemin did not appreciably affect the content of cytochrome P-450.
A full saturation of tryptophan pyrrolase with heme could also be achieved
by injection of a smaller dose of hemin (2 mg or 3 μmol/kg) although the
degree of the heme saturation began to decline in a few hr and returned to
near the control level at about 12 hr after the hemin injection (data not
shown).   At this dose of hemin, the activity of heme oxygenase was also

increased but only 3-4 fold.

Induction by Administration of Co^{2+} and Cd^{2+}

In view of the reported observations that Co^{2+} and Cd^{2+} were the effective
inducers of the hepatic heme oxygenase, the effects of subcutaneous administration of Co^{2+} and Cd^{2+} were studied in detail.   Fig. 3 shows the time
courses of the effects of administration of Co^{2+}.   The heme oxygenase activity began to increase within a few hr after the injection of 250 μmol of
Co^{2+}/kg and reached a maximum by 16-20 hr, then declined.   It should be
noted that the maximum activity obtained was about 45 fold of the basal level
in the control rat and was 3 times higher than the maximum activity attained
in the hemin-treated rat.   The activity of ALA synthase was also greatly
increased in these rats, showing an activity peak at about 12 hr after the
Co^{2+} administration.   These results are essentially similar to those reported by Maines and Kappas (1975).   On the other hand, the content of
cytochrome P-450 and the degree of heme saturation of tryptophan pyrrolase
decreased significantly, apparently in a reciprocal fashion to the increase
in the heme oxygenase activity.   Especially, the decrease of the degree of
heme saturation of tryptophan pyrrolase was remarkable.   The intracellular
heme pool may have been decreased due to enhanced degradation of heme as a
result of increased activity of heme oxygenase, although the decrease of
the intracellular heme pool may also be accounted for partly by the inhibition by Co^{2+} of de novo synthesis of heme at the step of insertion of iron
to protoporphyrin.

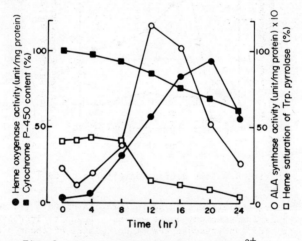

Fig. 3.   Time courses of effects of Co^{2+}.

        Considering the possibility that Co-protoporphyrin, which is not readily
broken down by the heme oxygenase system (Yoshida and Kikuchi, 1978b), may
have been responsible to the observed extensive induction of heme oxygenase
in the Co^{2+}-treated rat, in an experiment we have compared the effects of
administration of equimolar hemin, Co-protoporphyrin and $CoCl_2$ (10 μmol/kg),
and found that the inducing activity of Co-protoporphyrin was rather lower
than that of hemin.   Namely, the heme oxygenase activity in the liver of
rats treated with Co-protoporphyrin for 12 hr were 4.75-6.10 units/mg protein while the value in the hemin-treated rats were 7.74-8.26; the heme oxygenase activity in the Co^{2+}-treated rats was not appreciably increased.

All these observations strongly suggest that Co^{2+} has acted to increase
the heme oxygenase activity without mediation of either heme or Co-protoporphyrin, as proposed by Maines and Kappas (1977).
It is worth-noting that Co^{2+} also caused an extensive induction of ALA
synthase.   One possibility to account for this induction may be derepres-
sion of the enzyme synthesis due to the suspected decrease in the heme pool.
It should be noted, however, that Co-protoporphyrin, as same as iron-proto-
porphyrin, has been shown to be a potent inhibitor of the drug-induced increase of hepatic ALA synthase (Igarashi and others, 1978); the allyliso-
propylacetamide-induced increase of ALA synthase was also strongly suppressed when animals were pretreated with a large dose of $CoCl_2$ (about 250 µmol/
kg as used in the present study) (Maines and others, 1976; Igarashi and
others, 1978). In addition, as shown in Fig. 3, the once increased level
of ALA synthase declined rapidly after 12 hr of the experiment while the
degree of heme saturation of tryptophan pyrrolase still continued to decrease.   Thus the situations are quite controversial and further studies
are needed to account for the observed induction of ALA synthase by Co^{2+}.

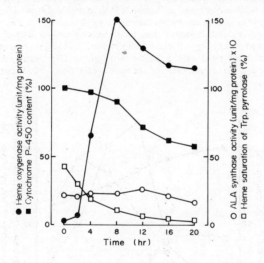

Fig. 4.   Time courses of effects of Cd^{2+}

Time courses of the effects of administration of Cd^{2+} (75 µmol/kg) are
shown in Fig. 4.   The heme oxygenase activity began to increase 2 hr after
the injection of Cd^{2+} and reached the highest level at about 8 hr, then fell
off gradually.   The maximum activity attained was even higher than the value
obtained in the Co^{2+}-treated rat.   The content of cytochrome P-450 and the
degree of heme saturation of tryptophan pyrrolase decreased progressively
with time, in a way similar to the case with Co^{2+}.   The activity of ALA
synthase was not much influenced by the Cd^{2+} treatment.   This is in contrast to the case with Co^{2+}.   In an experiment we examined the effect of
injection of a smaller amount of Cd^{2+}, i.e. 25 µmol/kg, considering that
other investigators usually employed this amount of Cd^{2+} (Maines and Kappas,
1976; Yoshida, Tak. and others, 1979; Eaton and others, 1980).   The activity
of heme oxygenase was also greatly increased in these rats and reached a
maximum which was 25-30 fold higher than the control level at about 4 hr
after the injection and then declined slowly (data not shown).

Induction by Administration of Bromobenzene

A single subcutaneous injection of 5 mmol bromobenzene/kg caused a progressive and extensive increase of the activity of heme oxygenase (Fig. 5).
The increase of the activity commenced after a short lag and reached a maximum at 20-24 hr after the injection, and the maximum activity attained was
comparable to that obtained in Cd^{2+}-treated rats. The degree of heme saturation of tryptophan pyrrolase was not increased but decreased progressively
with time, after a short lag, and the heme saturation was reduced to nearly
zero at 12 hr or later after the drug injection. This would reflect that
the heme pool may have been reduced to an extremely low level possibly as a
result of high activity of heme oxygenase in these rats. Nevertheless, the
level of heme oxygenase still continued to increase linearly even after 12
hr of the experiment. Thus, it is highly probable that the induction of
heme oxygenase by bromobenzene is not mediated by heme. The content of
cytochrome P-450 also diminished progressively, and the level at 24 hr after
the bromobenzene injection was about 60% of the basal level in the control
rat. The activity of ALA synthase, however, was not increased in spite of
that the heme pool may have been reduced to an extremely low level. This
is also in contrast to the case with Co^{2+}.

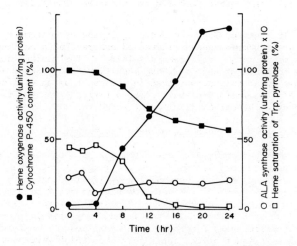

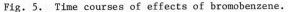

Fig. 5. Time courses of effects of bromobenzene.

Induction by Administration of Carbon Disulfide

Järvisalo and others (1978) reported that the administration of carbon disulfide to rats increased the activity of hepatic heme oxygenase to some
extent. In this case, heme is supposed to be liberated from cytochrome P-
450 and to act as a real inducer. Then, carbon disulfide would provide a
desirable system to demonstrate that heme functions as a true inducer. In
our own experiments, the content of cytochrome P-450 decreased to about 60%
of the control level within 2 hr after the intraperitoneal administration of
carbon disulfide (5 mmol/kg) and the level of cytochrome P-450 remained
reduced throughout the whole period of the experiment (Fig. 6). In contrast,
the heme saturation of tryptophan pyrrolase increased considerably, supporting the view that carbon disulfide promotes the dissociation of heme from
cytochrome P-450. The once increased level of the heme saturation, however,

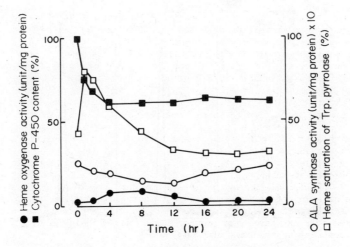

Fig. 6. Time courses of effects of carbon disulfide.

declined soon.   In reciprocal to the decrease in the cytochrome P-450 content, the activity of heme oxygenase increased and reached a maximum about 4 hr after the administration of carbon disulfide.   The maximum activity attained was 3-4 fold higher than the basal activity; the maximum activity attained is almost equal to that obtained in the rat treated with a relatively small dose of hemin (3 μmol/kg).   The activity of ALA synthase was slightly decreased in the carbon disulfide-treated rat.

Polysome-Directed Cell-Free Synthesis of Heme Oxygenase

In vitro synthesis of heme oxygenase was attempted in a rabbit reticulocyte lysate system using polysomes isolated from the liver of rats treated or untreated with inducers and using a combination of [^{3}H]leucine and a rabbit antibody (IgG) specific to the rat liver heme oxygenase. Rats were fasted for 24 hr, then injected with bromobenzene (5 mmol/kg) or Cd^{2+} (75 μmol/kg) subcutaneously 12 hr or 8 hr before being killed, respectively, or hemin (30 μmol/kg) intraperitoneally 8 hr before being killed.   The reaction was carried out using an aliquot of the total polysomes which were prepared from livers pooled from three rats.   Other experimental methods used were essentially similar to those employed by Yamauchi and others (1980).

When compared on the basis of incorporation of radioactivity into total protein, there was no significant difference in the protein synthetic activity between the polysomes prepared from the liver of control rat and those prepared from the rats treated with either hemin, Cd^{2+}, or bromobenzene. However, there was a large difference in the amount of radioactivity recovered in the immunoprecipitates in respective reaction systems.   Then, an aliquot of each sample was subjected to SDS-polyacrylamide gel electrophoresis and analyzed for radioactivity.   As shown in Fig. 7, the immunoprecipitates gave one major peak of radioactivity and the position of the peak coincided with the position of heme oxygenase (minimum molecular weight 32,000), and the radioactivity recovered in the heme oxygenase fraction was significantly higher in the induced rat systems than in the uninduced control rat system.   Moreover, the radioactivities recovered in the individual rat systems were apparently proportional to the activities of heme oxygenase in the livers from which polysomes were prepared.   These results indicate

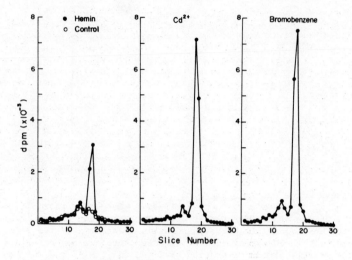

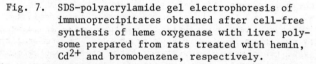

Fig. 7.   SDS-polyacrylamide gel electrophoresis of
immunoprecipitates obtained after cell-free
synthesis of heme oxygenase with liver poly-
some prepared from rats treated with hemin,
Cd^{2+} and bromobenzene, respectively.

that the functional mRNA for heme oxygenase was greatly increased in the
rats treated with inducers and suggest that Cd^{2+} and bromobenzene, as same
as hemin, enhanced the synthesis of mRNA for heme oxygenase, giving rise to
increased synthesis of heme oxygenase in the liver.

It has been reported that actinomycin D had little effect on the Cd^{2+}-
induced increase of the heme oxygenase activity in mouse liver (Yoshida Tak.
and others, 1979) and on the bromobenzene-induced increase in rat liver
(Guzelian and Elshourbagy, 1979).   We have found, however, that the induction of heme oxygenase by either of bromobenzene, Cd^{2+} and Co^{2+} was completely blocked by actinomycin D (a dose of 1.5 mg/kg 30 min before the administration of inducer and an additional half a dose at 3 hr of the induction; rats were killed 6 hr after the injection of inducer), as well as by
cycloheximide (data not shown).   These observations are in good accordance
with the view that the induction of heme oxygenase can be accounted for by
increased synthesis of the heme oxygenase-specific mRNA.

COMMENTS

The induction of heme oxygenase by non-heme inducers appears to involve two
apparently different mechanisms; the one, heme-mediated and the other, independent of mediation by heme.   The increase of the heme oxygenase activity caused by the administration of carbon disulfide is likely to be
mediated by heme, whereas those observed after the administration of Co^{2+},
Cd^{2+} and bromobenzene appear to be independent of mediation by heme.   In
the case with carbon disulfide, the degree of heme saturation of tryptophan
pyrrolase was significantly increased, though temporarily, and the extent of
induction of heme oxygenase was relatively moderate and was comparable to
that observed for rats treated with a reduced dose of hemin (3 μmol/kg).
On the other hand, in the induction with Co^{2+}, Cd^{2+} and bromobenzene, there

was no indication of the increase of heme pool as judged by the degree of
heme saturation of tryptophan pyrrolase and nevertheless, the extents of
the induction of heme oxygenase far exceeded the extents of induction observed after the injection of as much as 30 μmol/kg of hemin. These inducers may have acted directly to the regulatory site(s) for synthesis of
heme oxygenase without mediation by heme.   Precise mechanism of the action
of these inducers remains uncertain.

Several investigators pointed out that the increase in the heme oxygenase activity was accompanied by a decline of the cytochrome P-450 level in
rat liver (Maines and Kappas, 1975, 1976; Guzelian and Elshourbagy, 1979).
We have observed the same situation in the present study. However, interpretation for the decrease of the content of cytochrome P-450 in question
has been controversial (De Matteis, 1978).   One possibility is that this
is due to enhanced degradation of heme moiety of cytochrome P-450 resulted
by highly increased heme oxygenase activity; the heme moiety of cytochrome
P-450 appears to be exchangeable with heme in the heme pool (Abbritti and
De Matteis, 1973; Correia and others, 1979).   The other possibility is
that the inducing agent directly affects the apoprotein of cytochrome P-450,
or the heme moiety, or the both, thus causing reduction of the level of cytochrome P-450.   In an experiment not reported here, we have examined comparatively the effects of administration of Co^{2+}, Cd^{2+}, Ni^{2+} and Mn^{2+} on the
increase of the heme oxygenase activity and the decrease of the cytochrome
P-450 content, and found that there was no appreciable correlation between
them; for instance, while the activity of heme oxygenase at 16 hr of the
experiment was more than 10 times higher in the Co^{2+}-treated rat than in the
Mn^{2+}-treated rat, the degree of reduction of the content of cytochrome P-450
was about 20% in either rats.   In our experiments, metal ions seem to have
exerted some direct effect upon cytochrome P-450, although degradation of
the heme moiety of cytochrome P-450 may have also been enhanced more or less
by high activities of heme oxygenase in those rats.

ACKNOWLEDGMENT

We thank Dr. M. Yamamoto in this laboratory for his cooperation in the experiment of cell-free synthesis of heme oxygenase.   This work was supported
in parts by Grants 348117 and 568069 from the Ministry of Education, Science
and Culture, Japan, and by a grant from the Yamanouchi Foundation for Metabolic Studies, Japan.

REFERENCES

Abbritti, G., and F. De Matteis (1973). Effects of 3,5-diethoxycarbonyl-
1,4-dihydrocollidine on degradation of liver haem. Enzyme, 16, 196-202.
Correia, M.A., G.C. Farrell, R. Schmid, P.R. Ortiz de Montellano, G.S. Yost,
and B.A. Mico (1979). Incorporation of exogenous heme into hepatic cytochrome P-450 in vivo. J. Biol. Chem., 254, 15-17.
De Matteis, F. (1978). Loss of liver cytochrome P-450 caused by chemicals.
In F. De Matteis and W.N. Aldridge (Ed.), Handbook of experimental pharmacology, Vol. 44, Springer-Verlag, Berlin. pp. 95-127.
Eaton, D.L., N.H. Stacey, K.-L. Wong, and C.D. Klaassen (1980). Dose-response effects of various metal ions on rat liver metallothionein, glutathion, heme oxygenase, and cytochrome P-450. Toxicol. Appl. Pharmacol.,
55, 393-402.
Guzelian, P.S., and N.A. Elshourbagy (1979). Induction of hepatic heme
oxygenase activity by bromobenzene. Arch. Biochem. Biophys., 196, 178-185.

Igarashi, J., N. Hayashi, and G. Kikuchi (1978). Effects of administration of cobalt chloride and cobalt protoporphyrin on δ-aminolevulinate synthase in rat liver. J. Biochem., 84, 997-1000.
Järvisalo, J., A.H. Gibbs, and F. De Matteis (1978). Accelerated conversion of heme to bile pigments caused in the liver carbon disulfide and other sulfur-containing chemicals. Mol. Pharmacol., 14, 1099-1106.
Kikuchi, G., and T. Yoshida (1980). Heme degradation by the microsomal heme oxygenase system. Trends in Biochem. Sci., 5, 323-325.
Maines, M.D., V. Janoušek, J.M. Tomio, and A. Kappas (1976). Cobalt inhibition of synthesis and induction of δ-aminolevulinate synthase in liver. Proc. Natl. Acad. Sci. U.S.A., 73, 1499-1503.
Maines, M.D., and A. Kappas (1975). Cobalt stimulation of heme degradation in the liver. Dissociation of microsomal oxidation of heme from cytochrome P-450. J. Biol. Chem., 250, 4171-4177.
Maines, M.D., and A. Kappas (1976). Studies on the mechanism of induction of haem oxygenase by cobalt and other metal ions. Biochem. J., 154, 125-131.
Maines, M.D., and A. Kappas (1977). Metals as regulators of heme metabolism. Science, 198, 1215-1221.
Omura, T., and R. Sato (1964). The carbon monoxide-binding pigment of liver microsomes. I. Evidence for its hemoprotein nature. J. Biol. Chem., 239, 2370-2378.
Pimstone, N.R., P. Engel, R. Tenhunen, P.T. Seitz, H.S. Marver, and R. Schmid (1971a). Inducible heme oxygenase in the kidney: a model for the homeostatic control of hemoglobin catabolism. J. Clin. Invest., 50, 2042-2050.
Pimstone, N.R., R. Tenhunen, P.T. Seitz, H.S. Marver, and R. Schmid (1971b). The enzymatic degradation of hemoglobin to bile pigments by macrophages. J. Exp. Med., 133, 1264-1281.
Shibahara, S., T. Yoshida, and G. Kikuchi (1978). Induction of heme oxygenase by hemin in cultured pig alveolar macrophages. Arch. Biochem. Biophys., 188, 243-250.
Shibahara, S., T. Yoshida, and G. Kikuchi (1979). Mechanism of increase of heme oxygenase activity induced by hemin in cultured pig alveolar macrophages. Arch. Biochem. Biophys., 197, 607-617.
Tenhunen, R., H.S. Marver, and R. Schmid (1970). The enzymatic catabolism of hemoglobin: stimulation of microsomal heme oxygenase by hemin. J. Lab. Clin. Med., 75, 410-421.
Yamamoto, M., N. Hayashi, and G. Kikuchi (1981). Regulation of synthesis and intracellular translocation of δ-aminolevulinate synthase by heme and its relation to the heme saturation of tryptophan pyrrolase in rat liver. Arch. Biochem. Biophys., 209, June issue.
Yamauchi, K., N. Hayashi, and G. Kikuchi (1980). Cell-free synthesis of rat liver δ-aminolevulinate synthase and possible occurrence of processing of the enzyme protein in the course of its translocation from the cytosol into the mitochondrial matrix. FEBS Lett., 115, 15-18.
Welch, A.N., and A.A.-B. Badawy (1980). Tryptophan pyrrolase in haem regulation. Experiments with administered haematin and the relationship between the haem saturation of tryptophan pyrrolase and the activity of 5-aminolevulinate synthase in rat liver. Biochem. J., 192, 403-410.
Yoshida, Tak., M. Okamoto, Y. Suzuki, and Y. Hashimoto (1979). Cadmium-induced alterations in the activities of hepatic δ-aminolevulinic acid synthetase and heme oxygenase in mice. J. Pharm. Dyn., 2, 84-91.
Yoshida, T., and G. Kikuchi (1978a). Purification and properties of heme oxygenase from pig spleen microsomes. J. Biol. Chem., 253, 4224-4229.
Yoshida, T., and G. Kikuchi (1978b). Reaction of the microsomal heme oxygenase with cobaltic protoporphyrin IX, an extremely poor substrate. J. Biol. Chem., 253, 8479-8482.

Liver Haem as a Target for Drug Toxicity

F. De Matteis, A. H. Gibbs, P. B. Farmer, J. H. Lamb and C. Hollands

Medical Research Council, Toxicology Unit, Carshalton,
Surrey SM5 4EF, UK

ABSTRACT

Two distinct types of drug toxicity are illustrated, both with liver
haem as the main target. Drugs with unsaturated side chains and
certain dihydropyridines both convert liver haem into N-alkylated
porphyrins but the underlying mechanisms and biological properties of
the resulting pigments differ in the two cases. A monooxygenated
derivative of the unsaturated drugs becomes itself bound onto one of
the pyrrole nitrogen atoms of the haem of cytochrome P-450 and the
N-alkylated porphyrin which is produced does not inhibit the last
enzyme of haem biosynthesis, protohaem ferro-lyase. In contrast,
with 3,5-diethoxycarbonyl-1,4-dihydrocollidine only the 4-methyl substituent of the drug is transferred onto the pyrrole nitrogen atom and
the resulting porphyrin is a powerful inhibitor of protohaem ferro-
-lyase. The latter pathway involves transfer of the intact 4-alkyl
group onto the pyrrole nitrogen.

KEYWORDS

Haem; cytochrome P-450; N-alkylated porphyrins; inhibition of protohaem ferro-lyase; hepatic porphyria.

INTRODUCTION

Since the original discovery (Schmid and Schwartz, 1952; Goldberg and
Rimington, 1955; Solomon and Figge, 1959) that 2-allyl-2-isopropyl-
acetamide (AIA) and 3,5-diethoxycarbonyl-1,4-dihydrocollidine (DDC)
could both induce hepatic porphyria in experimental animals, these two
chemicals have been widely used to investigate the mechanisms by which
hepatic haem biosynthesis is regulated. Both drugs are powerful
inducers of the rate-limiting enzyme of the pathway, 5-aminolaevuli-
nate synthetase (ALA-S; E.C. 2.3.1.37) and numerous studies have
appeared in which these drugs have been used to stimulate ALA-S so
that its biosynthesis and regulation by haem, the end product of the
pathway, could be studied in detail. It has become apparent more
recently that with both chemicals the primary effect is probably an

irriversible modification of the structure of haem leading to a loss of
its function as a feedback regulator of ALA-S (and therefore to a com-
pensatory stimulation of the enzyme) and also to decreased activity of
certain liver haemoproteins, including cytochrome P-450 and catalase.
More and more attention has therefore been focused in the last few
years on the modification of the structure of haem caused by treatment
with these drugs and on the underlying biochemical mechanisms.
Modified porphyrins (or green pigments) have been isolated after treatment with both drugs and these arise from haem by irriversible modification of its structure.   However, as will be discussed below, there
are important differences between the two drugs in the mechanism by
which they convert haem into green pigments and also in structure and
biological properties of the resulting green pigments.

EFFECT OF UNSATURATED DRUGS ON LIVER CYTOCHROME P-450

AIA and several other allyl-containing drugs, including allyl barbiturates, cause destruction of liver cytochrome P-450. The original
findings (reviewed by Ortiz de Montellano and coworkers (1978a; and
by De Matteis, 1978) demonstrated that metabolic activation of the
allylic double bond was required before the haem moiety of the cytochrome could be converted into abnormal porphyrins or green pigments.
Similar findings have since been reported for unsaturated compounds
containing the acetylenic grouping, including ethynyl-substituted
steroids (White and Muller-Eberhard, 1977; White, 1978 and 1981; Ortiz
de Montellano and Kunze, 1980) and destruction of liver cytochrome
P-450 has also been reported after drugs with the unsaturated vinyl
grouping, such as vinyl chloride and fluroxene (2,2,2-trifluoroethyl
vinyl ether) (Ivanetich and coworkers, 1975; 1976; Guengerich and
Strickland, 1977).   More recently Ortiz de Montellano and collaborators (1978b; 1979) have made the important observation that a
reactive derivative of the effective drugs (of either the allylic or
the acetylinic group) becomes covalently bound onto the porphyrin
nucleus of haem; and work from our own laboratory has shown that the
various green pigments produced from the action of these unsaturated
chemicals on haem are all N-monosubstituted (De Matteis and Cantoni,
1979; De Matteis and coworkers, 1980a).   Additional evidence for
N-alkylation has been reported by Ortiz de Montellano and coworkers
(1981).   The exact nature of the alkylating metabolite of the unsaturated drugs and the detailed mechanism of the N-alkylation reaction
are still unclear but several lines of evidence point to a reactive
monooxygenated intermediate (De Matteis and coworkers 1980b; Ortiz de
Montellano and coworkers, 1981).   It can therefore be concluded that
these unsaturated drugs are metabolized by cytochrome P-450 into
reactive derivatives which alkylate one of the pyrrole nitrogens of
its prosthetic group and therefore inhibit the haemoprotein by a
suicidal type of inactivation.

As originally reported for AIA (De Matteis and Unseld, 1976) the green
pigments produced by treatment with either allylic or acetylenic compounds contain iron in their native form (White, 1981; De Matteis,
Gibbs and Unseld, 1981), are therefore present in the liver as alkylated haems, but readily lose iron on exposure to acid to generate the
corresponding N-alkylated porphyrins.   Green pigments of this group
do not inhibit liver protohaem ferro-lyase (E.C.4.99.1.1), the enzyme
which converts protoporphyrin into haem, neither *in vivo* nor *in vitro*
(De Matteis, Gibbs and Smith, 1980; De Matteis, Gibbs and Tephly, 1980)

and for this reason none of the unsaturated drugs responsible will
cause a very marked increase in liver protoporphyrin in vivo. The
accumulation of the intermediates of the pathway which has been described in the liver of animals given unsaturated drugs could simply
result from the large increase in liver haem turnover which in turn
stimulates markedly hepatic ALA-S; the supply of haem precursors would
then exceed the activities of the subsequent enzymes of the pathway,
even though the activities of these subsequent enzymes may all be
normal.

LIVER ACCUMULATION OF N-METHYL PROTOPORPHYRIN AFTER DDC AND GRISEOFULVIN

In clear contrast to the unsaturated drugs discussed above DDC, griseofulvin and isogriseofulvin produce accumulation in the liver of a
second type of green pigment with strong inhibitory properties toward
protohaem ferro-lyase in vitro (Tephly, Gibbs and De Matteis, 1979;
Tephly and coworkers, 1980; De Matteis and Gibbs, 1980). Marked
inhibition of liver protohaem ferro-lyase is also observed in vivo
after treatment with this second group of drugs (Onisawa and Labbe,
1963; Lockhead, Dagg and Goldberg, 1967) and because of this the liver
concentration of protoporphyrin (the substrate of the inhibited enzyme)
increases markedly, giving rise to the biochemical picture of hepatic
protoporphyria. The inhibitory pigment also appears to originate
from turnover of liver haem (Tephly and coworkers, 1980) and has been
identified as N-methylprotoporphyrin (De Matteis and coworkers, 1980;
Ortiz de Montellano, Beilan and Kunze, 1981).

Inhibition of the enzyme is thought to reflect tight binding of the
N-methylated porphyrin with the active center, as suggested by kinetic
studies carried out in vitro (De Matteis, Gibbs and Tephly, 1980) and
also by the structure required by a N-methylated porphyrin in order to
inhibit the enzyme. Protoporphyrin IX and mesoporphyrin IX, both of
which are substrates of protohaem ferro-lyase, when N-monomethylated,
become powerful inhibitors; whereas coproporphyrin III, which is not
a substrate, will not inhibit after N-methylation. The size of the
alkyl group present on the pyrrole nitrogen atom has also been shown
to be important for the inhibitory effect, N-ethyl mesoporphyrin being
less active than N-methyl mesoporphyrin (De Matteis, Gibbs and Smith,
1980). This may reflect steric hinderance by a large N-alkyl group
of the binding of the modified porphyrin at the active center, for
example by distortion of the tetrapyrrolic system so as to alter the
distance between (and spatial arrangement of) the two propionic acid
side chains in position 6 and 7 of the porphyrin: both of these are
known to be important for a porphyrin to be accepted at the active
center of the enzyme (Honeybourne, Jackson and Jones, 1979).
Similarly the large size of the alkyl group may play a part in the
lack of inhibition of the enzyme by the first group of green pigments,
those produced by unsaturated compounds. The detailed mechanism of
enzyme inhibition by N-methyl protoporphyrin has not yet been elucidated, but the following possibility has been considered (De Matteis
and Gibbs, 1980). The presence of a methyl group at one of the
pyrrole nitrogen atoms would be expected to interfere with a normal
(i.e. tetraco-ordinate) incorporation of a bivalent metal and a charged
metal complex will be produced (McEwen, 1946). The enzyme may then
be blocked in an intermediary stage of the enzymic reaction, unable to
release the "completed" metalloporphyrin product. More work is
required to clarify these points.

F. De Matteis *et al.*

TABLE 1 Absorption Spectra of the Green Pigments isolated from the Liver of Control Mice and of Mice given either DDC or its 4-Ethyl analogue. Comparison with synthetic N-Methyl and N-Ethyl protoporphyrin

Absorption maxima (nm)

Porphyrin	Dication			Zinc Complex			
	Soret	II	I	Soret	α	α	α'
Green Pigment (with DDC)*	412	560	604	431	547	596	633
N-Methyl protoporphyrin*	412	560	604	431	545.5	594.5	633
Green Pigment (with 4-Ethyl analogue of DDC)*	417.5	564.5	608	431.5	546	592	631.5
N-Ethyl protoporphyrin*	417.5	563	606	431	547	592	631.5
"Control" Green Pigment	413	563	603	431	545	592	632

The neutral spectrum of all porphyrins listed above is of an aetio type with very similar absorption maxima to those given elsewhere (De Matteis and Gibbs, 1980) for the DDC pigment. The dication and zinc complexes were prepared (De Matteis and Gibbs, 1980) and their spectra determined in $CHCl_3$, using the porphyrin methyl esters.

* From De Matteis and coworkers (1980b, 1981).

TABLE 2 Inhibitory Activity towards Protohaem Ferro-
         -lyase of Green Pigments isolated from the
         Liver of Control Mice and of Mice given
         either DDC or its 4-Ethyl analogue.
         Comparison with synthetic N-Methyl and
         N-Ethyl protoporphyrin.

Porphyrin	Inhibitory Activity (Units/nmol)
Green Pigment (with DDC)[*]	17.5, 15.5, 16.6
Green Pigment (with 4-Ethyl analogue of DDC)[*]	4.8, 5.7, 4.6
"Control" Green Pigment	16.2, 10.3
N-Methyl Protoporphyrin[*]	14.4, 12.4
N-Ethyl Protoporphyrin[*]	6.3, 6.6

[*] From De Matteis and coworkers (1981), where
reference is given to methods followed for isolation of pigments and assay of inhibitory activity.

It can be concluded that DDC and griseofulvin induce hepatic porphyria
by a multistage mechanism in which conversion of liver haem into
N-methylprotoporphyrin is apparently the first step. Marked inhibition of protohaem ferro-lyase and secondary stimulation of liver ALA-S
follow in turn. As a result of these last two effects protoporphyrin
accumulates in the liver and hepatic protoporphyria becomes
established. Support for this mechanism has recently been obtained by
injecting mice with authentic N-methylmesoporphyrin and by showing
that inhibition of protohaem ferro-lyase, stimulation of ALA-S and
accumulation of protoporphyrin were all demonstrable in their livers
(De Matteis, Gibbs and Smith, 1980).

MECHANISM OF PRODUCTION OF N-METHYL PROTOPORPHYRIN BY DDC

In contrast to the N-alkylated porphyrins produced by unsaturated
compounds, which all originate from the haem of cytochrome P-450, it
is not yet clear from which pool of hepatic haem N-methyl protoporphyrin originates. It is true that both DDC and griseofulvin have
been reported to cause a loss of cytochrome P-450 (Wada and coworkers,
1968) and DDC also causes a loss of haem radioactivity from fractions
of the liver homogenate resembling in distribution that seen after
AIA (Abbritti and De Matteis, 1973); however the evidence implicating
cytochrome P-450 as the source of N-methyl protoporphyrin is as yet
far from conclusive.

We have recently studied the mechanism of production of N-methyl
protoporphyrin in mice treated with DDC and have obtained evidence
that the methyl group on the pyrrole nitrogen atom originates from
the drug (De Matteis and collaborators, 1981). These experiments, to
be summarized below, were suggested by the report (Loev and Snader,
1965) that under relatively mild chemical conditions certain dihydropyridines lose their 4-alkyl substituent to suitable nucleophiles on
oxidation; and also by the findings (Cole and Marks, 1980) that in a
series of dihydropyridines tested the presence and nature of the
4-alkyl substituent affects the inhibitory activity on protohaem
ferro-lyase, the analogue lacking a 4-alkyl substituent being almost

Drug Administered   N̲ - alkylated porphyrin
                                          isolated

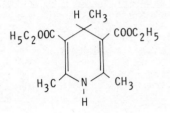

Protoporphyrin - N - CH₃

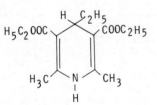

Protoporphyrin - N - C₂H₅

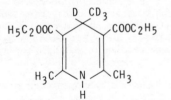

Protoporphyrin - N - CD₃

Fig.1. The N̲-alkyl substituent of protoporphyrin
       originates from the 4-alkyl grouping of a
       dihydropyridine (discussed in the text).
       Drugs shown are (from top to bottom):
       unlabelled DDC; its 4-ethyl analogue; DDC
       labelled with deuterium in its 4-methyl
       group.

completely inactive. We have compared 3,5-diethoxycarbonyl-1,4-
-dihydro-2,4,6-trimethylpyridine (DDC) with the corresponding 4-ethyl
analogue (3,5-diethoxycarbonyl-1,4-dihydro-2,6-dimethyl-4-ethylpyri-
dine) for their ability to produce accumulation of green pigments in
the liver of mice *in vivo*. The two drugs, henceforth referred to as
the 4-methyl and 4-ethyl dihydropyridines, cause accumulation of a
green pigment resembling (in spectral characteristics and in ability
to inhibit protohaem ferro-lyase *in vitro*, Table 1 and 2) N̲-methyl
protoporphyrin and N̲-ethyl protoporphyrin, respectively. The
electron impact mass spectrum of the two green pigment′ dimethyl
esters was also determined. A molecular ion at m̲/z̲ values of 604 and
618 was found for the pigments produced by treatment with 4-methyl and

4-ethyl dihydropyridine, compatible with a structure of N-methylproto-porphyrin and N-ethylprotoporphyrin, respectively. This suggested that in the N-alkylation reaction the 4-alkyl group of the dihydro-pyridine was donated to the pyrrole nitrogen.

Conclusive evidence that the alkyl group on the pyrrole nitrogen atom originates from the 4-alkyl substituent of the drug was obtained by using DDC labelled with deuterium in the 4-methyl substituent. The resulting green pigment was purified as the dimethyl ester and sub-jected to electron impact mass spectrometry, where it produced a molecular ion at m/z value of 607. The increase of 3 mass units (when compared with the molecular ion of the corresponding pigment produced by unlabelled DDC) is compatible with the methyl group being trans-ferred intact, possibly as a carbonium ion.

These findings, summarized in Fig.1, establish the source of the N-methyl grouping in the DDC pigment. They also provide an explana-tion for the inability of 3,5-diethoxycarbonyl-1,4-dihydro-2,6-di-methylpyridine to inhibit protohaem ferro-lyase (Cole and Marks, 1980), as this drug does not possess a 4-alkyl group which can be donated and, on account of this, cannot be expected to give rise to the N-alkylated protoporphyrin inhibitor. By analogy with the present results one of the methyl groups of griseofulvin or isogriseofulvin could be the source of the N-substituent of the green pigments pro-duced by these drugs.

An inhibitor of protohaem ferro-lyase (with similar chromatographic characteristics and Soret absorption to that produced by DDC) can be demonstrated in trace amounts in the liver of control mice which have received no treatment (Tephly and coworkers, 1979, 1980). This "control" pigment has now been purified (using the pooled livers of at least 200 mice) and characterized spectrally. Its inhibitory acti-vity on protohaem ferro-lyase has also been determined and compared with that of the pigment isolated after DDC treatment and with that of synthetic N-methyl protoporphyrin. The control pigment resembled both "natural" and synthetic N-methyl protoporphyrin in both respects (Tables 1 and 2). These findings suggest that N-methyl protoporphyrin occurs normally in the liver, that is independently of drug administra-tion. The source of the N-substituent in the "control" pigment is not known: more work is required to determine whether it originates from an endogenous methyl donor or from a component of the laboratory diet.

REFERENCES

Abbritti, G. and De Matteis, F. (1973) Enzyme, 16, 196-202.
Cole, S.P.C. and Marks, G.S. (1980) Int.J.Bioch., 12, 989-992.
De Matteis, F. (1978) Pharmac.Ther.A.2, 693-725.
De Matteis, F. and Cantoni, L. (1979) Biochem.J., 183, 99-103.
De Matteis, F. and Gibbs, A.H. (1980) Biochem.J., 187, 285-288.
De Matteis, F. and Unseld, A. (1976) Biochem.Soc.Trans., 4, 205-209.
De Matteis, F., Gibbs, A.H. and Smith, A.G. (1980) Biochem.J., 189, 645-648.
De Matteis, F., Gibbs, A H. and Tephly, T.R. (1980) Biochem.J., 188, 145-152.
De Matteis, F., Gibbs, A.H. and Unseld, A.P. (1981) In R.Snyder (Ed.) Biological Reactive Intermediates 2: Chemical Mechanisms and Bio-logical Effects, Plenum Publ.Co., New York, in press.

138   F. De Matteis *et al.*

De Matteis, F., Gibbs, A.H., Cantoni, L. and Francis, J. (1980a). In Ciba Foundation Symposium 76, Excerpta Medica, Amsterdam pp.119-131
De Matteis, F., Gibbs, A.H., Jackson, A.H. and Weerasinghe, S. (1980b) FEBS Lett., 119, 109-112.
De Matteis, F., Gibbs, A.H., Farmer, P.B. and Lamb, J.H. (1981) FEBS Lett., 129, 328-331.
Goldberg, A. and Rimington, C. (1955) Proc.Roy.Soc.B., 143, 257-280.
Guengerich, F.P. and Strickland, T.W. (1977) Mol.Pharmacol., 13, 993-1004.
Honeybourne, C.L., Jackson, J.T. and Jones, O.T.G. (1979) FEBS Lett., 98, 207-210.
Ivanetich, K.M., Marsh, J.A., Bradshaw, J.J. and Kaminsky, L.S. (1975) Biochem.Pharmacol., 24, 1933-1936.
Ivanetich, K.M., Bradshaw, J.J., Marsh, J.A., Harrison, G.G. and Kaminsky, L.S. (1976) Biochem.Pharmacol., 25, 773-778.
Lockhead, A.C., Dagg, J.H. and Goldberg, A. (1967) Brit.J.Derm., 79, 96-102.
Loev, G. and Snader, K.M. (1965) J.Org.Chem., 30, 1914-1916.
McEwen, W.K. (1946) J.Am.Chem.Soc., 68, 711-713.
Onisawa, J. and Labbe, R.F. (1963) J.Biol.Chem., 238, 724-727.
Ortiz de Montellano, P.R., Beilan, H.S. and Kunze, K.L. (1981) Proc. Natl.Acad.Sci.USA, 78, 1490-1494.
Ortiz de Montellano, P.R. and Kunze, K.L. (1980) J.Biol.Chem., 255, 5578-5585.
Ortiz de Montellano, P.R., Mico, B.A., Yost, G.S. and Correia, M.A. (1978a) In M. Seiler (Ed.), Enzyme Activated Irriversible Inhibitors, Elsevier/North-Holland, Amsterdam, pp.337-352.
Ortiz de Montellano, P.R., Mico, B.A. and Yost, G.S. (1978b) Biochem. Biophys.Res.Commun., 83, 132-137.
Ortiz de Montellano, P.R., Kunze, K.L., Yost, G.S. and Mico, B.A. (1979) Proc.Natl.Acad.Sci.USA, 76, 746-749.
Ortiz de Montellano, P.R., Beilan, H.S., Kunze, K.L. and Mico, B.A. (1981) J.Biol.Chem., 256, 4395-4399.
Schmid, R. and Schwartz, S. (1952) Proc.Soc.exp.Biol.(N.Y.), 81, 685-689.
Solomon, H.M. and Figge, F.H.J. (1959) Proc.Soc.exp.Biol.(N.Y.), 100 583-586.
Tephly, T.R., Gibbs, A.H. and De Matteis, F. (1979) Biochem.J., 180, 241-244.
Tephly, T.R., Gibbs, A.H., Ingall, G. and De Matteis, F. (1980) Int.J. Biochem., 12, 993-998.
Wada, O., Yano, Y., Urata, G. and Nakao, K. (1968) Biochem.Pharmacol. 17, 595-603.
White, I.N.H. (1978) Biochem.J., 174, 853-861.
White, I.N.H. (1981) Biochem.J., 196, 575-583.
White, I.N.H. and Muller-Eberhard, U. (1977) Biochem.J., 166, 57-64.

Toxic Effects of Metals on the Synthesis and Disposition of Heme

T. R. Tephly, B. L. Coffman, M. S. Abou Zeit-Har, R. Sedman,
E. West and I. Simon

Departments of Pharmacology and Biochemistry, The Toxicology
Center, University of Iowa, Iowa City, Iowa 52242, USA

ABSTRACT

The heme biosynthetic pathway is perturbed by many chemicals and metals, and
heme and hemoprotein biosynthesis may be disrupted as a result of exposure
to these agents. Cobalt treatment of rats leads to marked decreases in the
rate of heme biosynthesis and in the level of hemoproteins in hepatic
microsomes. Cardiac heme biosynthesis in isolated perfused rat hearts is
also decreased as a result of cobalt-induced decreases of δ-aminolevulinic
acid synthetase activity. Lead acetate does not inhibit either heme biosynthesis or δ-aminolevulinic acid synthetase activity in isolated perfused rat
hearts. Fasting of rats, which may lead to increases in hepatic δ-aminolevulinic acid synthetase activity, leads to a rapid and extensive decrease
in cardiac δ-aminolevulinic acid synthetase activity and a marked decrease
in the rate of cardiac heme biosynthesis. Friend erythroleukemic cells
which can be induced by dimethylsulfoxide to synthesize hemoglobin show an
increase in δ-aminolevulinic acid synthetase activity in response to cobalt
exposure, and mutant forms of these cells which cannot be induced to synthesize hemoglobin because of a deficiency in ferrochelatase activity display
an increase in δ-aminolevulinic acid synthetase activity when exposed to
cobalt. Therefore, cobalt treatment may lead to different effects on the
heme biosynthetic pathway in different tissues. This response may be
dependent on the physiologic function of the organ and the degree of control
imposed by the end product, heme, on the rate-limiting step of the pathway,
δ-aminolevulinic acid synthetase.

KEY WORDS

Heme, Cobalt, Lead, Heart, δ-Aminolevulinic acid synthetase, Friend cells,
Ferrochelatase, Fasting, Porphyrin, Toxicity.

INTRODUCTION

The heme biosynthetic pathway is a complex system involving many cellular
compartments; and as far as we know, it occurs in every organ and tissue in
the mammal. Aerobic cells require oxygen and hemoproteins are intimately

involved in oxidative processes including the transport of oxygen. The heme
prosthetic group is derived from glycine and succinyl-CoA, and the system is
subjected to efficient and fine control. After heme is formed, it is transported from the mitochondrion to other sites of the cell, including the
nucleus, where it may exert control at a genetic level.

The effects of chemicals on heme biosynthesis and catabolism are important
to understand since many steps of the heme biosynthetic pathway are subject
to regulation by these xenobiotics. In addition, many foreign chemicals and
metals appear to exert an inductive or repressive effect at the genetic
level, thereby promoting or inhibiting synthesis of rate-limiting steps in
the pathway leading to heme formation. In certain cases, these alterations
produced by xenobiotics are deleterious. In another sense, they help us to
understand the mechanism of reaction for many of the steps of the heme
biosynthetic pathway. This paper will deal with the effect of metals and
certain nutritional states as they interact with and perturb the heme
biosynthetic pathway in the liver, the heart and the Friend erythroleukemic
cell.

THE EFFECT OF METALS ON HEME BIOSYNTHESIS

Lead exerts a profound effect on heme biosynthesis. The inhibition of δ-
aminolevulinic acid (ALA) dehydratase and ferrochelatase is well known and
the hematologic effects produced by lead have been studied extensively.
Since lead toxicity occurs widely and is a major pediatric problem in urban
society, it is important to understand the mechanism of toxicity of this
metal. Studies in experimental animals, and recently in humans, have
demonstrated the effects of lead not only on the erythropoietic system but
on hepatic heme biosynthesis and hemoprotein synthesis. Alvares and Kappas
(1979) demonstrated the effect of lead on heme biosynthesis, catabolism,
hepatic microsomal cytochrome P-450 and associated enzymic activities in rat
liver. They showed that there was a decrease in ALA dehydratase activity,
microsomal heme content, cytochrome P-450 content, benzo(α)pyrene hydroxylase activity and ethylmorphine N-demethylase activity in rats administered
lead acutely. In this study, ALA synthetase activity was not altered
although microsomal heme oxygenase activity was dramatically increased.
They also showed the effect of lead on the metabolism of antipyrine in lead
workers and in acutely lead-poisoned children prior to and after chelation
therapy. Their work demonstrates that lead can alter the half-life of a
drug known to be metabolized by the hepatic microsomal cytochrome P-450-
dependent system. Thus, lead can exert marked effects in the hemopoietic
system and on hepatic systems.

We have recently studied heme biosynthesis in the isolated perfused rat
heart. This has been a convenient way to study a functional system outside
of the animal and to determine the effects of xenobiotics such as drugs and
metals on a metabolic system in a living tissue. Using this system, it has
been possible to monitor the viability of the organ as well as the heme
biosynthetic pathway. We have studied the rate of incorporation of ^{14}C-
glycine or ^{14}C-δ-aminolevulinic acid (ALA) into cardiac heme as a way of
determining the rate of heme biosynthesis.

Male Sprague-Dawley rats (200-250 g) were allowed food and water ad libitum
or fasted 24 hours prior to sacrifice. After sodium pentobarbital anesthesia,
600 units of heparin was administered via the tail vein. The hearts were
rapidly excised, chilled in iced 0.9% NaCl and perfused by the technique

described by Morgan and his colleagues (1971). Ten ml of perfusion medium
were passed through the heart; and when all visible blood was washed out,
the heart was cannulated. The hearts were allowed to recover from the
anoxia associated with the process of removal and cannulation. The perfusion media described by Morgan and his coworkers (1971) was employed. This
system included all the amino acids at plasma level values, 15 mM glucose,
25 milliunits/ml of insulin and 1% albumin at 37°C, pH 7.4. This media was
equilibrated with oxygen:carbon dioxide (95:5). Lead acetate or cobaltous
chloride were added to the incubation media. The heart rate was monitored
constantly and ATP and creatine phosphate levels were determined at various
times during the perfusion process. Cardiac ALA synthetase activity was
determined by a modification of the method of Briggs and coworkers (1976).
Glycine radioactivity and glycine content in the isolated perfused hearts
were determined by a modification of the method of Ohmori and coworkers
(1978).

Table 1 shows that lead has no effect on the rate of incorporation of ^{14}C-
glycine into cardiac heme. Concentrations of 2 and 100 μM lead acetate had
no significant effects on the rate of incorporation of ^{14}C-glycine into
cardiac heme.

TABLE 1 Effect on the Rate of Heme Synthesis in Rat Hearts

	Heme Biosynthesis (dpm/nmol heme)
Control	21,984 ± 3,489
Lead Acetate (2 μM)	17,216 ± 1,871
Lead Acetate (100 μM)	18,252 ± 1,581

Values represent the mean of 5 or more determinations ± SE. Those obtained for lead treatments were not significantly different from
controls (P > 0.05). Heme was isolated as
described by Baron and Tephly (1969).

δ-Aminolevulinic acid synthetase activities were about the same in hearts
perfused in the presence or absence of lead.

Piper and coworkers (1976) showed that purified erythrocytic or hepatic
uroporphyrinogen I synthetase activity is inhibited by lead in vitro.
These studies are interesting in that the enzyme is not inhibited in hepatic
cytosol preparations. Once the enzyme is dialyzed or purified, it becomes
sensitized to lead. Thus, a factor is present in normal hepatic cells which
is capable of protecting the uro I synthetase activity against the effects
of lead. Piper and van Lier (1977) have evidence which suggests that the
factor is a pteridine compound.

Cobaltous chloride administration in vivo has been demonstrated to produce
a marked decrease in hepatic microsomal heme concentrations and decreases in
hepatic microsomal cytochrome P-450 proteins (Tephly et al., 1973). A great
deal of work has been done using cobaltous chloride because of its usefulness
in titrating hepatic microsomal cytochrome P-450 to various levels in liver
and thereby associating the relationship between metabolism of drugs and the
cytochrome P-450 system. The mechanism of cobaltous chloride in decreasing
hepatic microsomal heme and cytochrome P-450 levels has been the subject of
a great deal of study recently. Tephly and colleagues demonstrated that

livers of rats treated with cobaltous chloride have a marked decrease in the
ability to incorporate ^{14}C-ALA into hepatic microsomal heme (Tephly et al.,
1973). Cobalt inhibits ferrochelatase activity and ALA synthetase activity
presumably by forming the cobalt-porphyrin complex (Igarashi et al., 1978;
Jones and Jones, 1968; Sinclair et al., 1979; Watkins et al., 1980).
Nakamura and colleagues (1975) and DeMatteis and Gibbs (1977) showed that
treatment of rats with cobaltous chloride leads to marked and rapid decreases
in hepatic ALA synthetase activity.

Cobalt produces a marked myocardial toxicity which often leads to death
(Kennedy et al., 1981). We have recently demonstrated that cobaltous chloride administration to rats leads to a marked decrease in both hepatic and
cardiac ALA synthetase activity. Indeed, the decrease in cardiac ALA synthetase activity that was produced established a state of low cardiac ALA
synthetase activity for a much longer duration of time than is usually seen
in rat liver (Sedman and Tephly, 1980). Cobaltous chloride addition to
mitochondria prepared from the hearts of rats did not decrease ALA synthetase
activity. Therefore, there is no direct inhibition of ALA synthetase
activity in vitro by the addition of cobaltous chloride to reaction mixtures.

TABLE 2   The Effect of Cobaltous Chloride on Cardiac ALA
Synthetase Activity in the Isolated Perfused Rat Heart

Treatment	ALA Synthetase Activity[a] (nmol/g heart/hour)
Control	10.0 ± 1.0
Cobalt (90 µM)	6.0 ± 0.5[b]
Cobalt (45 µM)	7.5 ± 1.0[b]

[a]Each value represents the mean $\pm$ standard
error of 4 hearts. ALA synthetase activity
was determined by Briggs and coworkers (1976).

[b]Denotes significant decrease from control
($P < 0.05$).

Table 2 demonstrates the effect of cobaltous chloride on cardiac ALA synthetase activity in the isolated perfused rat heart preparation. One hour
after perfusion, control values were essentially the same as those seen in
animal in vivo. However, when cobaltous chloride was added to the perfusate, a significant decrease in ALA synthetase activity was observed within
1 hour. It can be seen in Table 3 that cobalt produces a marked decrease
in the rate of ^{14}C-glycine incorporation into cardiac heme. This is consistent with the decrease in ALA synthetase activity observed (about 50%) in
this experiment. Control values ($\pm$ SE) of ALA synthetase were 7.8 ($\pm$ 0.8)
nmol ALA formed/g tissue/hr and ALA synthetase activity obtained in hearts
perfused with cobalt was 3.6 ($\pm$ 0.4) nmol ALA/g tissue/hr. In these experiments, there was no significant decrease in tissue glycine uptake or in free
glycine levels obtained in the hearts perfused as described. Therefore,
cobaltous chloride leads to a decrease in cardiac ALA synthetase activity
and a concomitant decrease in the rate of incorporation of ^{14}C-glycine into
cardiac heme. Similar experiments have been performed with ^{14}C-ALA substi-
tuted for ^{14}C-glycine. No difference in the rate of incorporation of ^{14}C-
ALA into cardiac heme was observed between control and cobalt perfused

hearts. Therefore, it would appear that ALA synthetase activity is the rate-limiting step in heme biosynthesis in the heart, and changes in the level of this enzyme lead to changes in rate of heme biosynthesis in the heart.

TABLE 3   The Effect of Cobalt on Heme Biosynthesis in the Isolated Perfused Rat Heart

Treatment	dpm/nmol Heme
Control	$22,000 \pm 3,500$[a]
Cobalt (90 μM)	$10,200 \pm 1,370$[b]

[a]Values represent the mean $\pm$ SE obtained from 4 hearts.

[b]Significantly different from control values ($P < 0.01$). ^{14}C-glycine (100 μCi) was added to perfusion media at zero time and hearts were removed 2 hours after perfusion. Heme was isolated as described by Baron and Tephly (1969).

THE EFFECT OF FASTING ON CARDIAC ALA SYNTHETASE ACTIVITY
AND HEME BIOSYNTHESIS IN THE HEART

It has been shown that when rats are fasted for 24 hours, marked decreases in cardiac ALA synthetase activity occur (Briggs et al., 1976). The time course of decrease of ALA synthetase activity once food has been removed from rats is demonstrated in Fig. 1. ALA synthetase activity fell eventually to about 20% of the activity detected in hearts of rats which were allowed food.

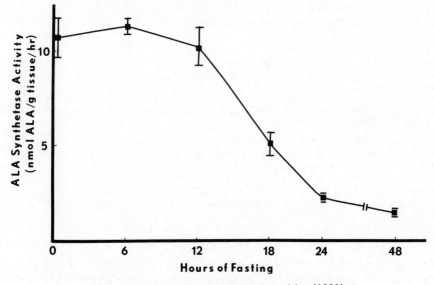

Fig. 1. Taken from Sedman and Tephly (1980).

Table 4 demonstrates that, over 3 hours of perfusion, there was no decrease
in cardiac ALA synthetase activity in hearts of fed or fasted rats. However,
it can be seen that there is a significant decrease in the ALA synthetase
activity in hearts obtained from fasted rats. Table 5 demonstrates that the
rate of incorporation of ^{14}C-glycine into cardiac heme b is also significantly reduced in hearts obtained from fasted rats. The decrease in glycine
incorporation into cardiac heme a was also decreased by about 50%. ^{14}C-ALA
incorporation into cardiac heme was not significantly different in isolated
perfused hearts obtained from fed or fasted rats. Therefore, ALA synthetase
activity appears to regulate the rate of heme biosynthesis in the heart.

TABLE 4   ALA Synthetase Activity in Isolated Perfused
Hearts Obtained from Fed and Fasted Rats

| | ALA Synthetase Activity (nmol/g heart/hr) | |
Time of Perfusion (Hours)	Fed	Fasted
0	13 $\pm$ 1.0	4.0 $\pm$ 0.1[a]
1	18 $\pm$ 2.5	4.0 $\pm$ 1.0
2	18 $\pm$ 2.2	5.0 $\pm$ 0.5
3	16 $\pm$ 2.0	5.0 $\pm$ 1.2

[a]Values represent the mean $\pm$ SE obtained from 4 hearts.
All values obtained from fasted hearts were significantly lower than those obtained from fed hearts.

TABLE 5   Incorporation of ^{14}C-Glycine into Cardiac Heme b

| | ^{14}C-Heme b (dpm/100 μmol heme b) | |
Treatment	Fed Rat	Fasted Rat
1 hour perfusion	723 $\pm$ 214	364 $\pm$ 102
2 hour perfusion	1196 $\pm$ 186	450 $\pm$ 91[a]

Values represent the mean $\pm$ SE obtained from 4 hearts.
Heme b was isolated as described by Sedman and Tephly
(In Press).
[a]Significantly different from values obtained from fed
hearts ($P < 0.05$).

EFFECT OF COBALT ON ALA SYNTHETASE ACTIVITY IN FRIEND
ERYTHROLEUKEMIC CELLS

Murine erythroleukemic cells (Friend cells) have been a useful model for
the study of the regulation of heme biosynthesis and the synthesis of
hemoglobin. Sassa (1976) has shown a sequential induction of enzymes of the
heme biosynthetic pathway during erythroid differentiation of Friend cells.
These cells are capable of synthesizing heme and the rate-limiting step in
the pathway appears to be the rate of formation of ALA as catalyzed by ALA
synthetase. Recently, it has been possible to study hemeless mutants which
when grown in the presence of dimethyl sulfoxide (DMSO) are incapable of
synthesizing hemoglobin and have an absence of ferrochelatase activity

(Rutherford et al., 1979). Rutherford and coworkers (1979) have shown that agents which normally induce Friend cells to make hemoglobin cannot induce heme biosynthesis in the mutant Friend cell. We have studied the effect of cobalt on Friend cells (F^+) which can be induced by DMSO to make hemoglobin and the effect of cobalt on a mutant cell line incapable of producing hemoglobin when treated with DMSO (R_3). These cells were grown in suspension culture and were supplemented with heat inactivated fetal calf serum at 37° in a 5% CO_2 atmosphere. After cells were grown for 4 days, cobalt was added to incubations and cells were allowed to grow for another hour. At the end of this time period, cells were disrupted by nitrogen cavitation and analyzed for ALA synthetase activity. It can be seen from Table 6 that there is an induction of ALA synthetase activity in these cells. This result came as a surprise since we expected that the inclusion of cobaltous chloride would have led to decreased ALA synthetase activity in the inducible cells, i.e. those with ferrochelatase activity. We had expected no effect in the DMSO-nonresponsive Friend cells, i.e. ferrochelatase-deficient cells.

TABLE 6   ALA Synthetase Activity After Treatment of Friend
          Erythroleukemic Cells with Cobalt

	ALA Synthetase Activity[a] (pmol/mg protein/hr)
F^+	300
F^+ + 25 µM Co^{++}	410
F^+ + 50 µM Co^{++}	420
R_3	110
R_3 + 25 µM Co^{++}	410
R_3 + 50 µM Co^{++}	390

[a]Values are the mean of two experiments.

ACKNOWLEDGMENT

Supported by NIH grant GM12675.

REFERENCES

Alvares, A. P., and A. Kappas (1979). Lead and polychlorinated biphenyls: Effects on heme and drug metabolism. Drug Metab. Rev., 10, 91-106.
Baron, J., and T. R. Tephly (1969). Effect of 3-amino-1,2,4-triazole on the induction of rat hepatic microsomal oxidases, cytochrome P-450 and NADPH-cytochrome c reductase by phenobarbital. Mol. Pharmacol., 5, 10-20.
Briggs, D. W., L. W. Condie, R. M. Sedman, and T. R. Tephly (1976). δ-Aminolevulinic acid synthetase in the heart. J. Biol. Chem., 251, 4996-5001.
DeMatteis, F., and A. H. Gibbs (1977). Inhibition of haem synthesis caused by cobalt in rat liver. Biochem. J., 162, 213-216.
Igarashi, J., N. Hayashi, and G. Kikuchi (1978). Effects of administration of cobalt chloride and cobalt protoporphyrin on δ-aminolevulinate synthase in rat liver. J. Biochem., 84, 997-1000.

Jones, M.S., and O. T. G. Jones (1968). Evidence for the location of
ferrochelatase on the inner membrane of rat liver mitochondria.
Biochem. Biophys. Res. Commun., 31, 977-982.
Kennedy, A., J. D. Dornan, and R. King (1981). Fatal myocardial disease
associated with industrial exposure to cobalt. Lancet, 8217, 412-414.
Morgan, H. E., D. C. Earl, A. Broadus, E. B. Wolpert, K. E. Giger, and L. S.
Jefferson (1971). Regulation of protein synthesis in heart muscle. 1.
Effect of amino acid levels on protein synthesis. J. Biol. Chem., 246,
2152-2162.
Nakamura, M., Y. Yasukochi, and S. Minakami (1975). Effect of cobalt on
heme biosynthesis in rat liver and spleen. J. Biochem., 78, 373-380.
Ohmori, S., M. Ikeda, Y. Watanabe, and K. Hirota (1978). A simple and
specific determination of glycine in biological samples. Anal. Biochem.,
90, 662-670.
Piper, W. N., R. B. L. van Lier, G. Rios, and T. R. Tephly (1976). Studies
on the role of a factor regulating lead inhibition of erythrocytic and
hepatic uroporphyrinogen I synthetase activity. Life Sci., 19,
1225-1234.
Piper, W. N., and R. B. L. van Lier (1977). Pteridine regulation of inhibition of hepatic uroporphyrinogen I synthetase activity by lead chloride.
Mol. Pharmacol., 13, 1126-1135.
Rutherford, T., G. C. Thompson, and M. R. Moore (1979). Heme biosynthesis
in Friend erythroleukemia cells: Control by ferrochelatase. Proc.
Natl. Acad. Sci. USA, 76, 833-836.
Rutherford, T. R., and D. J. Weatherall (1979). Deficient heme synthesis as
the cause of non-inducibility of hemoglobin synthesis in a Friend
erythroleukemia cell line. Cell, 16, 415-423.
Sassa, S. (1976). Sequential induction of heme pathway enzymes during
erythroid differentiation of mouse Friend leukemia virus-infected
cells. J. Exp. Med., 143, 305-315.
Sedman, R. M., and T. R. Tephly (1980). Cardiac δ-aminolevulinic acid
synthetase activity: Effects of fasting, cobaltous chloride and hemin.
Biochem. Pharmacol., 29, 795-800.
Sedman, R., and T. R. Tephly. Isolation and separation of heme a and heme b
from cardiac tissue by thin layer chromatography. Biochem. Pharmacol.
(In Press).
Sinclair, P., A. H. Gibbs, J. F. Sinclair, and F. DeMatteis (1979). Forma-
tion of cobalt protoporphyrin in the liver of rats. A mechanism for
the inhibition of liver haem biosynthesis by inorganic cobalt.
Biochem. J., 178, 529-538.
Tephly, T. R., C. Webb, P. Trussler, F. Kniffen, E. Hasegawa, and W. Piper
(1973). The regulation of heme synthesis related to drug metabolism.
Drug Metab. Disp., 1, 259-266.
Watkins, S. J., J. Beason, and T. R. Tephly (1980). Identification of
cobalt protoporphyrin IX formation in vivo following cobalt administration to rats. Biochem. Pharmacol., 29, 2319-2323.

The Heme Biosynthetic Pathway in the Prediction of Haloaromatic Hydrocarbon Toxicity

G. D. Sweeney

Dept. of Medicine, McMaster University, Hamilton, Ontario L8N 3Z5, Canada

ABSTRACT

Skin disease associated with abnormal porphyrin excretion (porphyria cutanea tarda; PCT) followed hexachlorobenzene poisoning in Turkey and also occurred in workers making trichlorophenol contaminated with 2,3,7,8-tetrachlorodibenzo(p)dioxin (TCDD). This led to the recognition that various halo-aromatic hydrocarbons (HAH's) can interfere with heme bio-synthesis. This biochemical lesion is confined to the liver and has been reported only after exposure to HAH's which include in their effects induction of the hepatic polysubstrate monooxygenase systems utilizing cytochrome P-448 as terminal oxidase. A consequence of exposure to such compounds is a selective decrease in activity of uroporphyrinogen decarb-oxylase (UD) leading to impaired conversion of uroporphyrinogen to copro-porphyrinogen and a characteristic accumulation of porphyrins with 8-4 (COOH) groups. Studies using TCDD (which is a specific inducer of P-448) have shown that (a) interaction with a regulatory gene product leading to induction of P-448 is necessary for UD to be inhibited, (b) TCDD has no direct effect on UD, (c) non-heme iron, probably ferritin, is involved in this process and (d) the antioxidant butylated hydroxyanisole provides partial protection against UD inhibition. In general, protection against porphyria is associated with protection against histological damage to the liver. Probably these findings apply to all HAH's which induce P-448 and cause porphyria. Because the abnormal porphyrin excretion is character-istic, it may provide a useful basis to examine human populations for exposure to compounds of this type.

KEYWORDS

Haloaromatic hydrocarbons; porphyria; TCDD; 2,3,7,8-tetrachlorodibenzo(p)-dioxin; dioxin; iron; antioxidant; uroporphyrinogen decarboxylase.

INTRODUCTION

The term "porphyria" has been used loosely to include different disorders of

147

heme biosynthesis caused by a variety of toxic substances. However, this
Symposium has stressed the diverse manner in which toxins may interact with
heme biosynthesis to cause similarly diverse, albeit characteristic, alterations in the synthesis or degradation of heme. This paper will discuss
the porphyria caused by certain halo-aromatic hydrocarbons (HAH) including
2,3,7,8-tetrachlorodibenzo(p)dioxin (TCDD).

Names for disturbances of heme biosynthesis can be confusing; any condition
where the production of porphyrins is increased may be called a porphyria
(Meyer and Schmid, 1978) and various names refer to the condition with which
this paper is concerned. The term "porphyria cutanea tarda" (PCT) has been
widely used but (a) this implies a chronic disease of the skin which need
not accompany the biochemical lesion and (b) the same term (PCT) has been
used to describe inherited human disorders which have quite different biochemical findings. Doss (1971) has used a better term,"chronic hepatic
porphyria" with subtypes A-D to denote severity. The time has perhaps come,
however, to refer to the specific disturbances of hepatic heme biosynthesis
caused by HAH's as "acquired uroporphyrinogen decarboxylase (UD)[1] deficiency."
The evidence is now fairly strong that reduced activity of this enzyme is a
necessary condition for a characteristic pattern of porphyrins to occur in
liver, urine or feces. Further, it seems appropriate to avoid using the
name of a skin disease which may never manifest itself. In this paper, the
abnormality of heme biosynthesis caused in mammalian (not necessarily avian)
systems by exposure to HAH's will often be referred to as "porphyria" for
the sake of simplicity. However, the reader should recognize that this
refers specifically to the porphyria resulting from acquired UD deficiency.

As a consequence of reduced activity of uroporphyrinogen decarboxylase, the
urine contains highly carboxylated porphyrins, mostly $(COOH)_8$ and $(COOH)_7$,
and coproporphyrin, while the feces contain relatively greater quantities
of less polar porphyrins. These porphyrins are derived from porphyrinogen
intermediates by nonenzymatic oxidation. In man, an inherited predispo-
sition to this disease can exist with affected individuals showing reduction
of UD activity in red cell hemolysate (Benedetto and others, 1978;
de Verneuil and others, 1978). Alcohol, synthetic estrogens and industrial
exposure to chlorinated aromatic hydrocarbons are also accepted as causative
agents. Study in animals of a similar biochemical condition has led to
some clarification of possible pathogenetic mechanisms and at present it is
reasonable to associate the acquired enzyme defect with induction of hepatic
polysubstrate monooxygenase (PSMO) activity characteristic only of certain
HAH's. However, the exact mechanism underlying the decline in UD activity
remains unknown.

The importance of UD deficiency acquired as a consequence of exposure to
HAH's is thus twofold. First, clarification of the pathogenetic mechanism
will increase understanding of the toxicity of these significant industrial
and environmental poisons. Second, the disturbance of heme biosynthesis
is characteristic, and analysis of urine and/or feces may yet prove to be
the most sensitive way to screen populations for evidence of significant
exposure to toxins of this type.

---

[1]Uroporphyrinogen carboxy-lyase: EC 4.1.1.37

The object of this paper will be (a) to review the history leading to our current understanding of this problem, (b) to describe some recent studies which reflect on pathogenetic mechanisms, and (c) to consider the practical implications of current concepts for screening programs. The history of our present knowledge of this problem involves two separate threads: the first begins with an epidemic of cutaneous porphyria in Turkey and the second with the recognition of porphyria and chloracne affecting workers in a factory manufacturing trichlorophenol.

THE TURKISH EPIDEMIC AND HEXACHLOROBENZENE PORPHYRIA

Between 1956 and 1960 more than 4,000 Turkish peasants developed cutaneous porphyria because they ate foods made from wheat which had been treated with the fungicide hexachlorobenzene (HCB) (Cam and Nigogosyan, 1963; Schmid, 1960). Ockner and Schmid (1961) successfully reproduced this biochemical disorder by feeding male rats a diet containing 0.2% w/w HCB and thus provided an animal model for further study. There have been many subsequent contributors to our present understanding of this disorder and the disturbance of heme biosynthesis characteristic of HCB is partly explained by reference to Fig. 1. San Martin de Viale and others (1970) documented the pattern of highly carboxylated porphyrins excreted in urine of HCB-poisoned rats. Feces of such animals contain large amounts of less polar porphyrins including isocoproporphyrins (Elder, 1975), best explained by the action of coproporphyrinogen oxidase on $(COOH)_5$ porphyrinogen. This pattern of porphyrin overproduction may be attributed to decreased activity of UD, the enzyme catalysing the stepwise decarboxylation of uroporphyrinogen (Jackson and others, 1976) and decreased activity of UD in HCB porphyria was demonstrated by Taljaard and others (1972) and Elder (1977). The activity of δ-aminolevulinic acid synthase (ALA-S), the regulatory enzyme for heme biosynthesis (Fig. 1) need not be increased in HCB porphyria, nor is there evidence of defective hepatic hemoprotein synthesis when porphyria first appears during HCB treatment. San Martin de Viale and others (1970) stressed the similarity of porphyria in rats treated with HCB to the human disease seen in Turkey and also on sporadically occurring cases of porphyria cutanea tarda.

HCB porphyria develops over weeks or months; the strain of rat used (Smith, Cabral and De Matteis, 1979) affects the rate at which the metabolic lesion develops and female rats are more susceptible (San Martin de Viale and others, 1970). There is marked induction of hepatic microsomal cytochrome with hypertrophy of the smooth endoplasmic reticulum but cell necrosis is also a feature. The morphological changes are greatest in the centro-lobular region which is also where porphyrin fluorescence is maximal (Sweeney and others, 1971). Most studies of HCB-induced porphyria have used technical grade material which is extremely impure (Lui, Sampson and Sweeney, 1976). One sample was found to contain dioxin (Villaneuva and others, 1974). However, Goldstein and others (1978) have used purified material and established that HCB can cause porphyria in the absence of detectable contaminants. Finally, three lines of evidence suggested a close relationship between hepatic iron and HCB-porphyria. (a) In 1962, Ippen reported that repeated venesection improved human subjects with PCT, (b) in 1972 Taljaard and others reported that siderosis accelerated the appearance of porphyria in rats given HCB, and (c) Kushner, Steinmuller and Lee (1975), using an in vitro system, reported iron-dependent inhib-ition of UD activity.

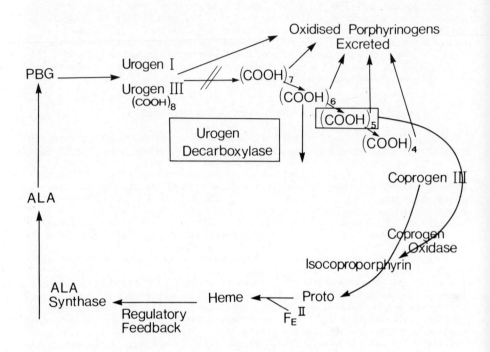

Fig. 1.   Features of heme biosynthesis of special relevance
          to PCT. δ-aminolevulinate (ALA) formation deter-
          mines flux through the pathway; this is regulated
          by ALA-synthase. 8-carboxyl uroporphyrinogen
          (UROGEN I, III) undergoes stepwise decarboxylation
          to 4-carboxyl coproporphyrinogen (COPRO III) which
          is further metabolized by coproporphyrinogen
          oxidase to protoporphyrin IX (PROTO). If 5, and
          possibly 6, carboxyl porphyrinogens accumulate,
          coprogen oxidase may catalyse sidechain modifica-
          tions. Isocoproporphyrins arise in this way (Elder,
          1975). Incorporation of iron into PROTO forms heme
          which, in various ways, regulates the activity of
          ALA-synthase.

PORPHYRIA DUE TO TCDD

The occurrence of PCT in a herbicide factory making trichlorophenol was noted
by Bleiberg and others (1964) and attributed to a contaminant arising during
the process.   Detailed analytical data is not available but animal studies
to be reviewed below make it reasonable to assume that the biochemical disturbance in these patients was comparable to that caused by HCB and was an
acquired deficiency of hepatic UD activity.   The possible contaminant in
trichlorophenol was identified as a chlorodioxin and having been involved
in the follow-up study of Bleiberg's patients, Poland and others (1971)

commenced a thorough study of the toxicity of 2,3,7,8-tetrachlorodibenzo(p)-
dioxin (TCDD). This chlorinated aromatic cyclic ether is formed when
trichlorophenol (TCP) is heated with sodium hydroxide; the reaction leading
to TCDD is exothermic, tends to get out of control and has led to many
serious industrial accidents in which humans have received significant
exposure (Hay, 1979).

Reviewing studies up to 1975, Poland and Kende (1976) focussed attention on
the extreme potency of TCDD.   Using the cultured chick embryo system they
had shown that TCDD induced ALA-S and the PSMO-activity, aryl hydrocarbon
hydroxylase (AHH).   As an inducer of PSMO activity, TCDD resembled 3-
methylcholanthrene (3MC) rather than phenobarbital (PB) inducing the cytochrome referred to as P-448 (see Nebert and others, 1981) as terminal
oxygenase.   Poland argued that this sensitive biological response should
be associated with a high affinity receptor site within the cell in order
for TCDD to be active at such low concentrations (ED_{50} for AHH induction
$\sim 1 \times 10^{-9}$ mole/kg).   Highly labeled ^{3}H-TCDD was prepared, and using
methodology similar to that used to demonstrate receptors for steroid
hormones, a high affinity binding site was defined in the cytosol of mouse
liver with a K_d of 10^{-12} M (Poland, Glover and Kende, 1976).

It was known that inbred strains of mice could be categorized as "AHH-
responsive" or "AHH-nonresponsive" depending upon whether treatment with
3MC would induce AHH activity.   Poland and Glover (1974) showed that TCDD
was sufficiently potent to induce this activity maximally even in the so-
called nonresponsive strains which lacked the high affinity binding site
but appeared to possess a binding site with lower affinity for TCDD (Poland,
Glover and Kende, 1976).   The nature of the site which binds TCDD and
permits induction to be expressed in "nonresponsive" mice remains controversial as Okey and others (1979) have failed to find evidence for specific
cytosol binding of TCDD in these animals.

Investigating the association between exposure to TCDD in TCP factories and
the occurrence of porphyria cutanea tarda (PCT), Goldstein and others (1973)
gave 25 µg/kg of TCDD to a responsive strain of mice and noted the development of hepatic porphyria.   They also noted in these experiments that the
porphyria could not be dissociated from histologically proven damage to the
liver.   In an ongoing study of the pathogenesis of porphyria caused by
HAH's we turned our attention from HCB to TCDD for a number of reasons.
First, we found it difficult to purify HCB and could not distinguish its
effects from the possible effects of many trace impurities (Lui, Sampson
and Sweeney, 1976).   Second, we had found HCB to be extensively metabolized
(Koss, Koransky and Steinbach, 1979; Lui, Sampson and Sweeney, 1976) with
the possibility that its effects could be due to reactive metabolites.
Finally, we recognized that all haloaromatic hydrocarbons known to cause
porphyria induced P-448, or were mixed inducers which exhibited the inducing
effects of both 3MC (P-448) and PB (P-450): it seemed probable that
induction of the PSMO systems with P-448 as terminal oxidase might be a
necessary condition for porphyria.   Poland's studies on the interactions
between TCDD and living systems encouraged us to use the properties of this
toxin for further exploration of the pathogenesis of acquired UD deficiency.

STUDIES ON THE MECHANISMS OF PORPHYRIA DUE TO TCDD

The first question we addressed was whether susceptibility to porphyria
would show the same inheritance as AHH-responsiveness in inbred strains of
mice.   We administered 25 µg/kg TCDD weekly to C57Bl/6J (AHH-responsive,

Ah/Ah), DBA/2J (AHH-nonresponsive, ah/ah), and measured the total urinary
excretion of porphyrins by each group of mice weekly. A clear-cut result
was obtained: nonresponsive animals did not develop porphyria whereas
animals possessing the Ah-gene did (Fig. 2A). We measured the activity
of UD in cytosol derived from mice used in this experiment and found a
significant decrease in UD-activity in AHH-responsive mice (C57Bl/6J) but
no decrease in AHH nonresponsive (DBA/2J) mice treated with TCDD. Next
we obtained progeny of a backcross between DBA/2J mice and the offspring
of a C57 x DBA cross. These animals would be either homozygous nonresponsive (ah/ah), or heterozygous (Ah/ah). After phenotyping we tested
groups of these mice for susceptibility to porphyria and found the Ah/ah
animals to be susceptible without any clear difference between these hetero-
zygotes and homozygous (Ah/Ah) C57Bl/6J mice tested previously (Jones and
Sweeney, 1980). We concluded that susceptibility to porphyria was
inherited with AHH-responsiveness and that susceptibility behaved as a
dominant character. Further, this experiment demonstrated that TCDD had
no direct effect on UD activity but that some product of the AHH-regulatory
gene was required for TCDD to produce porphyria. At the doses of TCDD
used, no difference was demonstrated among the various strains in the
extent to which PSMO activity was induced, so the basis for the difference
is not clear at this time. In keeping with the earlier observation of
Goldstein and others (1973), that porphyria and histological damage due to
HAH's were not separable, we noted that the histologic changes in the
livers of responsive mice were marked whereas the livers of nonresponsive
mice (DBA/2J) remained relatively normal despite 25 µg/kg weekly of TCDD.

In order to clarify the role of iron in the response to TCDD we prepared a
group of iron-deficient C57Bl/6J mice by repeated venesections while the
animals were fed a casein-based, low iron diet. The same dose of TCDD was
then administered as in the preceding experiment examining the role of AHH
responsiveness. Again a clear-cut result was obtained: iron-deficient
animals did not develop porphyria whereas animals eating regular laboratory
chow did (Sweeney and others, 1979). A legitimate criticism of this work
drew attention to the different diets consumed by the low iron and normal
iron animals. This work has been repeated using appropriately controlled
diets and with essentially similar results; we have repeatedly confirmed
that iron-deficient animals are protected against porphyria due to TCDD.
Further, in iron-deficient animals the activity of UD remains unaltered
during treatment with TCDD whereas in the animals which have not been
venesected or which have been venesected but have received supplementary
iron (Jones, Cole and Sweeney, in press) porphyria has occurred and the
activity of UD has been reduced. A comparison of urine porphyrin
excretion in iron-deficient and iron replete mice treated with TCDD is
shown in Fig. 2(B).

While urine porphyrin excretion provides a convenient quantitative endpoint
for these experiments, it has been less easy to compare histological changes
in low iron and normal iron animals. While considerable protection against
histological damage due to TCDD can be obtained with an iron-deficient state,
the protection is incomplete. A series of experiments was also performed
in groups of mice which had not been rendered iron deficient but which were
maintained on casein-based low-iron diet supplemented with varying amounts
of iron; subgroups of the groups fed different levels of iron received
varying doses of TCDD from 0.25 to 100 µg/kg/week. The results of this
experiment (Jones, Cole and Sweeney, in press) showed in general that
synergism exists between the amount of iron in the diet and the dose of
TCDD. This finding is in keeping with the finding (Taljaard and others,
1972) that siderosis predisposes to porphyria in rats fed HCB.

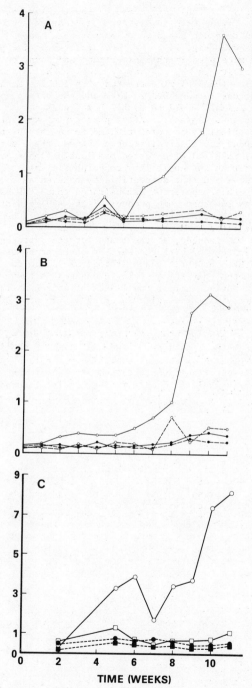

μg URINE PORPHYRIN/24 HOURS/MOUSE

TIME (WEEKS)

Fig. 2 (A-C).

Each of figures 2 A to C
show the total daily urine
porphyrin output of mice
studied in groups (n ≥ 6).
Measurements were made
weekly for 11 weeks and
porphyrin was measured by
first derivative spectro-
photometry (Jones & Sweeney,
1976).

(A) o—o C57Bl/6J and o--o
    DBA/2J mice treated
    with TCDD (25 µg/kg/wk).
    ●—● C57, and ●--●, DBA
    control groups treated
    with vehicle alone.

(B) Four groups of C57Bl/6J
    mice were fed regular
    laboratory chow (normal
    iron) or were made iron-
    deficient by repeated
    venesections combined
    with a casein-based low
    iron diet (low iron),
    o—o normal iron, and
    o--o low iron mice
    treated with TCDD (25
    µg/kg/wk). ●—● normal
    iron and ●--● low iron
    control groups.

(C) Four groups of C57Bl/6J
    mice were fed powdered
    laboratory chow with,
    or without 0.75% w/w
    of butylated hydroxy-
    anisole (BHA) added.
    o—o TCDD treated with-
    out BHA and □---□
    TCDD treated with BHA.
    ●--● BHA alone, and
    ■--■, no treatment.
    The dose of TCDD was
    10 µg/kg initially,
    followed by 2.5 µg/kg/wk.

The mechanisms whereby iron is synergistic remains unclear. From extensive measurements of the concentration of microsomal cytochrome in low iron
and normal iron animals and in the activity of the associated PSMO systems,
we have not found evidence that the protective effect of a low iron state
may be due to failure to induce microsomal cytochrome. We feel therefore
that the evidence suggests that it is storage iron not heme which is
necessary for the toxicity of TCDD and related compounds to be expressed.
We have postulated that the iron may be involved in a free radical mechanism
possibly leading to the formation of hydroxyl free radical formed by ferrous
iron interacting with hydrogen peroxide. This reaction would then initiate
lipid peroxidation.

To obtain evidence supporting lipid peroxidation as a mechanism involved in
the toxicity of TCDD and production of porphyria, we fed mice a diet with
or without 0.75% butylated hydroxyanisole (BHA). The mice were treated
initially with 10 μg/kg TCDD at weekly intervals and urine porphyrin was
measured as in the previous experiments. The antioxidant supplement to
the diet prevented the onset of porphyria during the duration of these
experiments (Fig. 2(C)) supporting the suggestion based on the role of iron
that lipid peroxidation or a related free radical mechanism is involved.
Further, BHA added to the diet provided considerable protection against
histologic damage occurring under these circumstances, particularly the
extent to which neutral fat accumulated when animals were sacrificed 3 weeks
after initiating treatment with TCDD.

The foregoing experiments demonstrate the importance of a product of the
Ah-gene locus in liver toxicity due to TCDD. We have shown that the toxic
process requires iron and that it is unlikely that this is heme iron.
Considerable protection against this process is afforded by incorporation
of the antioxidant BHA in the diet. Vitamin E at a dosage level of 0.01%
in the diet was without effect.

STUDIES OF PORPHYRIN METABOLISM: PREDICTION OF HEPATOTOXICITY

An important question is the extent to which the foregoing observations made
using TCDD are transferable to other substances. Goldstein and others
(1975) showed that the commercial polychlorinated biphenyls (PCB's; Aroclors
1242 and 1016) would cause porphyria in rodents; 1242 was more potent.
Subsequently, this laboratory (Goldstein and others, 1976) tested a series
of specially synthesized pure hexachlorobiphenyls and showed that those
isomers which were predicted to be 3MC-type inducers, according to rules
established by Poland and Glover (1977) were also toxic, and produced
porphyria. Studies with HCB, TCDD and PCB's suggest that two generaliza-
tions may be valid: first, that any HAH which interacts strongly enough
with the Ah-gene regulatory product (the TCDD receptor) will induce P-448-
dependent PSMO activity and second, that these compounds are also able to
cause porphyria and are hepatotoxic to rats, mice and humans.

Poland, Glover and Kende (1976) first defined structure-activity requirements for isomeric dioxins by measuring their potency as inducers of AHH
and affinity for the TCDD binding protein; they extended this concept to
certain PCB's, to azoxybenzenes and to chlorinated biphenylenes to conclude
that any planar molecule roughly 3 x 10 Å and halogenated at sites corresp--
onding to the corners of this rectangle, would interact with the TCDD
receptor. Parkinson, Cockerline and Safe (1979) described more limited
rules for PCB's: both *para* positions, a minimum of two *meta* positions, and
not more than one *ortho* position must be chlorinated for significant

induction of the 3MC type to occur. (No satisfactory rules exist to define
PB-type induction and additional patterns of induction have been reported
(Dent and others, 1978)).   If, indeed, histological damage to the liver
and acquired UD deficiency are not separable, these structure/activity
rules may define a very large number of hepatotoxic HAH's with effects
which could be screened for because of an effect on heme biosynthesis.

Some comment is necessary concerning the extensive data available regarding
accumulation of porphyrins in cultured avian liver, or liver cells.   The
studies of Poland and Glover previously cited in which induction of ALA-S,
or AHH were the chosen endpoints emphasized the great value of this system
in studies of structure-activity relationships. The work of various groups
(Debets and others, 1981; Kawanishi, Mizutani and Sano, 1978; Sinclair and
Granick, 1974) have demonstrated that HAH's alter porphyrin accumulation in
these in vitro systems.   However, this paper is concerned with a specific
porphyria in which decreased UD activity is associated with accumulation of
porphyrins of which $(COOH)_8$-, $(COOH)_7$-, $(COOH)_5$- and porphyrins and isocoproporphyrin (Fig. 1) are most characteristic.   This author is not yet
convinced that porphyrin accumulation in chick embryo liver systems meet
the same criteria specified above for mammalian systems. The chick
embryonic liver system tends to accumulate porphyrin in response to exposure
to a large number of foreign chemicals and xenobiotics which need not be
toxic to mammals and it is essential to distinguish this response from the
specific biochemical defect caused in intact animals by HAH's.

POPULATION SCREENING

The epidemic of porphyria in Turkey focussed attention on human intoxication
with HCB.   There have been many industrial accidents leading to exposure of
workers to TCDD (Hay, 1979), but porphyria as an overt medical problem has
only occasionally been encountered. Porphyria has so far not been reported
as a feature of the well-documented hepatotoxicity of PCB's in the Japanese
"Yusho" epidemic (Kuratsune and others, 1972).   Neither has significant
increase in porphyria been reported following the Seveso accident in 1976
involving TCDD (Pocchiari, Silano and Zampieri, 1979).   In contrast, chloracne which is probably also a specific consequence of a toxin interacting
with the Ah-gene product in skin, was reported in each of these situations.
However, an important report from Strik and others (1979) described studies
of porphyrin excretion in residents of Michigan whose tissues contained
residues of polybrominated biphenyls (PBB's).   This group was compared with
a control group of Wisconsin residents who had not been exposed to PBB's.
Total porphyrin measurements using an ion exchange method did not show a
significant difference between the two groups.   However, when esterified
urine porphyrins were examined by quantitative thin layer chromatographs,
47% of Michigan subjects, but only 8% of Wisconsin subjects showed $(COOH)_7$
> $(COOH)_5$.   This abnormal ratio could have reflected reduced hepatic UD
activity in the PBB- exposed group.   It is a common experience that when
HAH's are used to produce porphyria in laboratory animals, hepatic porphyrin
content initially increases faster than urine porphyrin and that the hepatic
porphyrin consists of the highly carboxylated products which are normally
present only as trace amounts in the urine.   Screening for this abnormality
would therefore require that $(COOH)_7$, and perhaps $(COOH)_8$, porphyrins be
separately identified.   The sensitive and rapid screening test available
for total urine porphyrins (Jones and Sweeney, 1979) indicates roughly
whether copro- or uro-porphyrin predominates but could overlook a significant increase if this affected only the $(COOH)_7$ porphyrin.   Quantitative
thin layer chromatography is tedious; recent methods using HPLC (e.g. Hill,

Sirmans and Needham, 1980) to quantify each porphyrin present in urine may
be applicable to mass screenings when confidence limits for normality have
been adequately defined. Elder (1975) reported that the ratio of isocoproporphyrin to coproporphyrin in feces served to distinguish patients with
PCT of the type associated with decreased UD activity from other types of
porphyria. Possibly absolute levels of fecal isocoproporphyrins might be
useful in screening patients for acquired UD deficiency but with presently
available methodology this appears unlikely because of the tedious sample
preparation required.

In summarizing the effects of HAH on heme biosynthesis it has been possible
to record significant advances in knowledge, but equally significant
questions remain unanswered. Various HAH's induce various patterns of
PSMO activity, such induction is associated with large increases in ALA-S
in avian systems, but not in mammalian systems; the reason for this
difference is unknown. Those HAH's with structures which, by virtue of
partially defined structure activity relations, bind to the "TCDD receptor"
and cause PSMO induction of the 3MC type, will cause an acquired UD
deficiency and are hepatotoxic. However, it is not known whether 3MC
itself will cause porphyria. Further, these statements rely excessively
on data from rats and mice and application to man must remain an open
question. Considerable evidence now points to a role for iron in hepatotoxicity due to TCDD and HCB; does this apply to all HAH's binding to the
TCDD receptor and what are the implications for dietary iron intake in
human populations exposed to HAH's? Do significant sex differences exist
in susceptibility to HAH's? Female rats are more susceptible than male
rats to HCB; is this because the male degrades the toxin faster, or for
more fundamental reasons? Finally, what is the value of our detailed
knowledge of disturbed heme biosynthesis in designing screening programs
for human population groups which have been exposed to HAH's?

ACKNOWLEDGEMENT

Supported by the Medical Research Council of Canada.

REFERENCES

Benedetto, A. V., Kushner, J. P. and Taylor, J. S. (1978). Porphyria
    cutanea tarda in three generations of a single family. New Engl. J. Med.,
    298, 358-362.
Bleiberg, J., Wallen, M., Brodkin, R. and Applebaum, I. L. (1964). Indust-
    rially acquired porphyria. Arch. Dermatol., 89, 793-797.
Cam, C. and Nigogosyan, G. (1963). Acquired toxic porphyria cutanea tarda
    due to hexachlorobenzene. J. Amer. Med. Assoc., 18, 88-91.
Debets, F. M. H., Reinders, J. H., Debets, A. J. M., Lossbröek, T. C. and
    Strik, J. J. T. W. A. (1981). Biotransformation and porphyrinogenic
    action of hexachlorobenzene and its metabolites in a primary liver cell
    culture. Toxicology (in press).
Dent, J. G., Elcombe, C. R., Netter, K. J. and Gibson, J. E. (1978). Rat
    hepatic microsomal cytochrome P-450 induced by polybrominated biphenyls.
    Drug Metab. & Disp., 6, 96-101.
De Verneuil, H., Nordmann, Y., Phung, N., Grandchamp, B., Aitken, G.,
    Grelier, M. and Noire, J. (1978). Familial and sporadic porphyria cuta-
    nea: two different diseases. Int. J. Biochem., 9, 927-931.
Doss, M. (1971). Suggested pathobiochemical development of chronic hepatic
    porphyrias. Klin. Wschr., 49, 941-942.

Elder, G. H. (1975). Differentiation of porphyria cutanea tarda symptomatica from other types of porphyria by measurement of isocoproporphyrin in faeces. J. Clin. Pathol., 28, 601-607.

Elder, G. H. (1977). Porphyrin metabolism in porphyria cutanea tarda. Seminars in Hematol., 14, 227-242.

Goldstein, J. A., Hickman, P., Bergman, H. and Vos, J. G. (1973). Hepatic porphyria induced by 2,3,7,8-tetrachlorodibenzo-p-dioxin in the mouse. Res. Commun. in Chem. Pathol. & Pharmacol., 6, 919-928.

Goldstein, J. A., Hickman, P., Burse, V. W. and Bergman, H. (1975). A comparative study of two polychlorinated biphenyl mixtures (Aroclors 1242 and 1016) containing 42% chlorine on induction of hepatic porphyria and drug metabolizing enzymes. Toxicol. & Appl. Pharmacol. 32, 461-473.

Goldstein, J. A., McKinney, J. D., Lucier, G. W., Hickman, P., Bergman, H. and Moore, J. A. (1976). Toxicological assessment of hexachlorobiphenyl-isomers and 2,3,7,8-tetrachlorodibenzofuran in chicks. II. Effects on drug metabolism and porphyrin accumulation. Toxicol. & Appl. Pharm., 36, 81-92.

Goldstein, J. A., Friesen, M., Scott, T. M., Hickman, P., Hass, J. R. and Bergman, H. (1978). Assessment of the contribution of chlorinated dibenzo-p-dioxins and dibenzofurans to hexachlorobenzene-induced toxicity, porphyria, changes in mixed function oxygenases, and histopathological changes. Toxicol. & Appl. Pharm., 46, 633-649.

Hay, A. (1979). Accidents in trichlorophenol plants: a need for realistic surveys to ascertain risks to health. Ann. N. Y. Acad. Sci., 320, 321-324.

Hill, R. H., Sirmans, S. L. and Needham, L. L. A rapid isocratic HPLC procedure for the determination of urinary porphyrins. J. High Res. Chromat. & Chromat. Commun., 3: 588.

Ippen, H. (1962). Porphyrin metabolism in porphyria cutanea tarda. Panmin. Med., 4, 381-382.

Jackson, A. H., Sancovich, H. A., Ferramola, A. M., Evans, N., Games, D. E., Matlin, S. A., Elder, G. H. and Smith, S. G. (1976). Macrocyclic intermediates in the biosynthesis of porphyrins. Phil. Trans. R. Soc. Lond. B., 273, 191-206.

Jones, K. G. and Sweeney, G. D. (1976). Measurement of urine porphyrins and porphyrinogens. Biochem. Med., 15, 223-232.

Jones, K. G. and Sweeney, G. D. (1979). Quantitation of urinary porphyrins by use of second-derivative spectroscopy. Clin. Chem., 25, 71-74.

Jones, K. G. and Sweeney, G. D. (1980). Dependence of the porphyrinogenic effect of 2,3,7,8-tetrachlorodibenzo(p)dioxin upon inheritance of aryl hydrocarbon hydroxylase responsiveness. Toxicol. & Appl. Pharm.,53, 42-49.

Jones, K. G., Cole, F. M. and Sweeney, G. D. (1981). The role of iron in the toxicity of 2,3,7,8-tetrachlorodibenzo-(p)-dioxin (TCDD). Toxicol. & Appl. Pharm. (in press).

Kawanishi, S., Mizuntani, T. and Sano, S. (1978). Induction of porphyrin synthesis in chick embryo liver cell cultured by synthetic polychloro-biphenyl isomers. Biochem. Biophys. Acta, 540, 83-92.

Koss, G., Koransky, W. and Steinbach, K. (1979). Studies on the toxicology of hexachlorobenzene. IV. Sulphur-containing metabolites. Arch. Toxicol. 42, 19-31.

Kuratsune, M., Yoshimura, T., Matsuzaka, J. and Yamaguchi, A. (1972). Epidemiologic study on Yusho, a poisoning caused by ingestion of rice oil contaminated with a commercial branch of polychlorinated biphenyls. Exp. Health Perspec., 1, 119-128.

Kushner, J. P., Steinmuller, D. P. and Lee, G. R. (1975). The role of iron in the pathogenesis of porphyria cutanea tarda. II. Inhibition of uro-porphyrinogen decarboxylase. J. Clin. Invest., 56, 661-667.

Lui, H., Sampson, R. and Sweeney, G. D. (1976). In M. Doss (Ed.), Porphyrins in Human Diseases, S. Karger, Basel, pp. 405-413.

158   G. D. Sweeney

Meyer, U. A. and Schmid, R. (1978). In J. B. Stanbury, J. B. Wyngaarden and
   D. S. Fredrickson (Eds.), The Metabolic Basis of Inherited Disease, 4th
   ed. McGraw Hill Book Co., New York, Chap. 50, pp. 1166-1220.
Nebert, D. W., Eisen, H. J., Negishi, M., Lang, M. A. and Hjelmeland, L. M.
   (1981). Genetic mechanisms controlling the induction of polysubstrate
   monooxygenase (P-450) activities. Ann. Rev. Pharmacol. Toxicol., 21, 431-
   462.
Ockner, R. K. and Schmid, R. (1961). Acquired porphyria in man and rat due
   to hexachlorobenzene intoxication. Nature, 189, 499.
Okey, A. B., Bondy, G. P., Mason, M. E., Kahl, G. F., Eisen, H. J.,
   Guenthner, T. M. and Nebert, D. W. (1979). Regulatory gene product of the
   Ah locus. J. Biol. Chem., 254, 11636-11648.
Parkinson, A., Cockerline, R. and Safe, S. (1980). Polychlorinated biphenyl
   isomers and congeners as inducers of both 3-methylcholanthrene and
   phenobarbitone-type microsomal enzyme activity. Chem.-Biol. Interact.,
   29, 277.
Pocchiari, F., Silano, V. and Zampieri, A. (1979). Human health effects from
   accidental release of tetrachlorodibenzo-p-dioxin (TCDD) in Seveso, Italy.
   Ann. N. Y. Acad. Sci., 77, 311-320.
Poland, A., Smith, D., Metter, G. and Possick, P. (1971). A health survey of
   workers in a 2,4D and 2,4,5,T plant. Arch. Environ. Health, 22, 316-327.
Poland, A. and Glover, E. (1974). Induction of monooxygenase activities and
   cytochrome P_1-450 formation by 2,3,7,8-tetrachlorodibenzo-p-dioxin in
   mice genetically "nonresponsive" to other aromatic hydrocarbons. J. Biol.
   Chem., 249, 5599-5606.
Poland, A. and Kende, A. (1976). 2,3,7,8-tetrachlorodibenzo-p-dioxin:
   environmental contaminant and molecular probe. Fed. Proc., 35, 2404-2411.
Poland, A., Glover, E. and Kende, A. S. (1976). Stereospecific, high affin-
   ity binding of 2,3,7,8-tetrachlorodibenzo-p-dioxin by hepatic cytosol.
   Evidence that the binding species is receptor for induction of aryl hydro-
   carbon hydroxylase. J. Biol. Chem., 251, 4936-4946.
Poland, A. and Glover, E. (1977). Chlorinated biphenyl induction of aryl
   hydrocarbon hydroxylase activity: a study of the structure-activity
   relationship. Mol. Pharmacol., 13, 924-938.
San Martin de Viale, L. C., Viale, A. A., Nacht, S. and Grinstein, M. (1970).
   Experimental porphyria induced in rats by hexachlorobenzene. Clin. Chim.
   Acta, 28, 13-23.
Schmid, R. (1960). Cutaneous porphyria in Turkey. New Engl. J. Med., 263,
   397-398.
Sinclair, P. R. and Granick, S. (1974). Uroporphyrin formation induced by
   chlorinated hydrocarbons (lindane, polychlorinated biphenyls, tetra-
   chlorodibenzo-p-dioxin). Requirements for endogenous iron, protein
   synthesis and drug-metabolizing activity. Biochim. Biophys. Res. Commun.,
   61, 124-133.
Smith, A. G., Cabral, J. R. P. and De Matteis, F. (1979). A difference
   between two strains of rats in their liver non-haem iron content and in
   their response to the porphyrogenic effect of hexachlorobenzene. Chem.
   -Biol. Interact., 27, 353-363.
Strik, J. J. T. W. A., Doss, M., Schraa, G., Robertson, L. W. von Tiepermann,
   R. and Harmsen, E. G. M. (1979). In J. J. T. W. A. Strik and J. H. Koeman,
   (Eds.), Chemical Porphyria in Man, Elsevier-North Holland Biomedical
   Press, pp. 29-53.
Sweeney, G. D., Janigan, D., Mayman, D. and Lai, H. (1971). The experimental
   porphyrias - a group of distinctive metabolic lesions. S. Afr. Med. J.,
   45, 68-72.
Sweeney, G. D., Jones, K. G., Cole, F. M., Basford, D. and Krestynski, F.
   (1979). Iron deficiency prevents liver toxicity of 2,3,7,8-tetrachloro-
   dibenzo(p)-dioxin (TCDD). Science, 204, 332-335.

Taljaard, J. J. F., Shanley, B. C., Deppe, W. M. and Joubert, S. M. (1972). Porphyrin metabolism in experimental hepatic siderosis in the rat. II. Combined effect of iron overload and hexachlorobenzene. Brit. J. Hematol., 23, 513-519.

Villaneuva, E. C., Jennings, R. W., Burse, V. W. and Kimbrough, R. D. (1974). Evidence of chlorodibenzo-p-dioxin and chlorodibenzofuran in hexachlorobenzene. J. Agr. Food Chem. 22, 916-917.

SYMPOSIUM

Delayed Toxic Effects of Pre- and Perinatal Drug Exposure

Chairmen: T. Balazs, B. I. Lyubimov

An Overview on Delayed Toxic Effects of Pre- and Perinatal Drug Exposure

T. Balazs

Bureau of Drugs, Division of Drug Biology, Food and Drug
Administration, Washington, D.C., USA

ABSTRACT

Pre- or perinatal exposure to certain drugs, primarily those which act on
the central nervous system or endocrine glands, can produce permanent
functional changes that are expressed only late in postnatal
development. Delayed effects may occur in any organ system because of
slowly developing degenerative or proliferative changes. Pre- or
neonatally acquired chemically induced changes can affect the next
generation via alteration in DNA or in other hitherto unknown ways.

KEYWORDS

Delayed toxicity; prenatal-perinatal drug exposure; functional changes;
delayed degenerative changes; proliferative changes; delayed CNS effects;
delayed autonomic effects; neuroendocrine effects; cross-generational
effects.

INTRODUCTION

The delayed effects of pre- and perinatal administration of drugs are
those that cannot be detected at birth or at the end of the treatment
period; they become evident later. These effects include functional,
pathophysiological, and structural degenerative or proliferative
changes. Functional changes are attributable to an interference with the
development of an anatomically normally formed system whose function is
expressed late postnatally. Slowly developing chronic pathological
changes may reach the level of clinical detectability at times far
removed from the exposure to the drug. Similarly, in utero-acquired
genetic changes may not be detected until adulthood or until the
subsequent generation. Some of the delayed functional changes and most
of the chronic pathological changes persist throughout the lifetime.

Teratologic effects develop during organogenesis, but delayed effects
develop in late pregnancy and the perinatal period, during maturation of
the organ systems. The nursing newborn is exposed through the mother's

163

milk to highly lipophilic xenobiotics that are very slowly eliminated.
The neonate is most vulnerable to certain effects of drugs. Therefore
examples of delayed effects that appear after solely neonatal
administration of drugs to experimental animals are included in this
review, although, in some of these examples, late effects were already
apparent at the end of long-term treatment.

The problem of delayed effects has seldom been considered in the context
of preclinical safety studies, with the possible exception of behavioral
teratology and transplacental carcinogenesis. Information on the subject
is given to provide background for planning studies of preclinical
toxicology of new therapeutic agents to be used perinatally.

Delayed Central Nervous System Effects

Maturation of the central nervous system (CNS) occurs both pre- and
postnatally, over a long period of time. The susceptibility of the
system to drugs increases with development of the components of specific
neurotransmission (Shoemaker, 1980). In experimental animals, impaired
development of the arousal processes, delay in the appearance of the
inhibitory system and altered pharmacological effects of CNS-active drugs
have been observed in the progeny of drug-treated dams.

Kellogg and associates (1980) reported that development of the arousal
processes was impaired in offspring of rats treated with diazepam (2.5 to
10 mg/kg, s.c.) from days 13 to 20 of their gestation. The progeny had
marked, dose-related alterations in their developmental pattern of
spontaneous motor activity and acoustic startle reflex. (The presence of
diazepam was not demonstrable in progeny after 2 days of age in these
experiments.) These findings indicated suppression of arousal during the
third postnatal week of the offspring. A withdrawal syndrome
characterized by sedation, hypotonia and sucking difficulties ("floppy
infant syndrome") in the neonates of benzodiazepine-treated mothers has
been described and may represent a clinical counterpart (Rementeria and
Bhatt, 1977).

Altered pharmacological responses were observed in the offspring of rats
treated orally with diazepam (10 mg/kg) from days 2 to 20 of pregnancy;
the offspring were fostered by non-treated dams. Onset of the convulsive
effects of isoniazid, picrotoxin, harmaline and caffeine was delayed up
to postnatal day 14. Administration of diazepam provided less protection
against the effects of these agents in the 9-day-old rats of
diazepam-treated dams than it did in appropriate controls (Massotti,
Alleva and Balazs, 1980a).

We have investigated some of the biochemical determinants of the
postnatal pharmacological changes in the offspring of diazepam-treated
rats (Massotti and co-workers, 1980b). The pregnant females received
large doses (100 mg/kg b.i.d., p.o.) of the drug from days 5 to 22 to
exaggerate the fetal effects. No differences were detected in the
postnatal development of [^{3}H]diazepam and [^{3}H]γ-aminobutyric acid
(GABA) GABA binding to brain plasma membranes in the offspring of treated
and control rats. To study the interaction between GABA and
benzodiazepine as a function of age and drug treatment, the effect of
muscimol, a GABA agonist which stimulates [^{3}H]diazepam binding, was
examined in cortical membranes of these rats. The capability of muscimol
to stimulate this binding was greatly reduced in the progeny of treated

rats. This finding can be interpreted as evidence of alteration in the coupling between the GABA and benzodiazepine receptors, and may explain some of the altered pharmacological effects observed in the progeny of drug-treated dams.

A delay in the maturation of an inhibitory system has been postulated to occur in the progeny of phenytoin-treated rats (Vernadakis and Woodbury, 1969). The anticonvulsant effect of phenytoin is correlated to the maturation of the inhibitory system by 17-21 days of age in the rat. However, the progeny of phenytoin-treated rats had a decreased electroshock seizure threshold and more severe seizures until they were 26 days of age.

Gallager and Mallorga (1980) showed that the anticonvulsant effects of phenytoin are associated with an increase in [^{3}H]diazepam binding in cerebral cortical membranes. In the membranes of 2- and 3-week-old rats exposed in utero to phenytoin (20 mg/kg daily from days 14 to 20), this binding was decreased compared with controls that received a single dose of phenytoin 1 hr before they were killed. The decreased binding was due to a decrease in the total number of binding sites and was transitory, since the 28- to 35-day-old offspring of treated mothers had values similar to those of the controls.

Adaptive changes develop in the mature organism during prolonged exposure to drugs. For example, receptor supersensitivity develops after withdrawal of neuroleptics, and is related to an increase in the number of dopaminergic receptors. In animals having this supersensitivity, a dopaminergic agonist elicits an accentuated response and a neuroleptic elicits an attenuated one. The opposite occurs in the progeny of neuroleptic-treated animals (Rosengarten and Friedhoff, 1979). Offspring of rats treated daily with haloperidol (2.5 mg/kg, i.p.) from days 4 to 20 of their pregnancy were tested for apomorphine-induced stereotypic behavior at about 1 month of age. They had significantly less activity than their controls. [^{3}H]Spiroperidol binding in the striatum was decreased, even when they were 2 months of age, compared with controls. Similarly, rats treated perinatally with haloperidol and tested as young adults had a decreased response to amphetamine and a more pronounced response to haloperidol when compared with their controls (Spear, Shalaby and Brick, 1980).

In contrast to the short duration in adult animals of dopaminergic supersensitivity, which develops after treatment with neuroleptics for several weeks, the dopaminergic subsensitivity described above was of long duration. This finding, as well as the delayed behavioral alterations (impaired conditioned avoidance) demonstrated by Ahlenius and co-workers (1973) in neonatally penfluoridol-treated rats, imply that these developmental changes are fundamentally different from those occurring in the neuroleptic-withdrawn adult.

Severe dysfunctions of the CNS in offspring have been attributed to maternal intake of narcotics and ethanol and subtle deleterious effects to various other CNS-active drugs. This topic is presented by Dr. B. Ljubimov.

The time immediately after birth is one of the most sensitive periods to the effects of CNS-active drugs. Dendritic proliferation and

myelinization occur perinatally in most mammals. Because of immaturity
of the excretory systems, the duration of drug effects is prolonged.

Delayed and long-lasting behavioral changes have been reported to develop
in children whose mothers received large doses of analgesics durings
labor. Meperidine is eliminated 2-7 times more slowly in the newborn
than in the mother (Morselli and Rovei, 1980) and can produce neonatal
depression. Brackbill and associates (1974) examined newborn children
whose mothers received meperidine (50 to 150 mg, i.m.) as a premedication
to epidural anesthesia of prilocaine and newborns of mothers who received
only prilocaine. They found no differences in values of the Apgar score,
a measure of viability. The neonatal behavioral assessment scale of
Brazelton was used to analyze the early behavior (mean age, 28.4 hr).
Examination of the habituation rate to repeated sensory stimuli (mean
age, 32.5 or 48 hr) revealed impairment in the newborn of
meperidine-treated mothers. A significant correlation was found between
meperidine dosage and the overall score of this test.

Woodson and daCosta-Woodson (1980) compared the effects of 100 mg
meperidine and 25 mg promazine with no analgesic; their data were
consistent with those of Brackbill and co-workers (at 22 hr) on the
Brazelton scale. However, the combined influence of the other variables
(maternal, labor and infant) was comparable to that of analgesia.
Tronick and associates (1976) demonstrated that effects on behavior of
newborns were minimal and transitory when analgesics (alphaprodine and/or
promazine) and lidocaine alone or in combination were given in carefully
controlled doses.

The possible long-term consequences of obstetrical drugs on the
psychophysiological development of children have been investigated by
Broman and Brackbill (1980). They followed the late effects of
obstetrical medication on physical and cognitive development through age
7 in 1,944 children born to mothers having uncomplicated pregnancies.
Inhalation anesthetics and six other obstetrical drugs were evaluated,
and periodic pediatric, neurologic and psychometric examinations were
performed. The results suggested that inhalant anesthetics were
associated with deficits in psychomotor and neuromotor functioning in the
first year and that oxytocin was associated with psychomotor deficit.
Children of mothers given scopolamine had slightly lower scores on some
cognitive tasks and children of those given oxytocin had lower
achievement test scores. The inhalant anesthetics scopolamine and
secobarbital were associated with palpable liver at 4 months of age.
These data are of great significance, provided the effects of other
variables (maternal, labor, infant, etc.) are separated from those of the
drugs.

Van den Berg and associates (1980) carried out a prospective
epidemiological study on the late effects of inhalation agents (trilene,
nitrous oxide), narcotics (meperidine and alphaprodine) and local
anesthetics. The cognitive development of 4,000 children was examined at
age 5 and at age 9 to 11. Preliminary data revealed no distinguishable
effects. Although data of this study do not substantiate those of Broman
and Brackbill (1980), they may not contradict them, considering the
possible differences in both the drugs used and the psychological tests.

Delayed Effects in the Autonomic Nervous System

Since the functional differentiation of the autonomic nerves is influenced by signals from the tissue to be innervated, drugs acting prenatally on autonomic receptors may affect this event.

Albino rats were treated s.c. with atropine sulfate at 0.1 or 0.5 mg/kg/day from 11 to 18 days of pregnancy (Gruenfeld and Balazs, 1980), and their progeny were cross-fostered. Bradycardia and an enhanced negative chronotropic response to an s.c. injection of 40 mg pilocarpine/kg were detected in the dam for about 1 week after the end of treatment; these findings are consistent with the development of receptor supersensitivity. In the progeny, tachycardia lasting for 2 weeks and mydriasis lasting for a week after eye opening were seen. Sensitivity to pilocarpine was not altered. This finding is consistent with the presence of an adrenergic preponderance and may represent a developmental effect.

A gradually developing systemic hypertension was observed by Grollman and Grollman (1962) in the offspring of rats treated with adrenal corticosteroids, progesterone, chlorothiazide, or low potassium or high sodium diets. Hypertension developed at about 1 year of age. Hypertension did not develop when treatments with the drug or diet were terminated about midway through the pregnancy, even if they were initiated before conception. Cardiac left ventricular hypertrophy and a moderate thickening of the walls in the arterioles were the major postmortem findings.

A recent investigation by Kimmel and Buelke Sam (1981) of sodium salicylate in rats showed the development of hypertension. Sodium salicylate was given orally to rats on days 8 to 10 of pregnancy in doses of 125 or 175 mg/kg. At 4 months of age, indirect systolic blood pressure was increased in female progeny at both dose levels and in male progeny at the high dose level. Norepinephrine challenge during anesthesia in these rats produced a greater response in both systolic and diastolic pressures than in controls. Increased spontaneous motor activity was associated with this condition.

Levin and associates (1978) showed that maternal ingestion of salicylates or indomethacin increased in the offspring the ratio of pulmonary arterial medial width to external diameter because of the increased muscular layer. This change was attributed to the effect of these drugs on prostaglandin synthesis. Csaba and co-workers (1978) reported that several cases of pulmonary hypertension have occurred in newborn children whose mothers received indomethacin as a tocolytic for the maintenance of their pregnancy. Another tocolytic agent, fenoterol, which is a β_2-adrenergic agonist, has been implicated in cardiac abnormalities of newborn children (Vogt, Schmidt-Redemann and Urbanek, 1979). Certain functional disturbances, including arrhythmia, lasted for 3 weeks postnatally. Since this drug is lipophilic and reaches the fetus in sufficient concentration to produce tachycardia, it may provoke perturbation in the developing heart, which is overly sensitive to adrenergic amines. A role of excessive prenatal adrenergic stimulation in the pathogenesis of hypertrophic cardiomyopathy has been speculated (Perloff, 1981).

Large doses of epinephrine hydrochloride (1.5 mg/kg) given i.p. to
pregnant rats during days 6 to 9 of pregnancy (organogenesis) increased
the susceptibility of the offspring to restraint-induced gastric ulcer at
45 days of age (Bell, Drucker and Woodruff, 1965). It is possible that
the nature of the primary effect was structural in these rats, since this
effect did not develop when the drug was given during days 12 to 15 of
pregnancy.

Lau and associates (1977) demonstrated delayed and long-lasting effects
in the biosynthesis of catecholamines in the progeny of rats treated with
1 mg reserpine/kg s.c. on days 12 to 14 of pregnancy. Adrenal tyrosine
hydroxylase and dopamine β-hydroxylase activities increased at about 2
weeks postnatally and the increases persisted into adulthood. In another
study (Dailey, 1978), an adrenergic deficit was detected in the progeny
of rats whose mothers were treated s.c. with 100 μg reserpine/kg from day
8 of pregnancy until the time of weaning. The progeny had a decreased
ability to respond to cold stress at 60 days of age.

Delayed Neuroendocrine Effects

The gonads are formed as an expression of the genetic sex during the
first trimester of the pregnancy. During the later part of pregnancy (in
guinea pigs, primates) or postnatally (in rats, hamsters), neuroendocrine
differentiation occurs under the influence of endogenous androgens
(Gorski, Harlan and Christensen, 1977). The result becomes evident only
at puberty, when the pattern of pituitary gonadotrophin release manifests
itself; it is cyclic in the female and constant in the male. The brain
of the neonatal rat, if not influenced by endogenous androgen, will
exhibit a female sexual pattern in adulthood. An estrogenic metabolite
of endogenous androgen masculinizes the brain; it acts on a hypothalamic
area and on the pituitary, since the effect does not develop after
disruption of the axis or hypophysectomy. Administration of an androgen
to female rats during postnatal days 4 to 6 eliminated the cyclicity and
resulted in a constant estrus syndrome postpubertally. Androgen given to
guinea pigs from 30 to 55 days of pregnancy prevented the development of
lordosis (the sign of receptivity) in their female progeny following
treatment with estrogen and progesterone. Thus, genetically female
animals did not exhibit feminine sexual function in adulthood, regardless
of how they were stimulated hormonally. Androgens permanently
masculinized the female rat or guinea pig.

Neonatal castration of male rats resulted in feminization of the adult
sex activity due to a cyclic release of gonadotrophin. These rats
exhibited lordosis following treatment with estrogen and progesterone.
Sex steroids permanently modified the synaptic connections in the area of
the hypothalamus that controls gonadotrophin secretion.

Certain CNS-acting drugs (barbiturates, reserpine, chlorpromazine,
cannabinoids, etc.) interfere with the masculinizing effect of androgens
(Gorski, Harlan and Christensen, 1977; Dalterio and Bartke, 1979). Male
hamsters treated with 50-100 μg of pentobarbital on postnatal days 2 to 4
showed sexual behavioral deficits (decreased mounts, intromission and
ejaculation) at 60 days of age. The female type lordosis could be
elicited (Clemens, Popham and Ruppert 1979). Barbiturates also blocked
the masculinizing effect of exogenous androgens in females (Gorski,
Harlan and Christensen, 1977).

Gupta and associates (1980) reported that administration of phenobarbital at an earlier period, i.e., during pregnancy, also had delayed effects on reproduction; 40 mg/kg given s.c. to rats from days 12 to 19 of pregnancy reduced fertility in their offspring. Plasma gonadotrophin (LH) levels were decreased in both sexes and cytoplasmic steroid receptors (uterus or seminal vesicle) were increased.

Phenobarbital and some other CNS-acting drugs given to adult rats or hamsters inhibit ovulation. However, Alleva and co-workers (1975) reported that tolerance develops to this effect, since ovulation returns with repeated administration of the drug. Such an adaptation, which is not related to an increased metabolism rate of the drug, does not occur in the fetus. This example characterizes the difference in drug effects even though the mechanism may be identical, i.e., on the hypothalamus, in the developing and the mature organism: the former effect is delayed and irreversible and the latter is immediate and reversible.

In primates, sexual behavior is determined by hormonal influences during the intrauterine period. Female offspring of rhesus monkeys receiving testosterone propionate from 39 to 70 days of their gestational age were pseudohermaphroditic (Goy and Phoenix, 1971). These animals had masculine behavior in their social interaction (mounting, playing, fighting, etc.) in adulthood. Neonatal gonadectomy did not influence the adult sexual behavior, since it was determined prenatally.

The human fetus is very sensitive to the effects of androgens. Small therapeutic doses of 17-methyltestosterone and/or 17-ethynylestradiol, as well as some other synthetic progestins, can virilize the female (Wilkins, 1960). Congenital adrenal hyperplasia androgenizes the human fetus. The external genitalia of the newborn females have to be feminized surgically. These females are treated with corticosteroids to suppress androgen production. Throughout childhood these females exhibit boyish behavior, which can be attributed to the prenatal effects of excess androgens (Ehrhardt and Meyer-Bohlburg, 1981).

The pre- or neonatal effects of androgens are also reflected later in some other phenomena of sexual dimorphism, such as the patterns of agonistic behavior, locomotor activity, body weight regulation and metabolic functions.

Sex differences in the rate of hepatic steroid and drug metabolism are well established in post-pubertal rats and mice, and in some other species of experimental animals. The effect of neonatal testosterone is expressed with an increase in the production of specific hydroxylated metabolites of xenobiotics and steroids.

Levin and colleagues (1975) reported that the rate of 6-β-hydroxylation of testosterone in immature rats is similar in both sexes; however, at adulthood, it is 20-fold higher in the male than in the female. The testosterone level in the male castrated at birth is similar to that of the female in adulthood. At least two forms of cytochrome P-450 exist in the steroid hydroxylating system, and they differ in their turnover rate. The ratio of the two forms appears to be a function of neonatal androgen exposure.

The activities of mixed-function oxidases and UDP-glucuronyl-transferase in the microsomes of liver are higher in adult male rats than in females. After administration of testosterone to neonatal female rats or after hypophysectomy, the post-pubertal sex differences in the drug-metabolizing enzyme systems are abolished (Lucier, Lui and Lamartiniere, 1979).

Development of adult sexual dimorphism in drug metabolism functions, as in the examples mentioned above, is under central regulation and is imprinted neonatally in the rat. Similar events also occur in mice and probably in other species.

Pre- or neonatal exposure to phenobarbital, a potent inducer of microsomal mixed-function oxidases, can produce long-lasting effects. Phenobarbital administration to mice from day 6 of pregnancy until parturition produced significantly increased activity of the microsomal drug-metabolizing enzymes in the cross-fostered male offspring at 45 to 50 days of age (Yanai, 1979). This was accompanied by a decrease in weight of the seminal vesicles, implying that an effect also had occurred on the metabolism of endogenous steroids.

In rats neonatally exposed to phenobarbital for 1 week postpartum via the milk of the nursing dam, the activity of ethyl morphine $\underline{N}$-demethylase was increased by 160% and aflatoxin-DNA adduct formation by $\overline{40\%}$ at 37 weeks of age (Faris and Campbell, 1981). The latter, a covalent interaction, is involved in the initiation of cancer.

Delayed Effects on Endocrine and Immune Systems

Neonatal administration of glucocorticoid, thyroxine, or estrogen can produce permanent endocrinopathies. This is most likely attributable to their effects on the central regulation of the endocrine system which is "set" at this period. Similarly, the immune system is most vulnerable during the neonatal period when the thymus and other factors determine its capability.

Sawano and co-workers (1969) reported that a single s.c. injection of 1 mg of cortisone given to newborn rats produced growth retardation. On reaching 5-6 weeks of age, the rats had no growth hormone-releasing activity in the hypothalamus and little growth hormone or thyrotropin activity in their pituitary. In other neonatal studies, activities of several organ systems were affected in adulthood (Taeusch, 1975). Circadian variation of blood glucocorticoid levels was abolished, and brain cholesterol decreased. Impaired growth of the cerebellum, associated with decreased fine motor control and tremor, was detected. The condition was similar in some respects to the runting seen in neonatal thymectomy, including the defective ability to produce antibodies.

These findings are of clinical interest in view of the use of glucocorticoids in infants with respiratory distress syndrome. Gunn and associates (1981), in a follow-up study of the infants who survived for the first year of life, found that the incidence of neurologic abnormalities was increased. The incidence of otitis and/or pneumonia was greater in the steroid-treated children between the ages of 1 and 5 years than in the placebo group, and the percentage of their T lymphocytes was diminished. The adrenocortical suppression syndrome has been reported to occur in infants following maternal steroid therapy during pregnancy (Pomerance and Yaffe, 1973).

Bakke and colleagues (1977) described another unique, neonatally induced endocrinopathy produced by thyroxine. Large doses of thyroxine given to neonatal rats inhibited secretion of TSH in adulthood, and produced persistent hypothalamo-pituitary, thyroidal and gonadal abnormalities.

Prenatally or neonatally administered estrogens can produce abnormal development of vaginal epithelium, leading to neoplastic transformation in adulthood (Takasugi, 1979). Neonatal administration of 17β-estradiol (5 to 20 µg up to 3 to 5 days of age) to mice, led to a persistent vaginal cornification. Ovariectomy a week after treatment, with or without adrenalectomy or hypophysectomy, did not abolish this effect. Neonatal treatment of mice with androgen produced similar changes. Estrogen treatment from postnatal days 8 or 11 did not induce vaginal cornification. A high incidence of neoplastic transformation developed in these neonatally (3 to 5 days) steroid-treated mice in their old age. The incidence of tumors was lower in the ovariectomized mice, implying a promoter role of this hormone.

Mice treated neonatally with diethylstilbestrol (DES) (2 mg injection on day of birth) had persistent vaginal cornification and developed vaginal and cervical epidermal carcinoma at 13 to 26 months of age (Takasugi, 1979).

Herbst and associates (1979) reported the development of vaginal adenocarcinoma in young women in association with maternal DES therapy. Other clinical findings also linked the use of this agent to other cervical and vaginal lesions. Studies in experimental animals reproduced most of these abnormalities, as presented by Drs. McLachlan and Fabro in this symposium.

The delayed immunological effects of DES in mice were investigated by Luster and co-workers (1980). Pregnant mice were given 0.1 mg DES/kg s.c. on day 16 of gestation. Offspring were tested at 2 and 8 months of age. The sensitivity to Escherichia coli lipopolysaccharide was suppressed in females and enhanced in males. Delayed hypersensitivity responses and in vitro mitogenic stimulation of lymphocytes were decreased in both sexes.

The immunosuppression induced by the antineoplastic drugs, among other agents, should be mentioned. These drugs increase the susceptibility to infectious agents in children long after discontinuation of therapy. The thymus or the bursa-equivalent tissue are affected. Long-lasting consequences, e.g., development of autoimmune diseases or cancer, have been postulated (O'Reilly, 1980).

To demonstrate the susceptibility of the fetus or the neonate to chemicals affecting the development of the immune system, the effects of several non-medicinal chemicals, e.g., chlorinated phenolic compounds and methylmercury, were studied by Thomas and Hinsdill (1979). For example, tetrachlorodibenzo-p-dioxin (TCDD) was given in the feed to pregnant mice at 1, 2.5 or 5 ppb. Offspring were tested at 5 weeks of age. Increased sensitivity to an endotoxin challenge and reduced contact sensitivity to a potent sensitizer was observed in the 1 and 5 ppb groups, respectively. Thymus cortex atrophy and reduced anti-sheep erythrocyte plaque-forming cell response were detected in the groups given TCDD at 2.5 and 5 ppb.

Delayed Degenerative and Proliferative Changes and Cross-Generational Effects

Delayed degenerative changes following pre- or neonatal treatment with antibiotics and antineoplastic agents have been detected. The best known example of a delayed drug effect is that induced by tetracycline antibiotics in infants. Maternal treatment with this calcium chelator can produce yellow or brown discoloration and enamel hypoplasia of the deciduous teeth. Tetracycline is also incorporated in bone and may cause transitory depression of skeletal growth (Cohlan, 1964). Similar effects may develop after administration of the drug to neonates. The immature organism appears to be most vulnerable to the ototoxicity of streptomycin and kanamycin. Robinson and Cambon (1964) have reported hearing deficits in newborn children after maternal treatment with these drugs. The incidence is low because fetal drug levels are lower than maternal levels. Neonatal treatment, however, e.g., with aminoglycoside antibiotics, may produce cochlear drug levels higher than those in the adult because of the low renal excretion. Federspil and co-workers (1980), in a study of several species, found that neonates were the most sensitive to the ototoxicity of these antibiotics.

Daily administration of large doses (200 to 300 mg/kg, s.c.) of streptomycin sulfate to neonatal rats produced deafness and extensive cochlear damage (Alleva and Balazs, 1980). No injury developed when the treatment started in the weaned animal, even though it was given for as long as 3 months. Evidence has been presented for delayed or progressive effects in rats treated from postnatal days 2 to 7 with 300 mg streptomycin/kg. The rats began to hear at the usual time of 11 to 14 days and became deaf, as evidenced by the lack of response (Preyer reflex) to the sound of a Galton whistle on postnatal days 27 to 35, which was 3 to 4 weeks after the end of treatment. Another late effect detected in rats treated neonatally with streptomycin consisted of hyperactivity, circling, head bobbing and backward gait (Alleva and Balazs, 1978). These effects lasted for a few months after the end of treatment. This disorder is not likely of vestibular origin, since microscopically the cristae, maculae and vestibular nerves appeared normal. Light microscopic examination of the brain failed to detect abnormalities. Increases in the cortical serotonin receptors and in the dopamine levels in the corpus striatum were measured during the peak effect. It is possible that a developmental abnormality of the neuronal connections is expressed by this stereotypic dyskinesia.

Delayed effects of maternal or neonatal treatments with cytotoxic drugs have been shown to occur in both germinal and somatic tissues. For example, male offspring of rats treated with a single i.p. dose of 10 mg busulfan/kg between 13 to 20 days of gestation were sterile. The ovaries of female offspring of mice treated with 6-mercaptopurine during pregnancy had only a few oocytes and follicles at 3 months of age. A large number of these mice were sterile (Hemsworth and Jackson, 1963). Eriksson and co-workers (1973) reported that aminopterin given to pregnant women produced retarded growth in their children.

A delayed degenerative change in muscle in rats after neonatal administration of 6-mercaptopurine was recently observed in our laboratory (Alleva and co-workers, 1980). Daily administration of this drug (2 mg/kg, s.c.) from days 2 to 22 of age produced fatty atrophy in skeletal muscle of the lumbar, the sacral region and the posterior extremities. The lesion was noticeable histologically only 4 months after the end of treatment. Electron microscopic examination revealed loss of myofilaments 5 weeks posttreatment.

Specific tissues (e.g., lymphatic) of the neonates are more susceptible to certain direct-acting carcinogens than those of the adult. In the experiments of Berenblum and associates (1966), groups of mice were treated with urethane (1 mg/kg, i.p.) weekly for 10 weeks, beginning within 24 hr or at 45 days after birth. At 60 weeks of age, 35% of the former group and 6% of the latter group had developed lymphatic leukemia. This phenomenon is of clinical interest, since leukemia and lymphoma are the most common tumors in children. The peak incidence occurs at 4 to 6 years of age, which suggests that the induction occurred much earlier in life.

Cross-generational carcinogenesis has been detected after treatment of rats with alkyl nitrosourea and of mice with dimethylbenzanthracene (Tomatis, 1979). Tumors identical to those occurring in the treated mother developed in the progeny, and also occurred in the second and third generations. It has been postulated that the tumors occur as a consequence of a mutation at a specific locus, which results in cancer at a particular site, or after interaction with environmental factors at a particular site in individuals made susceptible to neoplastic transformation by a heritable lesion that does not produce cancer by itself. The latter seems to represent the inheritance of an increased susceptibility to a promoter. In a discussion of the mechanism of inheritance of acquired immunologic tolerance, Gorczynski and Steele (1980) recently postulated that a process occurs in which mutated somatic genes enter the germ line.

Bakke and associates (1977) demonstrated that cross-generational endocrinopathies can occur after neonatal administration of 1-thyroxine in rats. Large doses of 1-thyroxine given to neonatal rats produced persistent hypothalamo-pituitary, thyroidal and gonadal abnormalities. When females were mated with untreated males, their offspring, cross-fostered to untreated mothers, had abnormalities similar to those of their treated mothers. For example, both had abnormal hypothalamic and pituitary TSH concentrations and delayed estrus. The female progeny were mated with normal males; their offspring of both sexes had increased thyroid and decreased gonadal weights. Abnormalities in this F_2 generation were more severe than those occurring in the preceding one.

Among possible mechanisms, paramutation has been considered. This involves alteration in the function of regulator genes in both somatic and germ cells. If thyroxine alters this function, the unimodal distribution and the progressive severity of the disorder in the offspring could be explained. Spergel and co-workers (1975) postulated that this mechanism also occurs in the inheritance of another endocrinopathy, alloxan-induced diabetes in rats.

The delayed toxic effect of greatest concern has been genetic damage in the gonads. The female fetus is most vulnerable, since their germ cells divide mitotically early in development and then remain in a meiotic phase, and the genetic damage persists. Mutagenic effects may become evident when the female offspring of treated mothers reproduce. Reimers and associates (1980) reported that a mutagenic effect caused by 6-mercaptopurine in mice was manifested in early fetal loss, which was related to the dose administered to the grandparents during their pregnancy.

In the context of mutagenesis (although it may not belong there), an example is given for a paternal effect. An increased mortality was detected at 2 weeks of age in the undrugged offspring of male rats treated with various narcotic analgesics before mating (Smith and Joffe, 1975). The mechanism remains to be explored.

The problem of chemical mutagenesis has been well recognized. It has been surmised that chemically induced genetic damage in humans would most likely result in a slight increase in the incidence of severe genetic diseases and a generalized decrease in genetic fitness over a greatly expanded period of perhaps 10 or 20 generations (Mayer and Flamm, 1981). The few examples of cross-generational effects cited are perhaps of heuristic value for recognition of the diverse effects of pre- and perinatal drug exposure to a subsequent generation.

REFERENCES

Ahlenius, S., R. Brown, J. Engel, and P. Lundborg (1973). Naunyn-Schmiedebergs Arch. Pharmakol., 279, 31-37.
Alleva, F.R., and T. Balazs (1978). Toxicol. Appl. Pharmacol., 45, 855-859.
Alleva, F.R., and T. Balazs (1980). Toxicol. Lett., 6, 385-389.
Alleva, F.R., T. Balazs, B.H. Haberman, M.A. Weinberger, and L.J. Slaughter (1980). 19th Annual Meeting, Society of Toxicolology, Washington, D.C. (Abstract 201).
Alleva, J.J., M.W. Lipien, F.R. Alleva, and T. Balazs (1975). Toxicol. Appl. Pharmacol., 34, 491-498.
Bakke, J.L., N.L. Lawrence, S. Robinson, and J. Bennett (1977). Biol. Neonate, 31, 71-83.
Bell, R.W., R.R. Drucker, and A.B. Woodruff (1965). Psychon. Sci. 2, 269-270.
Berenblum, T., L. Boiato, and N. Trainin (1966). Cancer Res., 26, 357-360.
Brackbill, Y., J. Kane, R.L. Manniello, and D. Abramson (1974). Am. J. Obstet. Gynecol., 118, 377-384.
Broman, S., and Y. Brackbill (1980). Obstetric medication and early development. Presented at Annual Meeting, American Association for the Advancement of Science, San Francisco, CA.
Clemens, L.G., T.B. Popham, and P.H. Ruppert (1979). Dev. Psychobiol., 12, 49-59.
Cohlan, S.Q. (1964). N.Y. State J. Med., 64, 493-499.
Csaba, I.F., E. Sulyok, and T.J. Erti (1978). J. Pediatr. 92, 484.
Dailey, J.W. (1978). Res. Commun. Chem. Pathol. Pharmacol., 19, 389-402.
Dalterio, S., and A. Bartke (1979). Science, 205, 1420-1422.
Ehrhardt, A.A., and H.F.L. Meyer-Bahlburg (1981). Science, 211, 1312-1318.
Eriksson, M., C.S. Catz, and S.J. Yaffe (1973). Clin. Obstet. Gynecol., 16, 199-224.
Faris, R.A., and T.C. Campbell (1981). Science, 211, 719-721.
Federspil, P.J., W. Schatzle, M. Kayser, K. Sack, and J. Schentag (1980). Proceedings 11th Int. Congr. Chemother., 1, 607. American Society for Microbiology, Washington, D.C.
Gallager, D.W., and P. Mallorga (1980). Science, 208, 64-69.

Gorczynski, R.M., and E.J. Steele (1980). Proc. Natl. Acad. Sci. USA, 77, 2871-2875.
Gorski, R.A., R.E. Harlan, and L.W. Christensen (1977). In M. Norvell and T. Shellenberger (Eds.), Hormone Research, Vol. 3. Hemisphere, Washington, D.C. pp. 97-123.
Goy, R.W., and C.H. Phoenix (1971). UCLA Forum Med. Sci., 15, 193-201.
Grollman, A., and E.F. Grollman (1962). J. Clin. Invest., 41, 710-714.
Grunfeld, Y., and T. Balazs (1980). Proceedings Fifth FDA Science Symposium, HHS Publ. No. (FDA) 80-1076, Washington, D.C. p. 170.
Gunn, T., E.R. Reece, K. Metrakos, and E. Colle (1981). Pediatrics, 67, 61-67.
Gupta, C., B.R. Sonawane, S.J. Yaffe, and B.H. Shapiro (1980). Science, 208, 508-510.
Hemsworth, B.N., and H. Jackson (1963). J. Reprod. Fertil., 5, 187-194.
Herbst, A.L., R.E. Scully, and S.J. Robboy (1979). Natl. Cancer Inst. Monogr., 51, 25-35.
Kellogg, C., D. Tervo, J. Ison, T. Parisi, and R.K. Miller (1980). Science, 207, 205-207.
Kimmel, C.A., and J. Buelke-Sam (1981). Toxicologist, 1, 11.
Lau, C., J. Bartolome, F.J. Seidler, and T.A. Slotkin (1977). Neuropharmacology, 6, 799-809.
Levin, D.L., D.E. Fixler, F.C. Morriss, and J. Tyson (1978). J. Pediatr., 92, 478-483.
Levin, W., D. Ryan, R. Kuntzman, and A.M. Conney (1975). Mol. Pharmacol, 11, 190-200.
Lucier, G.W., E.M.K. Lui, and C.A. Lamartiniere (1979). Environ. Health Perspect., 29, 7-16.
Luster, M.I., R.E. Faith, J.A. McLachlan, and G.C. Clark (1980). Proceedings Fourth FDA Science Symposium, HHS Publ. No. (FDA) 80-1074, Washington, D.C. pp. 263-266.
Massotti, M., F.R. Alleva, and T. Balazs (1980a). Proceedings Fifth FDA Science Symposium, HHS Publ. No. (FDA) 80-1076 Washington, D.C. p 181.
Massotti, M., F.R. Alleva, T. Balazs and A. Guidotti (1980b). Neuropharmacology, 19, 951-956.
Mayer, V.W., and W.G. Flamm (1981). In A.L. Reeves (Ed.), Toxicology: Principles and Practice, Vol. 1. Wiley and Sons, New York. pp. 144-154.
Morselli, P.L., and V. Rovei (1980). Eur. J. Clin. Pharmacol. 18, 25-30.
O'Reilly, R.J. (1980). Proceedings 11th Int. Congr. Chemother. 2, 1488, American Society for Microbiology, Washington, D.C.
Perloff, J.K. (1981). Am. Heart J., 101, 219-226.
Pomerance, J.J., and S.J. Yaffe (1973). Curr. Probl. Pediatr., 4, 3-60.
Reimers, T.J., P.M. Sluss, J. Goodwin, and G.E. Seidel (1980). Biol. Reprod., 22, 367-375.
Rementeria, J.L., and K. Bhatt (1977). J. Pediatr., 90, 123-126.
Robinson, G.C., and K.G. Cambon (1964). New Engl. J. Med., 949-951.
Rosengarten, H., and A.J. Friedhoff (1979). Science, 203, 1133-1135.
Sawano, S., A. Arimura, A. Schally, T. Redding, and S. Schapiro (1969). Acta Endocrinol., 61, 57-67.
Shoemaker, W.J. (1980). Proceedings Fifth FDA Science Symposium, HHS Publ. No. (FDA) 80-1076, Washington, D.C. pp. 7-14.
Smith, D.J., and J.M. Joffe (1975). Nature, 253, 202-203.
Spear, L.P., I.A. Shalaby, and J. Brick (1980). Psychopharmacology, 70, 47-58.
Spergel, G., F. Kahn, and M.G. Goldner (1975). Metabolism, 24, 1311-1319.
Taeusch, H.W. (1975). J. Pediatr., 87, 611-622.

Takasugi, N. (1979). Natl. Cancer Inst. Monogr., 51, 57-66.
Thomas, P.T., and R.D. Hinsdill (1979). Drug Chem. Toxicol., 2, 77-98.
Tomatis, L. (1979). Natl. Cancer Inst. Monogr., 51, 159-184.
Tronick, E., S. Wise, A. Heidelise, L. Adamson, J. Scanlon, and T.B.
    Brazelton (1976). Pediatrics, 58, 94-100.
Van den Berg, B.J., G. Levinson, S.M. Shnider, S.C. Hughes and S.J.
    Stefani (1980). Annual Meeting of Society for Obstetric Anesthesia
    and Perinatology, Boston, Mass. (Abstract 130).
Vernadakis, A., and D.M. Woodbury (1969). Epilepsia, 10, 163-178.
Vogt, J., B. Schmidt-Redemann, and R.R. Urbanek (1979). Pediatr.
Paedol.,
    14, 355-362.
Wilkins, L. (1960). J. Am. Med. Assoc., 172, 1028-1032.
Woodson, R.H., and E.M. daCosta-Woodson (1980). Infant Behav. Dev. 3,
205-
    213.
Yanai, J. (1979). Biochem. Pharmacol., 28, 1429-1430.

Improvements in the Postnatal Detection of Central Nervous System Defects

H. Tuchmann-Duplessis* and C. Amiel-Tison**

*Laboratoire d'Embryologie, Faculté de Médecine, 45, rue des
Saints Pères, 75006 Paris, France
**Clinique Universitaire Baudelocque, 123, bld du Port Royal,
75014 Paris, France

Since teratological investigations have been developed in recent years, we
will deal here with a problem which has been somewhat overlooked : the abnormalities induced during intra-uterine life which are only post nataly
recognized.

Reproduction can be impaired by various drugs as well by environmental
agents. According to the moment of exposure, from gametogenesis to the foetal period and eventually also during lactation, the adverse actions on the
conceptus are variable. They range from infertility to embryotoxicity gross
congenital malformations and a large variety of more subtile morphological,
biochemical and functional abnormalities.

In animal experiments, many of these disorders are often overlooked, since
the offspring appears otherwise normal at birth. They are revealed subsequently by intelectual and behavioural impairements, or by motility, endocrine and immune disturbances.

Numerous investigations are necessary to detect these defects, they can be
recognized few months after birth like heart anomalies, several years later
like kidney and central nervous system malformations or even later, like vaginal cancer. Some anomalies are only fully recognized in subsequent generations.

Although the mechanism of these accidents is not fully recognized it has
been shown that when animals receive subteratogenic doses which do not produce obvious morphological malformations, lesions of the C.N.S. can occur
which determine deficient performances in learning tasks, because in many
species, particularly in Rodents the differentiation of the C.N.S. is late
and continues during the post natal period.

In human studies, brain-behavior relationships are even more difficult to interpret, the experiments are natural, and so confounded. Moreover, because brain plasticity is operating during infancy, the late outcome might be very misleading, seeming poorly related to the initial insult. Therefore sophisticated diagnostic methods are necessary to show mild abnormalities in the neonatal period and during the first year of life in order to demonstrate the"continuum of reproductive casualty".

A - Animal data

1. Prenatal physiology

The physiological activity of the conceptus can be divided into 3 main periods : the embryonic, the fetal and the neonatal period.

Embryonic period

The fundamental cell components nucleic acids, proteins and lipids are synthetised by the embryo.

Differentiation is characterised by a dissimilarity in the protein content of two cells ; it results from a selective activation and inactivation of genes.

The fetal period is characterised mainly by differentiation of the primordium into definitive organs, general growth, and the storage of energy substrates. The morphological maturation of the organs are paralleled by an improvement in functional activities. The protein content increases more than the D.N.A. content.

Compared with neonatal physiology, the fetal functional activities are limited. The Central Nervous System does not play the important coordination role it assumes later.

However very important remodelling movements take place in the brain. The development of fundamental nervous structures proceeds at different rates and is not completed until puberty. Periods of active growth and differentiation represent critical stages in central nervous system development, because the fine structures have the highest susceptibility to environmental and internal factors.

While organ functions are quite restricted during the prenatal development, the second feature of fetal physiology, growth,plays a predominant role. Increase in growth, results from two phenomena : cell proliferation and cell size increase. Growth starts with an increase of DNA followed by an accelerated protein synthesis. Formation of intercellular substances occurs simultaneously, particularly in connective tissues and their derivatives. The growth is linear and continuous but its speed is not constant. After a sharp increase up to month 3, it decreases throughout gestation.

Enzymatic Activities

Among the causes of high fetal susceptibility to drugs, the lack of development of the enzyme systems necessary for detoxification seems to play an essential role. Most of the oxidative enzymes which are involved in drug metabolism and in the detoxification of substances like bilirubin, adrenal steroids and salicylates, only gradually reach their normal values after birth.

The poor ability of the fetus to form glucuronides also enhances the susceptibility of the nervous system to various drugs such as morphine and the
barbiturates. Again, the low reducing potential of the erythrocytes, as well
as the immaturity of the fetal kidney, constitute an additional handicap to
the fetus, which cannot detoxify and excrete drugs as rapidly as the adult.

In the human fetus however, the enzymatic activity is more developed than
in experimental animals. A liver microsomal drug oxydizing system is already functioning in the first part of pregnancy.

2.The newborn Period is characterised by an adaptation to extrauterine life.
It is important as a test in which metabolic anomalies acquired in the course of gestation may cause a dysfunction of the enzymatic systems required
for the autonomic life of the baby. At birth, respiration is regulated by
surfactant which prevents the small alveoli from collapsing after the first
expiration.

The general metabolism performs a transfer from an anabolic state to a catabolic one. Before birth, the metabolic flow was oriented from the mother
to the fetus which stored glycogen and lipids. (After birth, new needs of
energy appear for thermogenesis, respiratory work and motility.) This energy is supplied by the utilisation of stored glycogen and lipids. A fault in
the storage or utilisation processes may have a deleterious effect on the
survival of the newborn.

Consequently, alterations occuring during late intrauterine stages expresses themselves only postnatally.

The particular interest of the neonatal period lies in the fact that it col-
lects a great number of anomalies which originate from various periods of
the intrauterine life and which are not detected in the foetus.

3. Methodology

Post natal testing

In the selection of the tests, one has to take in consideration their simplicity, their flexibility and time necessary to perform them. A battery
of tests has to be used in order to determine the various parameters of the
post natal development such as the somatic, the sexual and behavioural characteristics.

To detect deviations from normal animals, a definition of normality has to
be established by a strict observation of the offspring of "untreated" animals.

It has to be born in mind that the development and the behaviour of untreated animals can differ according to the litter size. Therefore litters
should be standardized to groups of 8 pups per litter. Tests should take
in consideration individual and inter individual behaviour.

Physical development can give the first indication of adverse effects.

Growth retardation evidenced by underweight, as well as prematurity are
generally associated with impaired test performances and a high post natal mortality.

For the assessment of physical development, the following parameters are generally used in the rat.

a) pina detachment   - day 14
b) ear opening and quadruped
   stance with elevated pelvis   - day 14
c) eye opening   - day 17
d) testis descendus   - day 27
e) vaginal opening   - day 41
f) weight development separate
   in males and females for each animal
   as compared to the controls   - days : 0.4.7.14.21.

Function need

Behavioral development is assessed by the following tests :

	days
a) auditory function	14
b) homing response	14
c) air righting	14
d) papillary reflex	21
e) loco-motor coordination	21
f) learning capacity	27
g) memory	34

Tests of learning and memory have been designed for psychopharmacology problems. They are difficult to be used for teratology testing since the animals can not be trained before the tests.

Grauviller (1976) has used a T maze test. The test rat is given a reward after a successful performance instead of punishment after an incorrect result.During a short conditioning period the rat has to learn the way to find the reward food pellets. This gives an indication of the learning capacity. The test is than repeated after 0, 24, 48 and 72 hours.

4. Results

Influence of neuro drugs on the central nervous system (C.N.S.)

The Central nervous system behaves like an organ system in which the various cells have different proliferation and differentiation schedules. Therefore according to the stage and to the duration of treatment, the importance of the morphological and behavioural damage varies.

Generaly the C.N.S. has a higher sensivity than other tissues.

Langman et al (1975) have shown that when azacytidine is given to mice in late fetal stages, or post nataly, three time more cells are affected in the C.N.S. than in other organs like the lung, liver, skin etc...

a/ Anti-convulsivants

The gross malformation rate in the descendance of epileptic parents is 2 to 3 times higher than in the general population. The most frequent embryopathies are cleft lip, cleft palate, cardiac and squeletal abnormalities.

Beside these obvious malformations a specific pattern of postnatal abnormalities have been described in infants born to epileptic mothers treated during pregnancy.

Hanson and Smith (1975-1976) described the fetal hydantoine syndrome, while Seip (1976), Feldman and al. (1977) found evidence of a fetal trimethadione syndrome characterized by cranio-facial malformations, developmental and psycho-motor delay, pre and post natal growth deficiency, impaired intellectual performance associated or not with cardiac, genito-urinary and skeletal malformations.

Bethenod and Frederich (1975) have described a similar clinical syndrome termed "child of epileptics".

Although a large variety of malformations could be experimentally produced in rodents with anti-convulsivants it seemed difficult to establish a direct relationship between a specific anti-epileptic drug and human abnormalities.

Several epidemiological studies seem in favor of a drug induced teratogenecity.

A survey of congenital malformations in infants born to mothers in Cardiff over a 7-year period revealed a malformation-rate of 2.7%. When the mother had a history of epilepsy and had been on anticonvulsants during the first trimester the rate was 6.7% (Lowe, 1973).

Besides congenital anomalies, mental subnormality occurred in 1.5% of the epileptic mother's children, compared with 0.2% in a control group. The perinatal mortality rate was 42.5 per 1,000 for pregnancies in which anticonvulsants were taken, which was nearly twice the regional rate. The rate for all epileptic women was 28.6 per 1,000. The increased perinatal mortality was mainly due to congenital malformations and to spontaneous haemorrhage which occurred in 6 of 388 births.

Shapiro and al. (1976) analyzing data from a collaborative perinatal project, concluded that epilepsy, either maternal or paternal, is the decisive factor of malformations. The anticonvulsant drugs are considered to be not directly implicated in the etiology of malformations.

From a collaborative study in Japan in which use was made of prospective and retrospective cases, Nakane and al. (1980) concluded that anticonvulsants have a teratogenic action in humans. The malformation incidence in the non medicated group was 2.3% as compared to 11.5% in the medicated group.

When the trimethadione treated patients are excluded, the malformation rate drops to 6.75%. Therefore, the authors conclude that trimethadione represents the highest teratogenic risk, while barbiturates and their derivatives are less dangerous. Diphenylhydatoin appeared in this study the less dangerous drug.

A strong experimental indication of teratogenic drug etiology is suggested by the observations of Finnell (1981) in three imbred mouse strains ; S.W. V., C_3H and $C_{57}Be$ 6 J. The last strain having spontaneous, tonic clonic seizure disorders, which mimics the human condition of epilepsia.

Phenytoin in doses of 20 to 60 mg/kg was given two weeks before mating and
continued throughout gestation. Fetal weights decreased significantly in
all strains as the dosage of phenytoin increased. The incidence of malformations increased also in the 3 strains with the concentrations of phenytoin in maternal plasma.

The females whose seizure disorders were left untreated, produced normal
offspring ; even when seizures occurred daily throughout the entire gestation period. The author therefore concluded that the malformations are determined by the drug and not by the maternal seizure syndrome.

The animal model of the fetal hydaitoin syndrome duplicated the human condition ; growth deficiency with low fetal weight, ossification disorders
with digital hypoplasia,ocular neural, cardiac and skeletal malformations.
Ventricular septal defects and dilated cerebral ventricles were also observed.

b / Lysergic acid diethylamide (L.S.D.)

Studies on ^{14}C-Labelled LSD provide evidence that the drug crosses the pla
centa and enters into the fetus during different stages of gestation in
mice and hamsters. Metabolic studies have measured the half life of LSD as
175 minutes in man and only 7 minutes in mice.

The distribution of LSD in the rat has been determined after intravenous
administration. The drug accumulates rapidly in the brain within 15 to 20
minutes after injection. Free LSD is distributed generally in the cerebellum, hippocampus choroidal plexus, pituitary and pineal glands. Bound LSD
is localised in the cortex, the midbrain and in the medulla.

Despite several claims, no definite dysmorphogenetic actions was observed
in L.S.D. treated animals.

The analysis of various human data suggests that there is an increased
risk of spontaneous abortion in users of illicit LSD (Long, 1972).

However Dishotsky and al. (1971) concluded that pure LSD ingested in moderate doses does not produce chromosome damage detectable by available methods, does not cause detectable genetic damage and is not teratogen or
cancerigen in man. A similar opinion has been reached by Long (1972).

c/ Narcotics

They are often used as premedicants in anaesthesia, and are also widely
utilised in pregnancy.

Obstetrical complications in addicted women are significantly higher than
in the general population. They include prenaturity, toxaemia and precipitated labour. Half of the neonates are premature and show evidence of retarded intrauterine growth. Over 70% of them show congenital neonatal addiction with clinically recognisable withdrawal symptoms suggesting hyperactivity of the autonomic nervous system and irritability of the central
nervous system. In addition, diarrhoea, rhinorrhoea, and shrill cry are
frequently present. The relative frequency of all of the symptoms observed have been listed by Stone et al. (1971). Symptoms start in the first
3 days of life, usually within 24 hours of delivery. A correct diagnosis

is essential because these babies if not recognised, proceed to convulsions, coma and death.

Zelson et al. (1971) surveyed 384 infants born of 382 heroin addicted mothers. Half of these children were under 2,600 g in weight and 40% were small-fordate infants. Among these children, 70% developed signs of withdrawal which required treatment.

Length of maternal addiction was directly correlated with the occurrence of withdrawal signs in the infants. With increased maternal intake of heroin there was a higher incidence of neonatal withdrawal symptoms. In addition, the closer to delivery the last dose of heroin was taken, the higher and earlier was the occurrence of withdrawal signs in the neonate. The incidence of congenital malformations was no higher than in the general newborn population.

However on of the most striking effects of drugs used in obstetric is an impairement of the infant ability to suck.Babies born to heroin or methadone addicted mothers or barbiturate treated were found to have greatly impaired sucking behaviour.

Follow-up of babies born to mothers maintained on methadone indicates that up to an age of 4 years the offspring show normal physiological and mental behaviour. In animals, Davis and Lin (1972) examined the influence of opiate administration during pregnancy on the behaviour of the offspring during post-natal maturation. Rats injected from days 5 to 18 of pregnancy with doses ranging from 15 mg/kg to 45 mg/kg had no difference in litter numbers, but the morphine offspring weighed significantly less at birth and their perinatal mortality was much greater. Postnatal behaviour of the offspring was not significantly modified.

Addiction symptoms have been observed in infants born of mothers taking large doses of barbiturates throughout pregnancy or in the last trimester. The symptomatology is quite similar to those observed in heroin addiction : hyperexcitability, overactivity, excessive crying, tremors, hyperphagia and outburst of screaming. However, the infants with barbiturate addiction differ from babies with congenital heroin addiction ; they are fully grown and show no respiratory depression in the perinatal period.

d/ Meprobamate

The difficulties to ascertain the influence of psycho active drugs on the postnatal behaviour is illustrated by the conflicting results of two groups of investigators.

Werboff and Havlena (1962) reported that reserpine, chlorpromazine and meprobamate, administered to pregnant rats from days 5 to 8, from days 11 to 14 or from days 17 to 20 of pregnancy respectively, produced alterations in postnatal development and general behaviour of the offspring. These effects amounted to a reduction of learning capacity which was apparent in all tests carried out at 25,55 and 120 days of age. These results were interpreted as reflecting a non specific effect of these drugs on the fetal nervous system.

Several years later, the problem of meprobamate was investigated by
Klezkin et al. (1966.1971) who had previously studied the effects of
this drug on embryogenesis. Having found no body weight deficiency
in the litters of animals treated with large doses of meprobamate,and
taking into consideration the apparently strange fact reported by Werboff and Havlena, that the observed nervous system disorders were not
related to the timing and duration of treatment, Kletzkin started off
by repeating Werboff's experiments in exactly the same conditions,
and likewise testing the learning capacity at 25,55 and 120 days after birth. No significant differences between the offsprint of treated animals and the controls was found. Caldwell and Spille (1964)
and Hoffeld and Webster (1965) also failed to verify the results published by Werboff and his group. Caldwell and Spille treated 3
groups of animals throughout pregnancy with 3 dosage levels of meprobamate, namely 32,64 and 128 mg/kg daily.

Werboff's conclusions on meprobamate appear to be in conflict with
pharmacological data that indicate that this drug has little or no
effect on the cerebral cortex. No alterations of learning capacity
have been reported in adult animals. And clinically, the experience
gathered in the last 15 years, during which thousands of women have
been treated with meprobamate at some time or other during pregnancy, is quite reassuring. No ill-effects have been reported and statistical observations involving several hundred cases do not indicate that there is an increased incidence of malformations in the babies of mothers treated with this drug.

e/ Azacytidine

Langman et al. (1975) have shown that when mice are treated with azacytidine at different stages of foetal and postnatal life, subtile
alterations of the neuro-anatomy occur which modify the behaviour.

Examination of azacytidine treated mice on day 15 shows an extreme reduction in the size of the brain due to reduction of the cerebral cortex.

The location of the damage of the C N S is determined by the area where
cells are proliferating at the time of treatment.

There is also a small weight difference between treated and control
new-born which persisted until adulthood.

The behaviour was modified : locomotor coordination and general activity was altered.

Treatment involving the cerebellum led to pronounced intentional tremors, the first week of life.

The difference between the groups must be dependent on loss of specific cells not on general damage.

Some of the behavioral effects are transient, normal righting reflexes
appear in all animals in the second week of life and all tremors disappear in all animals in the second week of life and all tremors disappear by weaning. However, certain anomalies like differences in acti-

vity persist in adult animals. A variety of congenital brain damages
can be related to cell loss late in pregnancy.

Similar observations have been made by Rodier et al. (1979).

In mice treated with 5 AZACYTIODINE on days 12 or 14, two injections of
4 mg/kg at a 6 hours interval, a general and a C.N.S. weight reduction
is observed. As a consequence, the behavior is impaired.

There is a permanent modification of the righting reflex and a deficit
in the loco-motor coordination.

Treatment on the 14th day of gestation led to decreased passive avoidance, increased active avoidance and hyperactivity. Similar reactions were also observed in mice treated the 18th day. Each treatment
time produced a different set of structural and functional abnormalities. The late fetal period and the early post natal period - 3th day
post nataly - are particularly susceptible.

Treatments on the 12 and 14 days were made with 0.5 mg/kg AZACYTIDINE.
Cell loss occurs only in locations where a high level of proliferation
prevails at the time of treatment.

Two righting response tests were employed ; on 6th day after birth and
16th day. The later was ascertained by the ability to right in air.

The general weight and the brain weight decrease was more important in
the 12 day treated group than the 14th day group. The earlier the treatment the greater the noxious effect.

The righting reflex was much more impaired in the 12 day treated group.

Passive avoidance performance was also altered by the treatment, as
well as the general activity. The 12 day group had hypoactivity while
later treatment showed hyperactivity.

The pattern of deficits in the early treatment group is consistent with
the idea that the cerebellar injury is a major factor in the behaviour
of the group.

There seems to be some recovery after cell loss on days 12-14. However,
the recovery when it occurs is far from complete.

f/ Hydroxures

BUTCHER and al. (1977) investigated the behaviour of rats receiving
subteratogenic or marginally teratogenic doses of drugs capable to
cause malformations of the C.N.S.

Learning deficits were found in animals receiving sodium salicylate or
an excess of vitamine A.

Hydroxurea (H U) which is a D.N.A. synthesis inhibitor, when given at
a dose of 375 to 500 mg/kg on the 12th day of gestation determines cell
death in limb buds and in the ependymal layer of the neural tube. However, in foetuses removed on the 20th day no apparent lesions are found.

The newborns are devided in two groups, one cross fostered, the other are normally nursed.

These rats are tested at 30-40 days of age in an open field. Ten days later, the animals were tested by their ability to swimm and were than required to learn the route of escape from a water filled multiple T. maze.

All subjects were weighted before being maze tested.

In the 500 H U treated animals there was a significant weight reduction. However, no differences in weight between cross fostered and non cross fostered subjects was found.

The main results can be summarized :

A/During the open field testing many treated subjects lacked normal neuro-muscular control of the hind limbs resulting in unsteady locomotor pattern.

B/Significantly more errors were made by all groups in learning the backward path through the maze than in forward path testing.

Cross fostering had not influence in the maze error results.

From this experiment it can be concluded that when animals receive sub-teratogenic doses of a drug known to produce prenatal malformations of the C N S, they can determine deficient performance in learning tasks.

Small doses can produce functional malformations in the absence of gross malformations.

A somewhat similar experiment has been made by Fritz (1980) who administered 500 mg/Kg hydroxurea from day 12 to 14 and performed in these rats behavioural tests on day 14 and 41.

The group treated on day 14 had a 72% post natal mortality and a reduced weight gain. Most of the behavioral tests were normal however the loco motor pattern particularly climbing on a wire mesh, was impaired in the treated group.

In this information, the lack to find abnormal behaviour may be related to the high mortality of the group.

g/Miscellaneous drugs

In a second experiment Butcher and al. examined the postnatal behaviour of prenatal treated acetazolamide (Diamox). This drug usually determines ectrodactyly and ulnar hemimelia.

Diamox was given subcutaneously on days 10 and 11 at a dosage of 500mg/Kg the treated subjects had 40% limb malformations. At 30-35 days of age, no difference in the test of the open field was found, neither in the swimming speed at 50-55 days differences were noted.

The performance of the Diamox animals was as good as either of the control groups prepared, while the hydroxurea subjects made substantially more errors.

Diamox which induces a high proportion of limb anormalies can determine locomotor defects but no learning impairements.

These observations demonstrate or at least suggest, that agents which cause malformations or damage of the foetal nervous system will produce behavorial impairments in the offspring when given in moderate quantities. While substances which produce obvious congenital malformations like Diamox, but which do not have a major effect upon the foetal nervous system will not produce behavioral modifications.

Mice exposed to polychlorinated bihenyls like T.C.B. during gestation (an isomer present in some P.C.B. mixtures) exhibit a long lasting neuro behavioral syndrome, consisting of stereotypic head movements rotational behavior increased motor activity, impaired neuro-muscular strength and coordination and learning deficits.

Tilson and col.(1979) Lucier et col (1978) observed also that the in utero exposure to T.C.B. produces hyperactivity starting at 2 weeks of age and lasting up to 8 month of age. Therefore also in adulthood modifications of the hepatic enzyme activity.

Agrawal et al (1981) reported that mice exposed orally to 3,4, 3,4, tetrachlorodiphenyl (T.C.B.) 32 mg/kg from day 10 to 16 showed in the offspring at the age of one year elevated levels of motor activity, associated with decreased dopamine levels and dopamine receptor sites.

These results suggest that in utero exposure to T.C.B. might permanently alter the development of striatal synapses. The hyperactivity exhibited by T.C.B. spinning mice consisted of repetitive lobbing of the head and rapid circular movement.

T.C.B. interfers with the synaptogenesis of dopaminergic systems.

The long term behavioral alterations of T.C.B. might be related to a permanent structural alteration of the dopaminergic system produced by the perinatal presence of the chemical.

Hyperactivity of the spinning mice was associated with large decreases in dopamine levels and receptor binding in the T.C.B. spinners.

Parabendozal, a antiparasitic drug used in veterinary medecine constitutes an interesting example of the complexity of pre and post natal teratogenic problems (Mercier-Parot 1976).

In the rat, the mouse and the sheep parabendazol has a high teratogenic potential, inducing a large variety of central nervous system and skeletal anomalies.

In contrast in other species, rabbits, hamsters, pigs and cattle even high doses of parabendozal are devoid of teratogenecity.

The post natal reactions are also unusual.

While prenatally treated sheep show a highly impaired behaviour, they
are often unable to suckle and lack most of the normal reflexes (Lapras
et al 1973). Rats treated in late periods of pregnancy and during lactation have a normal offspring (Mercier-Parot 1976). The growth curve,
the survival time, the somatic and sexual development as well as the
general behaviour are not impaired by the parabendozal treatment.
Tuchmann Duplessis and col. with Hiss and Legros (1976), we investigated a hypolipemic agent 2 (p.2.2. dichlorocyclopropyl) phenoxy 2-me-
thyl propionic acid.

When the drug was given orally at three doses levels 2, 10 and 50 mg/kg
in the mouse or in the rat, no embryotoxic or teratogenic effect was
found in either of these two species.

The peri and post natal toxicity studies yielded most interesting results in the rat. When the drug was given during the last third of pregnancy and through the lactation period to weaning, delivery was normal
pregnancy lasting 21 days and 12 hours.

However a high post natal mortality mainly during the 48h following delivery was observed. As compared to the 95%, survival rate of the control group, the average survival was 84% in the group receiving 2 mg/kg
33% in the group of 10 mg/kg no survival was obtained with the highest
dose 50 mg/kg.

The mortality was probably due to a post natal vascular thrombosis and
to an impairment of the liver which was enlarged and had a low glycogen
content.

In a second experience 3 pups of each surviving litter were allowed to
grow up in order to test their reproductive capacity.

Despite of existing thrombus formations in some of the pups their
growth and reproductive performance were normal.

This compound although devoid of teratogenecity induces intra uterine
lesions which restrict more or less the survival of neonates.

h/Cross generational effects

As pointed out by Alleva and Balazs (1981) some chemically induced changes in neonates can be transmitted to the next generation either through
mutation or to persistant effects on the hypothalamus or endocrine receptors.

We had such an experience with reserpine.

Experiments with reserpine which involved 3 generations of rats, gave
results which revealed an important fertility decrease without an apparent morphological modification.

Nulliparous Wistar female rats were treated with reserpine in a dose
of 100 ug/kg daily, the drug being mixed with their food. They were mated with untreated males after 3,7, and 12 months of this treatment.

In the group mated at 3 months of treatment, fertility was practically
the same as in untreated controls, but in the group mated at 7 months

there was a 50% reduction of fertility, and in the group mated at 12 months, only 5% of the animals produced young.

Then, although the litters were apparently normal and their development was quite similar to that of untreated controls, observations was continued to the third generation, the rats being given reserpine 100 ug/kg daily as soon as they were weaned. Fertility remained satisfactory after 3 months of continuous treatment, but decreased 27% at 8 months, and the groups of animals treated for 14 or 15 months had no descendants at all. Fertility percentage was a little lowered in animals of the third generation, but their body growth and behaviour remained normal (Tuchmann-Duplessis and Mercier-Parot 1962).

B. Human data

I. Methods of investigations

. Cranio-Facial morphology : size, shape, sutures, bone defects are carefully evaluated.

. Neurological evaluation : Clinical examination is based on passive and active tone status, primary reflexes, reactivity (Amiel-Tison 1979). The normal aspect and mild deviations from normal are defined. More than 80% of the cohort of full term newborns have stricly normal responses in the very first hours of life ; mild abnormalities within the first 3 days of life are common ; conversely, any kind of neurological abnormalities which are persisting at the end of the first week must be studied and followed.

. Evolving patterns during the first weeks of life ; the manner with which these neurological abnormalities are changing within the first weeks of life suggests an etiological orientation : when the symptoms are related with a recent insult during late pregnancy or birth process, they usually are rapidly changing, different from one day to the next. Conversely, when the symptoms are related with a more remoted insult in early pregnancy, they seemed very stable through the first weeks of life ; precise and repeated clinical evaluations are therefore necessary to detect these differents patterns.

. Complementary observations of neonatal behavior ; habituation, environmental interaction have been described in the first days of life (Brazelton, 1973). These observations may helps to better define expected behavior in the neonatal period.

. Other investigations ; they are indicated according to clinical findings. Electro encephalography, ultra sonography, computerized axial tomography.

. Elective timing for these investigations ; it might be crucial for the precise determination of the causal insult to perform these investigations very early, i.e. in the first postnatal days ; the exemple of status epilepticus is particularly demonstrative ; beginning a few hours after birth it may be related with intra partum fetal distress, which has actually been the main etiology until the general use of fetal heart rate monitoting. However very early C.A.T. scan or ultrasonography have shown that an identical clinical picture can very well be related with well organized vascular lesions such as Sylvian softening or multikystic encephalomalacy, having occured weeks or months before.

If radiological explorations are performed a few weeks after birth, their contribution to the etiological diagnosis becomes much less valuable.

Specific difficulties related to prematurity and intra utering growth retardation. Neurological symptoms are easier to elicit in full term compared to premature or small-for-dates newborns. Moreover, adaptation to extra uterine life is more stormy with respiratory and circulatory problems which may cause secondary brain insults. Poor caloric intake too may add post natal damage to these newborns. Finaly, in this group, the high percentage of malformations in small for dates infants may increase the etiologic uncertainties.

II. Results

At the moment, screening for perinatal brain damage can be summarized as follows :

1°/ Reliability of clinical screening of full term newborns :
With repeated clinical evaluations performed on every newborn, high or low risk, it is very unlikely that many cases of brain damage will escape this screening tool. A few cases of isolated mental retardation only will not be diagnosed in the first weeks of life.

Cerebral malformations are in the majority of the cases associated with cranio-facial defects, therefore they can be recognized with radiological explorations in early post natal life. Only cytoarchitectonic abnormalities will then escape this screening.

2°/ Necessity of first year follow-up with low birth weight newborns
In high risk infants, mostly premature or small for dates newborns neuromotor testing within the first year of life may allow to recognise some cases brain damage which was questionable in the neonatal period. This method of surveillance allows classification of the infants, at one year into three groups :

a) some children have shown normal development during the first year this is statistically reassuring.

b) in other cases, it has been possible to identify early motor abnormalities. If these mild or severe abnormalities persist at one year of age, they will be permanent.

c/ Finally there is an intermediate group with transistory motor deficiencies. These children, despite their apparent normality at one year will still be at risk of showing further moderate consequences at school-age. This classification which has no value in accurate diagnosis of the individual infant is of overall importance for the obstetrician and the pediatrician. (Amiel-Tison and Grenier, 1980).
Evaluating this group at 5-6 years of age, our preliminary data suggests that the clinical expression of the underlying pathological lesions may change with time, and that a pronostic value is attached to transient neurologic signs detected during the first year.

3°/ Social and environmental influences on the developing nervous
system.
The importance of social and cultural conditions is very great at all
ages.

Socially disavantaged children will suffer not only from poorer prenatal care, but also from poor social conditions after birth. It has been
perfectly demonstrated in the category of minot handicaps, grouped under the term "Minimal Brain Dysfunction", that cultural conditions are
as important as perinatal lesions. These influences have been reviewed
by Sameroff (1980).

4/ Neurological plasticity and recovery from brain insult.
The various models of recovery processess have been recently reviewed
in animal experiments and human studies. (St James Roberts, 1980). Neurological plasticity operates in a way that after a brain insult in fetal or neonatal period, the late outcome may be surprisingly good. After some degree of neurophysiological recuperation along with adaptive
behavior, the outcome will poorly correlate with early brain insult.

5/ Efficiency of modern perinatology
Prenatal prevention recently used in developped countries has be proven
efficient in reducing the occurence of severe mental retardation (Gustavson 1980) and cerebral palsy (Hagberg et al 1980). Analysing the
changing panorama of cerebral palsy in Sweden Hagberg has shown that an
association of risk factors is responsible of most of the cases of cerebral palsy. Common combination of "fetal deprivation of supply" and as-
phyxia and/or cerebral hemorrhage suggests that the brain is more susceptible to perinatal complications after negative intra-uterine influences.
Analysing the etiology of severe mental retardation, prenatal factors
(half of them being chromosomal) have shown to have a predominating res-
ponsability, compared to intra partum and post natal factors.

C/ Physiopathological considerations
A few recent topics are adding complementary informations to what has
been stated above :

a/ "Dysrythmia" in visceral maturation in relation with unfavorable
intra-uterine conditions.

First described by Gould, Gluck and Kulowich (1972), this phenomenan
is particularly clear in cases with maternal hypertension (Amiel-
Tison, 1980).

Evidence of an advance in neurological maturation of 4 weeks or more
was detected in 16 infants with gestational ages between 30 and 37
weeks. These infants were all from pregnancies in which it is fair to
conclude that one form or another of intra uterine stress was in operation, such as chronic hypertensive disease, pregnancy-induced hypertension, uterine malformation, or multiple pregnancy. The influence of unfavorable intra uterine conditions in accelerated maturation may not be
confined to the central nervous system. Gould and associates (1977) reported an advance in both pulmonary surfactant and neurological development in eight of 51 infants from high-risk pregnancies. They also reported that 25 infants with accelerated surfactant development also had
signs of neurological advancement.

The hypothesis is advanced that unfavorable intra uterine conditions can induce an acceleration of neurologic development. We may speculate whether corticosteroid secretion by the fetus, in response to stress may play a role in the induction of these effects.

This acceleration in cell differentiation might be associated with a decreasing rate in cell division, therefore a final cell loss. There is no data on late outcome and at this point there probably is nothing to be expected from long term follow up studies.

b/ Intrapartum infection in relation with cytoarchitectonic abnormalities.
The pathogenesis of microgyria is not yet well understood. Various factors may be causative (Larroche 1977). Mycrogyria has been described with intrapartum infections such as cytomegalic inclusion disease (Bignami 1964). It has been described too in association with congenital toxoplasmosis (Deleon 1972).

c/ Determination of sensitive periods and consequences of cerebral lesions.
In experiments on the rhesus monkey (Goldman-Rakic, 1980), bilateral cortical dysgenesis is observed after unilateral prenatal resection, if performed before 119 embryonic days (E 119), not observed if performed after E 119. Thus in the rhesus monkey there appears to be a 2 week period of gestation between E102 and E119 during which an insult to the brain can have profound effects on the formation of its sulcal and gyral pattern.

In the same time, this study shows that the primate brain does have a considerable capacity for reorganization of connections following certain kinds of brain injury.

SUMARY AND CONCLUSIONS

Certain anomalies induced during the intra uterine development are not obvious at birth. Sophisticated investigations are necessary to detect mild brain abnormalities during the neonatal and early postnatal period.

Histogenesis of the CNS which starts during the fetal period continues post natally in the newborn.

It has been shown that when animals receive subteratogenic doses of an agent which does not produce obvious morphological malformations, lesions of the C.N.S. can occur which determine deficient performances in learning tasks.

The C.N.S. behaves like an organ system in which the various cells have different proligeration and differentiation schedules.

Therefore according to the stage and to the duration of the treatment, the importance of the morphological and functional damage varies. The C.N.S. has generally a higher susceptibility than other organs.

Before analyzing some experimental and clinical data a short review of prenatal and neonatal physiology is presented.

The fetal functional activities are limited as compared with neonatal physiology. The C.N.S. does not play the important coordination role it assumes later. Important remodling mouvements take place in the brain before birth. However, the definite structures are only completed several years later.

The high susceptibility of the fetus to drugs and other environmental agents is mainly due to lack of development of the enzyme systems necessary for detoxification of substances like bilirubin, adrenal steroids ans salicylates. The poor ability of the fetus to form glucuronides enhances the sensivity of the C.N.S. to drugs like morphine or barbiturates.

The adaptation to the extra uterine life is characterized by the shift of metabolism with a transfer from an anabolic state to a catabolic one.

After birth, the new needs of energy, for thermogenesis, respiratory and motility functions are supplied by the utilisation of stored glycogen and lipids during pregnancy. Impairments of these processes can have deleterious effects on the survival of the newborn. Consequently other alterations occuring during late intra uterine stages expresses themselves only after birth.

The postnatal detection of minor abnormalities requires a rigourous methodology. In the selection of tests in experimental animals, one has to take in consideration their simplicity, their flexibility and the time necessary to perform them.

A large variety of chemicals when administered during the intra uterine development determine behavioral defects which can be transient or definitif. Azacytidine for example when given at various stages of the fetal period determines in the mouse a modification of the righting reflex and a deficit of the locomotor coordination. Each treatment time produces a different set of functional abnormalities. The late fetal and the early post natal period are the most susceptible.

Hydroxyurea, when administered in subteratogenic doses, determine functional impairments of the C.N.S. and deficient performance in learning tasks, without producing gross malformations. Similar observations have been made with Acetazolamide (Diamox).

Mice exposed to polychlorinated biphenyls like T.C.B. showed in their offspring at the age of one year elevated levels of motor activity, associated with decreased dopamine levels.

Important species differences exist in the susceptibility to a given agent. For example, parabendozal, an antiparasitic drug, when given during pregnancy determines in the sleep a highly impaired behaviour. The newborn are unable to suckle and lack most of the normal reflexes. Rats treated in late periods of pregnancy and during lactation have a normal offspring. Occasionnaly some changes induced in the neonate can be observed in the next generations.

Reserpine treated rats show a decreased fertility rate in subsequent generations.

Animal data show the high susceptibility of the developing C.N.S. The offspring of animals exposed during pregnancy to subteratogenic environmental agents including drugs even apparently normal at birth can present transient or definitif behaviour anomalies.

In the human baby, neurological investigations have recently progressed. The methods for clinical evaluation are more refined and more objective. Testing the behavioral competency of the newborn has enriched the definition of neurologic integrity.

Further more, new radiological investigations such as Computerized Axial Tomographies and ultra sonography are providing unvaluable information on the exact lesions and their evolution.

With this approach early detection and etiological classification of brain damage becomes possible at birth in a high percentage of cases. This is not simply of academic interest but extremely important for genetic counseling and preventive medecine.

Following these clinical and technical advances, the aims and methods of evaluating late outcome have to change too. As the plasticity of fetal and neonatal brain appears to act in various ways, the link between perinatal insult and unfavorable late outcome remains poorly defined. This cause-effect relationship is easier to demonstrate on neuromotor evaluation within the first year of life, that it is at school-age. Such a short term evaluation, though it has little value in the individual case allows medico-social and pedagogic efforts to be concentrated on a selected high risk-group and enables the progresses in perinatal medecine to be closely monitored.

BIBLIOGRAPHIE

AGRAWAL A.K. Tilson H.A. Bondy S.C. 1981
3.4.3.4. Tetrachlorophenyl given to mice prenatally produces long term decreases in striatal dopamine and receptor binding sites in the candate nucleus.
Toxicology letters 7. 417-424

ALLEVA F.R., BALAZS T. 1980 : Age dependent sensivity of the rat to neurotoxic effects of streptomycin. Toxic. Lett. 6. 385

ALLEVA F.R., BALAZS T., HABERMAN B.H., WEINBERGER B.A., SLAUGHTER L.J. 1980 ; Muscular degeneration in rats after post-natal treatment with 6 Mercaptopurine. Annual meeting Soc. Tox. Washington Abstract 201.

AMIEL-TISON, C. (1979)
Birth injury as a cause of brain dysfunction in full term newborns in "Advances in perinatal neurology".
Korobkin and Guilleminault (Eds).
Spectrum Publ. New-York p. 57-83

AMIEL-TISON, C. (1980)
Possible acceleration of neurological maturation following high risk pregnancy. Am. J. Obstet. Gynecol. 138 : 305 - 306.

BETHENOD M., FREDERICH A. 1975 : les enfants des antiépileptiques.
Pédiatrie 30 ; 227-248.

BIGNAMI, A. and APPICIUTOLI, L. (1964)
Micropolygynia and cerebral calcification in cytomegalic inelusion disease.
Acta neuropath (Berl.) 4 : 127 - 137.

BRAZELTON, T.B. (1973)
Neonatal behavioral assessment scale.
Clinics in developmental medecine n°50.
Heineman Medical Books - Philadelphie pp 66.

BUTCHER R.E., HAWVER K., BURBACHER T., SCOTT W. 1974 ;
Behavioural effects from antenatal exposure to teratogens.
Proc. of the Gatlingburg Conf. on Mental retardation N. Ellis Edit.

CALDWELL M.B., SPILLE D.F., 1964 : Effect on rat progeny of daily
administration of mepromabate during pregnancy and lactation. Nature
(London) 202 : 832 - 833.

DAVIS W.M., LIN C.H. 1972 : Prenatal morphine effects on survival
and behaviour of rat offspring. Research Communications in Chemical
Pathology and Pharmacology 3 : 205-214.

DELEON, G. (1972)
Observations on cerebral and cerebellar microgyria
Acta neuropathe (Berl.) 20 : 278-287.

DISHOTSKY N.I., LOUGHMAN W.D., MOGAR R.E., LIPSCOMB W.R. 1971 :
LSD and genetic damage. Science 172 : 431-440.

FELDMAN G.L., WEAVER D.D., LOVRIEN F.W. 1977 : The fetal trimethadione
syndrome Am.J. Dis. Child 131 ; 1389-1392.

FINELL R.H. 1981 : Phenytoin induced teratogenesis : a mouse model.
Science vol.211 ; p. 483-484.

FRITZ H. 1980 : Effects of prenatal treatment of female rats with hydroxyurea on growth and behaviour of the progeny. Symposium Paris Droit
et Pharmacie ; in Press.

GOLDMAN - RAKIC, P.S. (1980)
Plasticity of the primate telencephalon.
In "Neonatal Neurological assessment and outcome" Report of the 77th
Ross Conference on Pediatric Research.
Columbus, Ohio, Ross Laboratories : p 55 - 64.

GOULD, J.B., GLUCK, L., and KULOVICH, M.V. (1972)
The acceleration of neurological maturation in high stress pregnancy
and its relation to fetal lung maturity, Pediatr. Res. 6 : 276.

GOULD J.B., GLUCK L. and KULOVICH M.V. (1977)
The relationship between accelerated pulmonary maturity and accelerated
neurological maturity in certain chronically stressed pregnancies,
Am.J. Obstet. Gynecol. 127 : 181 - 186.

GRAUWILLER J., LEIST K.H. 1976 : The development of postnatal tests in
the safety evaluation of new drugs. Proceed 5th Conf. Europ. Terat.
Soc. pp. 79-86.

GUSTAVSON, K.H. (1980)
Epidemiology of severe mental retardation.
In "XVI International Congress of Pediatrics".
Abstracts of symposia and colloquia. Ballabriga and Gallart (Eds).
Barcelone p 198.

HAGBERG, B., HAGBERG, G. and OLOW, I. (1980)
The changing panorama of cerebral palsy.
In "XVI International Congress of Pediatrics".
Abstracts of symposia and colloquia. Ballabriga and Gallart (Eds).
Barcelone. p 281.

HANSON J.W., SMITH D.W. 1975 : The fetal hydaintoin syndrome J. PEDIAT
87 ; 285-290.

HOFFELD D.R., WEBSTER R.D. 1965 : Effect of injection of tranquilli-
zing drugs during pregnancy on offspring. Nature (London) 205 : 1070-
1072.

KLETZKIN M., BERGER F.M. 1971 : Influence of meprobamate on the fetus,
fertility and postnatal development ; in Tuchmann-Duplessis : Malformations congénitales des mammifères p. 55-272 (Masson, Paris).

KLETZKIN M., WOJCIECHOWSKI H., MARGOLIN S. 1966 : Tranquillizers in
pregnancy and behavioural effects on the offspring Nature 210 : 1290-
1291.

LANGMAN J., RODIER P., WEBSTER W. et al. 1975 : The influence of teratogens and tissue behaviour during the second half of pregnancy and
their effect on postnatal behaviour. Second Symposium on prenatal development. G. Thieme Edit. pp. 439-468.

LAPRAS M., DESCHANEL J.P., DELATOUR 1973 : Accidents teratologiques
chez le mouton après administration de parbendazole Bull. Soc. Sci.Vet.
Lyon 75 ; 53-61.

LARROCHE, J.C. (1977)
Cytoarchitectonic abnormalities.
In "Hand book of clinical neurology".
Vol 30 - VINKEN, P.J. and BRUYN, G.W. (Eds) ; North Holland Publishing
Cie - Amsterdam p 479-506.

LONG S.Y. 1972 : Does LSD induce chromosomal damage and malformations ?
A review of the litterature. Teratology 6 : 75-90.

LOWE C.R. 1973 : Congenital malformations among infants born to epileptic women. Lancet 1 : 9-10.

LUCIER G.W. DAVIS G.Y. Mc LACHIAN (1978)
Transplacental toxicology of the polychlorinated and polybrominated biphenyls. Handford Symposium NITS. Richland Washington.

MERCIER-PAROT L. 1976 : A propos de l'action tératogène du parbendazole.
Therapie 31 ; 491-503.

NAKANE, TERNO, OKUMA and 12 other associated authors-1980 : - Multi-
institutional study on the teratogenecity and fetal toxicity of antiepi-

leptic drugs. A report of a collaborative study group in Japan. Epilepsia 21 ; 663-680 Raven Press, New-York.

RODIER P.M., REYNOLDS S.S., ROBERT W.N. 1979 ; Behavioural consequences of interference with C.N.S. development in early fetal period. Teratology 19. 3 327-336.

SAINT JAMES ROBERTS, I : (1979)
Neurological plasticity, recovery from brain insult, and child development. In avances on child development and behavior Vol 14 - Reese, H.W. and Lipsitt, L.P. (Eds). Academic Press. Publ. New-York p. 253 - 319.

SEIP M. 1976 : Growth retardation, dysmorphic facies and minor malformations following massive exposure to phenobarbitane in utero. Acta Pediatr. Scand. 65 ; 617-621.

SHAPIRO S., STONE D., HARTZ S.C., ROSENBERG L., SISKIND V., MONSON R.R. MITCHELL A.A., HEINONEN O.P. 1976 ;
Anticonvulsants and prenatal epilepsy in the development of birth defects. Lancet 1 ; 272-275.

SAMEROFF, A.J. (1980)
Social and environmental influences on the developing nervous system. In "Neonatal neurological assessment and outcome". Report of the 77th Ross Conference on Pediatric Research. Columbus, Ohio, Ross Laboratories. p. 55-64.

STONE M.L., SALERNO L.J., GREEN M., ZELSON C. 1971 ;
Narcotic addiction in pregnancy. Amer. J. of Obst. and Gynec. 109 ; 716-723.

TIJO J.H., PAHNKE W.N., KURLAND A.A. 1970 ; LSD and chromosome :
A controlled experiment. Journal of the Amer. Medic. Association 210. 849-856.

TILSON H.A. DAVIS G.Y. Mc. LACHLAN J.A. LUCIER G.W. 1979.
The effects of polychlorinated biphenyls given prenatally on the neuro behavioral development of mice.
Environ. Res. 18 466-474.

TUCHMANN-DUPLESSIS H., MERCIER-PAROT L. 1962 ; Influence de traitements chroniques de réserpine sur la fertilité des partents et de leurs descendants. Comptes rendus des séances.
La Société de Biologie et de ses filiales. 156 : 587-590.

TUCHMANN-DUPLESSIS H., MERCIER-PAROT L. 1973 : Risque tératogène des anticonvulsivants. Bulletin de l'Académie Nationale de Médecine. Séance du 26 Juin.

TUCHMANN-DUPLESSIS H., HISS D., LEGROS J. 1976 :
Teratological and prenatal toxicity evaluations of a new hypolipemic agent. Proceedings of the 5th Conf. of the Europ. Terat. Soc. pp. 235-240.

WERBOFF J., HAVLENA J. 1962 ; Postnatal behavioural effects of tranquillizers administered to the gravid rat. Experimental Neurology 6 ; 263 - 269.

ZELSON C., RUBIO E., WASSERMAN E. 1971 ; Neonatal narcotic addiction 10 year observation Pediatrics 48 ; 178-189.

Maldevelopment of CNS Induced by Perinatal Metabolic Insults and Possibilities of Its Regulation

O. Benešová* and A. Pavlik**

*Dept. of Physiology, Medical School of Hygiene, Charles University,
Prague, Czechoslovakia
**Inst. of Physiology, Czechoslovak Acad. of Sci., Prague,
Czechoslovakia

ABSTRACT

Metabolic insults in the period of "brain growth spurt" in rats
(long-term malnutrition on days 1-40, short-term protein synthesis inhibition by cycloheximide on day 7) resulted in structural
and biochemical brain deviations and behavioral disorders in a-
dulthood. Pyritinol, a nootropic drug, administered for 7-10 days
following the noxious intervention, prevented the brain maldevelopment and functional disturbances in both behavioral teratology
models. Favourable regulatory effects of early and long-term pyritinol treatment on neuropsychopathological sequels of perinatal
distress were confirmed in clinical controlled prospective study
of 128 high-risk newborns.

KEYWORDS

Behavioral teratology models; perinatal distress; brain growth
spurt; high-risk newborns; nootropic drugs; pyritinol.

INTRODUCTION

Perinatal ontogenesis is characterized by growth acceleration
of some organs, in the first place of the brain. The perinatal
period of the "brain growth spurt" (Dobbing 1970) in which the
final histogenesis and differentiation of the brain structures
take place, is known as a sensitive "vulnerable" period of CNS
development. Whereas noxious insult during the early embryonic
stage causes gross malformations, noxious insult in the perinatal period of the fastest brain development leads - according
to its intensity, specificity and timing - to a variety of morphological and biochemical disturbances at cellular or subcellular level. Simultaneously, the brain developmental processes
may be disorganized in their regular sequence and linkage and,
being of once-and-for-all nature, can be compensated only in
limited extent. Thus, the mentioned microstructural and bioche-

mical alterations are transformed during further development
to delayed consequences manifesting themselves as permanent
functional abnormalities. This functional pathology which becomes apparent gradually during maturation and adolescence as
various behavioral deviations is studied by a branch of experimental teratology - behavioral teratology (Werboff and Gottlieb,
1963, Barlow and Sullivan, 1975). An example of such behavioral
teratology syndrome in clinical medicine is the "minimal brain
dysfunction" in children having suffered from perinatal
distress.

The period of "brain growth spurt" is involved in perinatal ontogenesis, but its maximum may be shifted predominantly before
or after birth in dependence on the animal species. In precocial
animals, i.e., those whose youngs are born relatively mature
(e.g., guinea pig, pig, sheep), the phase of rapid brain growth
is the component of prenatal development, whereas in altricial
animals whose youngs are born very immature (e.g., rat, mouse,
rabbit, dog) this phase is shifted postnatally. In man, the period of accelerated brain growth is a real perinatal event: it
begins in the third trimester of gravidity, attains its maximum
just before birth and continues, especially concerning myelination, during first two years of life. (Fig. 1). Thus disturbing
factors interfering at this time represent the greatest danger
for normal development of the human brain.

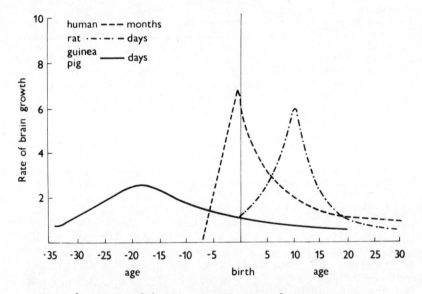

Fig. 1. Rate of brain growth in relation to
        birth in rat, guinea pig and man.
        Adapted from Dobbing (1970).

Fig. 2 illustrates in more details the sequence of three important phases of brain growth, i.e., neurogenesis, gliogenesis
and myelination in man in comparison with two animal species,
mostly used in teratological studies (rat, chicken). Regarding
these relations, its is evident that the full-term human brain

at birth corresponds to a rat brain at a postnatal age of 7-10
days. When a perinatal noxious insult effect, mode of action
and consequences in human are to be studied, an advantageous
model is provided by using the rat in which the critical period
of brain development occurs postnatally so that the investigation need not to be carried out in fetus in utero, but in a
better accesible, already born organism.

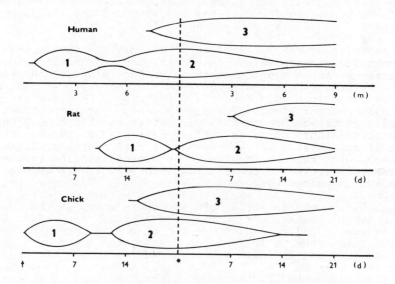

Fig. 2. Sequence of neurogenesis (1), gliogenesis
        including microneurogenesis (2) and
        myelination (3) in the brain of man, rat
        and chicken. (m) months (d) days ↑con-
        ception * birth

These considerations were the reason of choosing the rat as an
experimental animal for our studies of perinatal distress in
highrisk fetuses and high-risk newborns. In these perinatal
risk situations, the main pathophysiological role is played by
the disturbed function of the utero-placental unit (placental
insufficience or abnormality, premature placenta abruption, um-
bilical cord complications, abnormal fetus posture, irregular
uterine activity, prolonged labour etc). In all cases, the fetus
suffers from decreasedsupply of nutrients and oxygen, resulting
in acidosis and other metabolic disturbances which endanger predominantly the susceptible brain cells. Thus the primary risk
factors are nutrients and oxygen deficits.

BEHAVIORAL TERATOLOGY MODELS

1. Long-term Neonatal Malnutrition

Twelve years ago, we have started our studies in rats with the
model of early malnutrition because it had already been described as the cause of brain maldevelopment and delayed deviations of CNS functions by several authors (Barnes and others,
1966; Dobbing, 1968, 1970; Fraňková, 1968; Smart, 1971). But
the aim of our investigation was different from the basic
pathophysiological aspects of mentioned physiologists: we intended to study the possibility of preventing neuropsychopathological consequences of neonatal protein malnutrition by
convenient pharmacological treatment. For this purpose, we decided to use psychotropic drugs from a new group o neurodynamic
agents which are now denoted as "nootropics" (Giurgea 1972).
The main characteristic of their action is the increase of
mental efficiency based on the activation of the bioenergetic
metabolism of the nerve cell (Giurgea, 1977; Benešová, 1979).
In that time, i.e., in the seventies, we had only pyritinol
(Encephabol Merck) and meclophenoxate (=centrophenoxine,
Lucidril Bracco) at disposal. Thus, the model experiments were
carried out using these drugs.

Methodically, the following procedure was used. On the day
after birth, lactating dams with their pups were divided into
two groups: the first group was fed a normal diet with 25cal%
protein, the other a low protein diet containing only 5-8cal%
protein (LP). Litter size was adjusted to 8 pups. All pups
were weaned on day 28. The LP dietary regimen was continued
until day 40. Then LP rats were switched gradually, within 3
days, to normal diet so that from this day, all rats were fed
normal diet until the end of the experiment (250-280 days).
The drug treatment was given in ten doses (40 mg/kg/day, i.p.)
between days 40 and 50, i.e., in the period of nutritional
rehabilitation. The controls were injected by saline. The behavioral and electrophysiological tests were carried out in
adult rats (age 4-7 months), biochemical analysis of the brain
after decapitation at the age of 8 months. Altogether 250 male
and 185 female rats were used.

Adult rats which experienced protein deficit during first 40
postnatal days revealed significant behavioral, electrophysiological and biochemical deviations. They had lower body and
muscle weight (with decreased muscle glycogen concentration).
Their behavior was characterized by hyperactivity with the
features of stereotypy, increased emotionality and enhanced
aggressivity. They displayed higher intertrial reaction rate,
aimless and chaotic movements during conditioning without
significant change in registered criteria of active avoidance
learning. Electrophysiological studies showed sleep disorders
and decreased reactivity in cortical and transcallosal evoked
potentials. Decreased adaptability and deviations in metabolic
stress reaction were recorded in experiments with emotional
stress. Rest levels of nonesterified fatty acids in blood were
significantly higher. Brain biogenic amines (noradrenaline,
dopamine, serotonin) were increased; an exceptionally high
rise was ascertained with 5-hydroxyindolacetic acid, the

principal metabolite of serotonin.

In rats treated with pyritinol in the period of nutritional
rehabilitation (days 40-50), all these behavioral, electrophysiological and biochemical deviations were significantly
reduced, mostly normalized except for anatomical parameters
as body size and muscle fibre diameter (Benešová and others,
1977; Benešová, Pětová and Vinšová, 1980). But when the same
10 day pyritinol treatment was applied later on, at the age of
100 days, it was ineffective. The effects of other drugs tested (meclophenoxate, pyridoxine) were not convincing.

2. Short-term Protein Synthesis Inhibition

The described experimental model of prolonged neonatal malnutrition is, however, not convenient for a more detailed analysis of behavioral teratology mechanisms. The reason lies partly
in multifactorial nature of the insult used, partly in repeated and long-term interference with complex spatio-temporal
pattern of developmental processes. The harmful potential of
the noxious intervention and its dependence on the developmental stage ("vulnerable period") may be more clearly analyzed
in a model with single factor-single application design.

Therefore, behavioral teratology model was established (Pavlík
and Jelínek, 1979; Pavlík and Teisinger, 1980) based on short-
term inhibition of protein synthesis by cycloheximide. Why the
inhibition of protein synthesis? The protein synthesis is an
elementary metabolic process, important especially during development, the alteration of which is more or less the final
common pathway in action of all perinatal risk factors - hypoxia, malnutrition, acidose, intoxication etc. We have shown
that single injection of cycloheximide in rats at the time of
maximum postnatal brain growth, i.e., 7th day, induced reversible and reproducible protein synthesis inhibition which - in
spite of lasting only 12 hours - resulted in morphological,
biochemical and behavioral deviations in adulthood. Using this
experimental model, the corrective activity of nootropic drugs
pyritinol and piracetam (Nootropil UCB) on disturbed brain
development was studied.

Methodically, the experiments were carried out on 60 male rats
divided into 4 groups: a control group injected saline and 3
experimental groups injected cycloheximide (CHX: 0,6 mg/kg, s.
c,) on the 7th postnatal day. From the 8th to 14th day, two
experimental groups were administered pyritinol (30 mg/kg/day,
s.c.) or piracetam (100 mg/kg/day s.c.) while the remaining
groups received saline. The rats were weaned on the 28th day.
They were tested behaviorally between days 100-180 and sacrificed by the age of 6 months. The brains were dissected and the
olphactory bulbs, cerebellum, cerebral cortex and subcortical
structures including basal ganglia, hippocampus, thalamus and
hypothalamus were used for biochemical determinations of protein and nucleic acids. Such dissection of brain structures respects the different speed of their postnatal development. Since
the endocrine system and skeletal muscles undergo also a fast
development in the early postnatal period, the weight of

adrenals and their ascorbic acid concentration, plasma level
of thyroxine and triiodothyronine were assessed, together
with the weight and glycogen concentration of m. biceps
brachii.

Short-term inhibition of protein synthesis induced the retardation of body growth which persisted still in adult rats and
was not influenced by nootropic drugs. The growth of the brain
was also retarded, most markedly in the cerebellum and subcortical structures (data summarized in Table 1). The weight reduction was significantly abolished by pyritinol in the subcortical structures and by both pyritinol and piracetam in the
cerebellum. Reduced protein content in the cerebellum was normalized by both nootropic drugs. The content of DNA which may
be regarded as an indicator of cell number was decreased in
the subcortical structures, cerebellum and olphactory bulbs of
CHX rats. In CHX-pyritinol and CHX-piracetam animals, the cell
numbers in these structures attained the control values. The
changes of RNA were of similar trend (Kubík, Benešová and
Pavlík, 1981).

TABLE 1   Biochemical Changes in the Brain

Group	Weight(mg)	Protein cont.(mg)	DNA cont.(μg)	RNA cont.(μg)
Cerebral cortex:				
Control (saline)	1077+22.4	88.2+6.9	885+42.2	283+5.4
Cycloheximide (CHX)	1057+13.4	94.7+7.2	917+33.5	272+11.8[b]
CHX-pyritinol	1070+10.1	90.4+4.1[b]	963+32.9	312+7.4[b]
CHX-piracetam	1062+14.4	75.2+3.5[b]	917+23.1	282+10.8
Subcort. structures:				
Control (saline)	307+12.5	21.3+1.5	180+6.2[aa]	116+3.4
Cycloheximide (CHX)	265+8.3[aa]	21.0+1.6	153+7.1[aa]	107+2.9[a]
CHX-pyritinol	291+7.0[b]	21.5+1.1	168+5.2	113+2.6
CHX-piracetam	283+7.4	19.7+1.3	165+8.4	111+3.6
Cerebellum:				
Control (saline)	290+7.7[a]	28.5+0.7	1183+17.7[aa]	577+11.4
Cycloheximide (CHX)	270+5.1[a]	26.5+0.5[b]	1077+30.2[aa]	547+12.9
CHX-pyritinol	284+4.2[b]	28.4+0.5[b]	1146+14.4[b]	571+6.9
CHX-piracetam	290+7.7[b]	28.0+0.5[b]	1155+25.2	576+11.5
Olfactory bulbs:				
Control (saline)	97+4.8	8.6+0.4	115+7.3	188+9.9
Cycloheximide (CHX)	91+3.2	8.6+0.3	108+3.0	178+4.0
CHX-pyritinol	93+1.2	9.0+0.2	115+1.9[b]	185+2.4
CHX-piracetam	93+1.7	9.0+0.1	117+2.9[b]	184+2.3

a(aa)...P < 0.05(0.01) vs control group, b... P < 0.05 vs CHX gr.

The maldevelopment of endocrine system was apparent in the reduction of adrenal weight after cycloheximide administration
and was not influenced by nootropic drug treatment. On the
other hand, the decreased concentration of adrenal ascorbic

acid in CHX animals was normalized in both nootropic treated groups. Concerning thyroid hormones, a trend to thyroxine increase and triiodothyronine decrease in plasma was noticed in CHX rats. Significant fall of triiodothyronine level was found in CHX-piracetam group as compared to CHX-pyritinol group (Pavlík and others, 1981).

The open field behavior of CHX group was characterized by hyperactivity with abnormal pattern of behavioral act sequence. These behavioral deviations were not seen in both nootropic treated groups (Fig. 3).

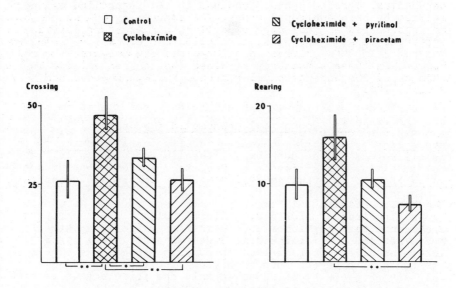

Fig. 3. Horizontal (crossing) and vertical (rearing) activity of male rats in open field (∅ 50 cm) assessed in five 3 min sessions. Statistically significant differences:＊P < 0.05;＊＊P < 0.01

In the test of 24 h retention of passive avoidance (withdrawal of entering shock compartment), the control rats exhibited good long-term memory in 83% animals, while CHX rats only in 46%. The score of CHX-pyritinol group approached control values (70%), but the CHX-piracetam rats (29%) performed even worse than the untreated CHX group. In the 1 h retention test of passive avoidance, as well as in the active avoidance test (two-way shuttle box), no statistically significant difference between groups was found, probably due to unimpaired function of short-term memory.

In motor coordination test (balancing on horizontal rod), 43% of control rats did not reach the criterion, whereas in CHX group 77% of animals. Both pyritinol and piracetam treatment reduced significantly the proportion of failures (39% and 25% resp.). These results correspond to similar differences in the

weight of m. biceps brachii: control = 312.3 + 8.6 mg; CHX-
saline = 265.7 + 7.5 mg; CHX-pyritinol = 287.3 + 8.6 mg; CHX-
piracetam = 295.3 + 4.4 mg. Muscle glycogen concentration was
significantly elevated in CHX-pyritinol group, this result resembling our previous findings in malnutrition model (Benešová
and others,1977, 1980).

The results gained with cycloheximide-induced model of behavioral teratogenesis characterize the extent of long-term consequences at the structural, biochemical and functional (behavioral) level. Further confirmation of regulatory effects of pyritinol on disturbed brain development indicated the usefulness
of this experimental model both for the elucidation of the mechanisms of behavioral teratogenesis (Pavlík, Jelínek and
Teisinger, 1981) and for the testing of development-regulatory
action of nootropic drugs.

PERINATAL DISTRESS IN HIGH-RISK NEWBORNS

Both our model experiments which could be considered to simulate the perinatal distress in high-risk newborns revealed the
favourable effect of pyritinol in the prevention of brain maldevelopment after early noxious metabolic insult. Basing on
these findings and on both experimentally and clinically proved
absence of any toxic effects of pyritinol, a long-term prospective controlled clinical study was carried out in 128 newborns
with high degree of morbidity due to high-risk pregnancy, high-
risk labour or both. All these infants were born in maternity
ward of the Prague University Obstetric Clinic, the same peri-
natological team participating in their prenatal and intranatal
care. The common etiopathological denominator in all cases
(light-for-dates after serious chronic intrauterine distress,
prematures with severe respiratory difficulties and infants
after severe acute hypoxia, saved only due to intensive reanima-
tion and special care in Intensive Neonatal Care Unit) was high
degree of hypoxia, malnutrition and acidosis with signs of
brain disturbance (Table 2). In addition to the special intensive neonatal and subsequent rehabilitation care, pyritinol (increasing dosage 16-80 mg daily, p.o.) was administered in 66
infants starting on the 3rd day after birth up until the age of
4-12 months, according to the neurological findings. The psychomotor development of the treated group in comparison with the
control group (62 cases) was followed up by the team of child
neurologist, paediatrician and psychologist. At the age of 5
years, the neurological evaluation revealed significant differences between both groups (Table 3).

Normal neurological findings were found in 88% of cases in the
treated group, but only in 47% of the control, the rest having
various neurological disorders. The percentage of severe handicaps (cerebral palsy, epilepsy, mental deficiency) was 7.5 in
the treated group in comparison with 38.7 in the controls
(Benešová, Pětová and Vinšová, 1980, Pětová, Vinšová and
Benešová, 1980).

Pyritinol treatment, given to another group of 50 babies with
similar perinatal histories, but started at the age of over

TABLE 2   Perinatal Characteristics of High-Risk Newborns

	Group 1 pyritinol n=66		Group 2 control n=62	
	n	%	n	%
High-risk pregnancy	62	93.9	55	88.7
Risk labour:	63	95.4	58	93.5
premature	48	72.7	40	64.5
hypoxia	50	75.7	42	67.7
Newborns:				
low birth-weight (1-2.5 kg)	41	62.1	43	69.4
Apgar score < 7 points: 1st min	51	77.3	50	80.6
10th min	27	40.9	25	40.3
Postnatal complications:				
hyaline membrane disease	55	83.3	47	75.8
cerebral oedema	14	21.2	8	12.9
intracranial haemorrhage	8	12.1	6	9.7
convulsions	18	27.3	10	16.1
alteration in muscle tone	45	68.2	40	64.5

TABLE 3   Neurological Evaluation at the Age of 5 Years

	Group 1 pyritinol n=66		Group 2 control n=62	
	n	%	n	%
Normal	58	87.9	29	46.8
Cerebral palsy - spastic form	3	4.5	11	17.7
Cerebral palsy - spastic form + epilepsy			3	4.8
Cerebral palsy - spastic form + exitus*	1	1.5		
Cerebral palsy - hypotonic form + oligophrenia	1	1.5	4	6.5
Cerebral palsy - hypotonic form + oligophrenia + epilepsy			1	1.6
Minimal brain dysfunction	1	1.5	4	6.5
Epilepsy			4	6.5
Mental deficiency (IQ 70)			1	1.6
Retardation of speech development	2	3.0	5	8.1

* exitus from intercurrent infection at the age of 15 months

6 months when the pathological neurological picture was already
developed, was effective only in disorders of speech development, but not in motor and mental defects (Pětová, 1970).

CONCLUSION

Summing up our results, it was proved, both experimentally and
clinically, that there exists the possibility of pharmacological intervention helping in prevention of brain maldevelopment
after perinatal metabolic insults. It may be assumed that
pyritinol acts as a neurodynamic stimulus for the disturbed
nerve cell metabolism. It activates the cell bioenergetic processes and increases the macromolecule synthesis, potentiates
the utilization of nutrients offered and accelerates recovery,
thus eliminating the danger of continuing destructive processes
and/or disorganization in the sequence and spatial linkage of
developmental events. In this way, the deficit in development
and maturation of the brain may be still caught up and brain
maldevelopment prevented. The important condition of sucessful
intervention is, however, the early commencement of pyritinol
administration. Treatment started later on when the metabolic
disturbance resulted already in cell damage and tissue defect
can hardly help - as it was evident both in animal experiments
and clinical trial.

Described experiments illustrate some ways and aims of the research in behavioral teratology. The basic task of this scientific branch is obviously the elucidation of behavioral teratology mechanisms. The findings of some authors (Mabry and Campbell, 1977; Lundborg and Engel, 1978; Engel and Lundborg, 1979;
Kellogg and others, 1980; Rosengarten and Friedhoff, 1980;
Coyle and others, 1980; Johnston, Carman and Coyle, 1981) indicate the possibility to interfere with the development of defined brain structures, distinct receptors and neurotransmitters by using specific drugs and timing. Such models of impaired
CNS functions may be perspectively employed in psychopharmacology or basic neuropsychiatry research. Our experiments modell-
ing brain damage induced by perinatal distress and investigating the maldevelopment-regulatory action of drugs confirmed the
usefulness for the neonatological practice.

REFERENCES

Barlow, S.M., and F.M. Sullivan (1975). Behavioral teratology.
    In C.E. Berry and D.E. Poswillo (Eds), Teratology - Trends
    and Application, Springer, Berlin, pp. 103-120.
Barnes, R. H., J. Robertson-Cunnold, R. R. Zimmermann, H. Sim-
    ons, R. B. MacLeod, and L. Krool (1966). Influence of nutri-
    tional deprivations in early life on learning behavior of
    rats measured by performance in water maze. J. Nutr., 84,
    399-410.
Benešová, O. (1979). Pharmacology of nootropic drugs. In O.
    Benešová and Q. Kümpel (Eds), Nootropic Drugs, UCB, Brussels.
Benešová, O., K. Tikal, J. Hvizdošová, S. Franková, V. Beneš,
    J. Mysliveček, and L. Puzanová (1977). Effect of pyrithioxine
    and pyridoxine on late consequences of early malnutrition in

rats. Activ. nerv. sup. (Praha), 19, 131-133.
Benešová, O., J. Pětová, and N. Vinšová (1980). Perinatal Distress and Brain Development, Avicenum, Prague.
Coyle, J. T., M. Beaulieu and M. V. Johnston (1980). Fetally-induced cortical lesions with a mitotic disruptor: effects on synaptic chemistry. Prog. Neuro-Psychopharmacol., Suppl. p. 116.
Dobbing, J. (1968). Effect of experimental undernutrition on development of the nervous system. In N. S. Scrimshaw and J. E. Gordon (Eds), Malnutrition, Learning and Behavior, MIT Press, Cambridge, pp. 181-202.
Dobbing, J. (1970). Undernutrition and the developing brain. In W. A. Himvich (Ed.), Developmental Neurobiology, Thomas, Springfield, pp. 211-261.
Engel, J. and P. Lundborg (1979). Increased mesolimbic ^{3}H-spiroperidol binding in 4 week old offspring of nursing rat mothers treated with penfluridol. Europ. J. Pharmacol., 60, 393-395.
Franková, S. (1968). Nutritional and psychological factors in the development of spontaneous behavior in the rat. In N. S. Scrimshaw and J. E. Gordon (Eds), Malnutrition, Learning and Behavior, MIT Press, Cambridge, pp. 312-326.
Giurgea, C. (1972). Vers une pharmacologie de l'activité intégrative du cerveau. Tentative du concept nootrope en psychopharmacologie. Actual Pharmac., 25e série, Masson, Paris, pp. 115-156.
Giurgea, C. and M. Salama (1977). Nootropic drugs. Prog. Neuro-Psychopharmacol, 1, 235-247.
Johnston, M.V., A. B. Carman and J.T. Coyle (1981). Effects of fetal treatment with methylazoxymethanol acetate at various gestational dates on the neurochemistry of the adult neocortex of the rat. J. Neurochem., 36, 124-128.
Kellogg, C., R. K. Miller, J. Chisholm and R. Simmons (1980). Benzodiazepine exposure: influence on neural and behavioral development. Prog. Neuro-Psychopharmacol., Suppl., 202.
Kubík, V., O. Benešová and A. Pavlík (1981). Protein and nucleic acid changes in the brain of adult rats injured by neonatal short-term inhibition of protein synthesis and the effect of nootropic drugs. Activ. nerv. sup. (Praha), 23, 51-53.
Lundborg, P. and J. Engel (1978). Neurochemical brain changes associated with behavioral disturbances after early treatment with psychotropic drugs. In A. Vernadakis, E. Giacobini and G. Filogamo (Eds), Maturation of Neurotransmission, Karger, Basel, pp. 226-235.
Mabry, P. D. and B. A.Campbell (1977). Developmental psychopharmacology. In L. L. Iversen, S. D. Iversen and S. H. Snyder (Eds), Principles of Behavioral Pharmacology, Plenum Press, New York, pp. 393-444.
Pavlík, A. and R. Jelínek (1979). Effect of cycloheximide administered to rats in early postnatal life: correlation of brain changes with behavior in adulthood. Brain Res., 167, 200-205.
Pavlík A., and J. Teisinger (1980). Effect of cycloheximide administered to rats in early postnatal life: prolonged inhibition of DNA synthesis in the developing brain. Brain Res., 192, 531-541.

210   O. Benešová and A. Pavlík

Pavlík, A., R. Jelínek and J. Teisinger (1981). In S. Trojan
   and F. Šťastný (Eds), Ontogenesis of the Brain, Tom 3,
   Charles University, Prague, in press.
Pavlík, A., O. Benešová, V. Kubík, S. Stoilov, M. Vávrová,
   A. Hankeová and J. Nedvídková (1981). Late consequences of
   neonatal short-term inhibition of protein synthesis in adult
   rats and the effects of nootropic drugs: a biochemical and
   behavioral study. Activ. nerv. sup. (Praha), 23, in press.
Pětová, J. (1970). Experiences with Encephabol therapy in
   children with CNS damage. Conference on Encephabol, Prague.
Pětová, J., N. Vinšová and O. Benešová (1980). Psychomotor
   development of high-risk newborns and its modification by
   early and long-term pyritinol administration. Activ. nerv.
   sup. (Praha), 22, 107-108.
Rosengarten, H. and A. J. Friedhoff (1980). Critical factors
   in prenatal neuroleptic effect on dopamine receptor maturation. Prog. Neuro-Psychopharmac., Suppl., 301.
Smart, J. L. (1971). Long-lasting effects of early nutritional
   deprivation on the behavior of rodents. Psychiatrie, Neuro-
   logie, Neurochirurgie, 74, 443-452.
Werboff, J. and J. S. Gottlieb (1963). Drugs in pregnancy:
   behavioral teratology. Obstetric. Gynec. Survey, 18, 420-425.

Altered Postnatal Development Following Intrauterine Exposure to Hormonally Active Chemicals

J. A. McLachlan* and S. E. Fabro**

*Transplacental Toxicology Section, Laboratory of Reproductive
and Developmental Toxicology, National Institute of Environmental
Health Sciences, Research Triangle Park, NC 27709, USA
**Department of Obstetrics and Gynecology, Georgetown University
Medical Center, Washington, DC, USA

ABSTRACT

Prenatal exposure to many drugs and other chemicals is associated with functional or structural defects which may only be expressed later in postnatal
life (transplacental toxicology). Such induction of long-term effects by
intrauterine chemical exposure has been reported for many organ systems including the immune system, central nervous system, and hepatic drug metabolizing enzymes. Of special interest is the developing reproductive system
in which exposure to foreign compounds, such as alkylating agents and polycyclic aromatic hydrocarbons, is associated with depletion of germ cells and
subsequent infertility of the mature individual. Prenatal exposure to hormonally active environmental chemicals such as diethylstilbestrol (DES) is
associated with impaired reproductive capacity in the male and female offspring of both mice and humans. In mice, intrauterine exposure to DES is
associated with congenital defects of the ovary and oviduct (developmentally
arrested oviduct) which are obvious at birth. Progressive changes in other
genital tissues (cervical enlargement, uterine squamous metaplasia, cystic
endometrial hyperplasia) following prenatal DES treatment may contribute to
the observed infertility. These long-term late effects induced by DES in
utero seem to require a secondary postnatal stimulus by estrogen for their
expression. These results suggest that late teratogenic effects may have
multiple critical periods.

KEY WORDS

Prenatal chemical exposure; transplacental toxicology; oviductal teratology;
diethylstilbestrol; infertility; critical periods; environmental estrogens.

INTRODUCTION

Many drugs and other chemicals enter our environment every year. Concern
has developed over the years regarding exposure of pregnant women to these

agents and the subsequent effects on their offspring. It has been known for
some three decades that the mammalian conceptus can be damaged by exposure
to chemicals during development. The resultant damage may be expressed at
birth (early teratogenic effect) or may only be expressed later in life
(late teratogenic effect or transplacental toxicity). The best known example of the early teratogenic effect is thalidomide, which caused malformations in fetuses (and observed in newborns) with little or no demonstrable
toxic effects on the mother (Fabro and Smith, 1966). There are many other
examples of teratogenic agents in animals as well as humans (Shepard, 1973).

TRANSPLACENTAL TOXICOLOGY

Only a few chemicals have been studied for their prenatally associated effects on postnatal development. Thus, structural or functional defects may
be induced by chemicals at any stage of gestation and expressed or detected
later in life. For example, abnormalities of the immune system in adult
animals have been reported following their intrauterine exposure to lead
(Luster and others, 1978), TCDD (Vos and Moore, 1974), PCBs (Luster and
others, 1980), hexachlorobenzene (Vos and coworkers, 1979) or diethylstilbestrol (Luster and coworkers, 1979).

It has been well known for many years that the sex behavior of adult laboratory animals can be irreversibly modified by perinatal exposure to estrogenic or androgenic hormones (Gorski, 1971). Moreover, it was recently reported that prenatal exposure to synthetic progestins increased the potential for physical aggression in both male and female offspring (Reinisch,
1981). Less well known are experiments which demonstrate that common environmental chemicals including ,p'-DDT (Nelson and others, 1978) or kepone
(Gellert, 1978) have long lasting effects on sex behavior which may be
attributed to their weak estrogenic effects (McLachlan, 1980). Prenatal
exposure to a single PCB isomer has been associated with behavioral abnormalities in the offspring (Lucier and coworkers, 1978) and related ultrastructural lesions in the central nervous system (Chou and others, 1979).

Similar long term effects on hepatic function have been reported following
developmental exposure to TCDD (Lucier and coworkers, 1975) or PCBs (Lucier
and McDaniel, 1979). This developmental imprinting of hepatic enzymes may
play an important role in altering the postnatal response to other xenobiotics and, thus, may have a more general biological significance. In the
rat, at least, developmental exposure to specific PCB isomers resulted in
altered hepatic steroid metabolism in the adults (Dieringer and others,
1979).

Another example of an altered postnatal response associated with prenatal
chemical exposure is the report of Alexandrov and colleagues (1980) that glucose utilization in the oral glucose tolerance test of 3 month old female
rats treated on the 21st day of pregnancy with N-nitrosomethylurea was significantly decreased when compared to untreated controls.

TRANSPLACENTAL TOXICOLOGY: INFERTILITY IN OFFSPRING

It is clear from these few examples that the induction of long-term alterations in postnatal function by prenatal exposure to diverse chemicals is an
important toxicological problem. Moreover, these examples also demonstrate
that many developing organ systems may be at risk. However, when considering

these long-term consequences or latent expression of toxic effects induced during the prenatal period, certain developing organ systems may be at particular risk.

For example, the development of the genital tract and subsequent attainment of fertility is a process which is extremely vulnerable to disruption by environmental agents. In most eutherian mammals, including mice and humans, the female fetus is extremely vulnerable to germ cell toxicants since the development of the oocyte occurs prenatally with no new germ cells formed after birth (Zuckerman, 1962). Therefore, any change induced in the fetal oocyte by chemicals during the prenatal period may result in decreased reproductive capacity of the offspring which will not be evident until much later in the animal's life when sexual maturity is reached. Reduced fertility in the offspring may be the most obvious consequence of prenatal exposure to toxic environmental chemicals. It could also include the possibility of long-term genetic damage to the developing germ cell or transplacental carcinogenic changes in fetal genital organs. Recently, several compounds have been shown to alter reproductive tract function following prenatal exposure to them (Table 1). Reduced fertility is commonly observed in each case of genital tract dysfunction.

Cytological and biochemical evidence show that the mitotic activity and DNA synthesis of female germ cells (oocytes) ceases by birth in both the mouse (Peters and Crone, 1967) and human (Baker, 1971) and resumes again only at the time of ovulation and fertilization of the mature egg. Therefore, chemicals which affect the female germ cell during oogenesis may be expected to have a lasting effect of the fertility of the female. Especially chemicals which alter DNA synthesis, such as alkylating agents (e.g. procarbazine, cyclophosphamide, and busulfan, Table 1), can be expected to interfere with germ cell replication and development. When female mouse fetuses are exposed to procarbazine during the peak of oocyte DNA synthesis (day 12-13) their fertility as adults was decreased more than females exposed before (day 10) or after (day 17) this critical period (McLachlan and colleagues, in press). Severe alterations in gonadal morphology were apparent in these mice.

Another alkylating agent, busulfan, has been reported to result in gonadal dysplasia in both male and female rats exposed to it in utero (Forsberg and Olivecrona, 1966). It is interesting that Diamond and colleagues (1960) had already reported marked ovarian hypoplasia in a small-for-gestational-age infant whose mother was treated for leukemia with busulfan.

Fetal ovaries may also be a target site for the action of some environmental pollutants, particularly polycyclic aromatic hydrocarbons (PAH); PAH are known to deplete primordial germ cells in rodents and primates (Dobson and colleagues, 1978). In fact, exposure of mice in utero to dimethylbenzanthracene results in depletion of both male and female germ cells at birth, and infertility after maturation (Davis and others, 1978). Similar results have been obtained with benzo(a)pyrene (MacKenzie and others, 1979).

TABLE 1   Some Compounds Which Alter Reproductive Tract Function After
Prenatal Exposure

Compound Given to Mother	Major Effects in Offspring	Species	
Dimethylbenzanthracene (DMBA)	Gonadal dysplasia and reduced fertility	Mouse	(1)
Benzo(a)pyrene	Gonadal dysplasia and reduced fertility	Mouse	(2)
Methoxychlor	Reduced fertility	Rat	(3)
Diethylstilbestrol (DES)	Genital tract abnormalities and reduced fertility in females	Mouse	(4)
	Genital tract abnormalities and reduced fertility in females	Human	(5)
	Genital tract abnormalities and reduced fertility in males	Mouse	(6)
	Genital tract abnormalities including semen pathology	Human	(7)
Clomid	Reproductive tract alterations	Rat	(8)
Methyl methanesulfonate	Sterility in males	Rat	(9)
Procarbazine	Gonadal dysplasia and reduced fertility in females	Mouse	(10)
Cyclophosphamide	Reduced fertility	Mouse	(11)
Busulfan	Gonadal dysplasia	Rat	(12)
	Ovarian hypoplasia	Human	(13)
Cyanoketone	Altered estrous cycles	Rat	(14)
Phenobarbital	Altered reproductive tract function in females	Rat	(15)

This list is not comprehensive but represents some examples of chemicals
reported to alter fertility after prenatal exposure.

(1) Davis, et. al., 1978
(2) MacKenzie, et. al., 1979
(3) Harris, et. al., 1974
(4) McLachlan, 1977.
(5) Herbst, et. al., 1980.
(6) McLachlan, et. al., 1975.
(7) Bibbo, et. al., 1975.
(8) McCormack and Clark, 1979.
(9) Lang, 1977
(10) McLachlan, et. al, in press.
(11) Sotomayer and Cumming, 1975
(12) Forsberg and Olivecrona, 1966.
(13) Diamond, et. al, 1960.
(14) Shapiro, et. al., 1974.
(15) Gupta, et. al., 1980.

Exposure to hormonally active chemicals during gestation should be expected to alter reproductive performance in offspring. Congenital defects have been associated with glucocorticoids (Salomon and Pratt, 1979) and synthetic progestins (Matsunaga and Shiota, 1979), but few long-term effects have been described. Recently Jones and Pacillas-Verjan (1979) have described the induction of cervicovaginal tumors in mice treated neonatally with progesterone suggestive of lesions induced with estrogens.

TRANSPLACENTAL TOXICOLOGY OF DIETHYLSTILBESTROL (DES)

The long-term effects of developmental exposure to estrogens has been extensively studied in animals and humans. Moreover, as shown in Fig. 1, this is a functional class of chemicals with widely diverse structures. Thus, many drugs and other environmental chemicals have the potential for estrogenic activity. Among these compounds, diethylstilbestrol (DES) has special interest for our laboratory.

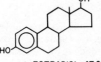
ESTRADIOL-17β

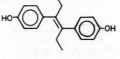
DIETHYLSTILBESTROL

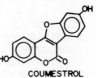
COUMESTROL

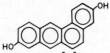
3,9-DIHYDROXYBENZ[a]ANTHRACENE

O,P-DDT

TETRAHYDROCANNABINOL(Δ⁹-THC)

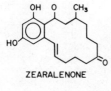
ZEARALENONE

KEPONE

2,8-DIBENZYLCYCLOOCTANONE

Fig. 1. Chemicals of diverse structure reported to be estrogenic. Detailed references are given in McLachlan, 1980.

DES was extensively used for over two decades as a drug to treat threatened abortion in women. The association of such treatment with a low incidence of vaginal malignancies (vaginal adenocarcinoma) in the offspring of such DES treated pregnancies is well known (Herbst and others, 1971). Other abnormalities of the vaginal epithelium such as adenosis or cervical hooding have been much more common in young women exposed prenatally to DES (Herbst and colleagues, 1975). Only recently, Herbst and others (1980) have reported altered reproductive capacity in DES-exposed women (Table 1). Similarly, genital tract abnormalities and semen pathologies in males have been associated with in utero exposure to DES (Bibbo and colleagues, Table 1).

Studies in our laboratory have focused on developing a mouse model in which vaginal adenosis or vaginal adenocarcinoma is observed in the female offspring of mice exposed during gestation to DES (McLachlan and colleagues, 1980).

As seen in Table 1, both male (McLachlan and colleagues, 1975) and female (McLachlan, 1977; McLachlan and colleagues, in press), offspring of DES-treated mice have decreased fertility. Genital tract lesions observed in the human males as well as in male mice treated in utero with DES include epididymal cysts, retained testes, sperm abnormalities, and prostatic inflammation; these lesions are inconsistent with normal fertility.

Ovarian-Oviductal Teratology

The mechanisms underlying the dose-related infertility seen in female mice exposed prenatally to DES is as yet unclear. However, at least two components of the postnatal alteration in reproductive function induced by prenatal exposure to DES can be described; one is observed early, the other late.

Altered differentiation of the ovary and oviduct is obvious at birth in gestationally DES exposed mice (McLachlan and colleagues, 1980); the oviduct retains a fetal anatomical position and has been termed developmentally arrested. Ovaries from DES treated mice also are congenitally defective with tubule-like structures in the medulla of the organ which are apparently of mesonephric duct origin. The ovaries of young treated animals have similar numbers of follicles as those in untreated control females but, following stimulation with exogenous gonadotropins, fewer ova are ovulated (McLachlan and colleagues, in press).

Postnatal Stimulation of Prenatally-induced Abnormality

The defects noted in the ovaries and oviducts of mice treated in utero with DES may be considered as early teratogenic effects. In fact, grafts of fetal ovaries from DES treated mice into the kidney capsules of untreated hosts expresses the structural abnormalities observed in the ovaries of DES treated adult mice. Other lesions of the reproductive tract observed in DES treated mice, including cervical enlargement, cystic endometrial hyperplasia and squamous metaplasia of the uterine epithelium of DES treated mice, seem to be progressive changes (McLachlan and colleagues, 1980) and thus, are appropriately considered late effects. As with the ovarian and oviductal changes, these genital tract lesions contribute to the decreased fertility in DES-exposed mice, which, at the highest doses (10 or 100 μg/kg/day), result in essential sterility throughout their reproductive life (McLachlan and colleagues, in press).

The contribution of secondary cues or stimuli to the expression of latent, long-term abnormalities induced prenatally is of great theoretical and practical interest. Are structural or cellular defects (including neoplasia) observed in adults following prenatal exposure to foreign chemicals mediated

by a second postnatal stimulus? A classical example in chemical carcinogenesis suggests that this may sometimes be the case. The work of Goerttler and Loehrke (1976) demonstrated that prenatal exposure to the potent
carcinogen, dimethylbenzanthracene (DMBA), at critical periods of pregnancy
in the rat was associated with skin tumors in the offspring only when their
skin was painted postnatally with the tumor-promoting phorbal ester, TPA.
The length of time between prenatal and postnatal chemical treatments and
the relationship of the critical period for embryonic induction to the presence of specific fetal skin stem cells (T. Slaga, personal communication)
points up the importance of temporal factors in the induction and subsequent
stimulation of expression of these skin lesions.

Similar considerations seem to apply to animals exposed developmentally to
DES. Boylan and Calhoon (1979) have demonstrated that when rats were exposed in utero to DES, postnatal treatment with DMBA resulted in a significantly greater yield of mammary tumors than in rats which were treated with
DMBA but received no prenatal treatment with DES.

Our laboratory has studied whether a second postnatal stimulus with estrogen
is required for the expression of the genital tract lesions which follow
prenatal exposure to DES. This is especially interesting since DES lesions
seen in human females have been associated with puberty. The role of postnatal exposure to estrogen in the final expression of the genital tract
tumors observed in mice exposed in utero to DES is not yet clear. However,
earlier lesions associated with infertility in this group of mice appear
to require a second exposure to estrogen for their expression. For example,
squamous metaplasia of the uterine epithelium is a common feature of adult
female mice whose mothers had been given DES (Fig. 2). However, if similarly DES exposed females are ovariectomized before puberty, no squamous
metaplasia is observed (McLachlan and colleagues, in preparation). Then if
the prepubertally ovariectomized mice are given injections of DES on days
22-24 of age, squamous metaplasia is observed in all the animals. Moreover,
this lesion persists in the absence of ovaries or additional estrogen treatment. Similar results were obtained for cervical enlargement and cystic
endometrial hyperplasia. Experiments to determine the contribution of
postnatal estrogen treatment to prenatal induction of genital tract tumors
are currently underway.

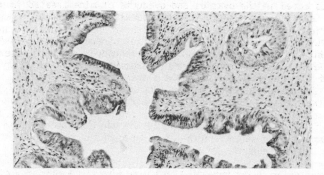

Fig. 2.   Squamous metaplasia of the uterine epithelium. The mouse
was treated prenatally with DES (100μg/kg/day on days 9-16 of gestation) and postnatally ovariectomized and treated with DES (100μg/
kg/day on days 22-24).

Similar studies using neonatally estrogen-treated mice reported that secondary estrogen treatment of ovariectomized adults did not appreciable affect the promotion of vaginal lesions when compared to ovariectomized mice which received neonatal estrogen treatment alone (Kawashima and co-workers, 1980). However, ovariectomy in this series of animals was done long after puberty and irreversible secondary stimulation may have already occurred. Thus, prenatally induced abnormalities observed later in life may not only require a second promotional stimulus for their expression but the time at which the postnatal stimulus occurs may also be critical.

These results suggest that for some functional defects induced by chemicals in utero which persist into postnatal life, there may be at least two critical periods: one for induction, the other for stimulation. Both are required for expression of the abnormality. Thus, the life experience of an individual may help to fix into its functional or structural repertoire, defects induced during development.

ACKNOWLEDGEMENT

The contribution to this work of R.R. Newbold is gratefully acknowledged. The authors thank Ms. Susan DeBrunner and Ms. Dawn Tabon for artful manuscript typing.

REFERENCES

Alexandrov, V. A., V. N. Anisimov, N. M. Belous, I. A. Vasilyeva, and V. B. Mazon (1980). The inhibition of the transplacental blastomogenic effect of nitrosomethylurea by postnatal administration of buformin to rats. Carcinogenesis, 1, 975-978.

Baker, T. G. (1963). A quantitative and cytological study of germ cells in human ovaries. Pro. Roy. Soc. Biol., 158, 417-433.

Bibbo, M., M. Al-Nageeb, I. Baccarini, W. Gill, M. Newton, K. M. Sleeper, M. Sonek, and G. L. Wied (1975). Follow-up study of male and female offspring of DES-treated mothers. A preliminary report. J. Reprod. Med., 15, 29-31.

Boylan, E. S., and R. E. Calhoon (1979). Mammary tumorigenesis in the rat following prenatal exposure to diethylstilbestrol and postnatal treatment with 7, 12-dimethylbenz(a)anthracene. J. Toxicol. Environ. Health, 5, 1059-1071.

Chou, S. M., T. Miike, and G. J. Davis (1979). Experimental induction of Werdnig-Hoffmann-type neuroglial peninsulas by prenatal PCB intoxication. In, T. Tsubaki, and Y. Toyokura (Ed.), Amyotrophic Lateral Sclerosis, University of Tokyo Press, Tokyo, pp. 239-262.

Davis, G. J., J. A. McLachlan, and G. W. Lucier (1978). The effect of 7, 12-dimethylbenz-a-anthracene (DMBA) on the prenatal development of gonads in mice. Teratology, 17, 33A.

Diamond, I., M. M. Anderson, and S. R. McCreache (1960). Transplacental transmission of busulfan (Myleran) in a mother with leukemia. Pediatrics, 25, 85-90.

Dieringer, C. S., C. A. Lamartiniere, C. M. Schiller, and G. W. Lucier (1979). Altered ontogeny of hepatic steroid-metabolizing enzymes by pure polychlorinated biphenyl congeners. Biochemical Pharmacology, 28, 2511-2514.

Dobson, R. L., C. G. Koehler, J. S. Felton, T. C. Kwan, B. J. Weubbles, and D. C. L. Jones (1978). Vulnerability of female germ cells in developing mice and monkeys to tritium, gamma rays, and polycyclic aromatic hydrocarbons. In, D. D. Mahlum, M. R. Sikov, P. L. Hackett, and F. D. Andrew (Ed.), Developmental Toxicology of Energy-Related Pollutants., Technical Information Center, U. S. Department of Energy, pp. 1-14.

Fabro, S. E., and R. L. Smith (1966). The teratogenic activity of thalidomide in the rabbit. J. Pathol. Bacteriol., 91, 511-519.

Forsberg, J. G., and H. Olivecrona (1966). The effect of prenatally administered busulfan on rat gonads. Bio. Neonate, 10, 180-192.

Gellert, R. J. (1978). Kepone, mirex, dieldrin, and aldrin: estrogenic activity and the induction of persistent vaginal estrus and anovulation in rats following neonatal treatment. Environmental Research, 16, 131-138.

Goerttler, K., and H. Loehrke (1976). Diaplacental carcinogenesis: initiation with the carcinogens dimethylbenzanthracene (DMBA) and urathane during fetal life and postnatal promotion with the phorbol ester, TPA, in a modified 2-stage Berenblum/Mottram experiment. Virchows Arch. (Pathol. Anat.), 372, 29-38.

Gorski, R. A. (1971). Gonadal hormones and the perinatal development of neuroendocrine function. In, L. Martini, and W. F. Ganong (Ed.), Frontiers in Neuroendocrinology, Oxford University Press, New York, pp. 237-282.

Gupta, C., B. R. Sonawane, S. J. Yaffe, and B. H. Shapiro (1980). Phenobarbital exposure in utero and alterations in female reproductive function in rats. Science, 208, 508-510.

Harris, S. J., H. C. Cecil, and J. Bitman (1974). Effect of several dietary levels of technical methoxychlor on reproduction in rats. J. Agr. Food Chem., 22, 969-973.

Herbst, A. L., H. Ulfelder, and D. C. Posknazer (1971). Adenocarcinoma of the vagina: association of maternal stilbestrol therapy with tumor appearance in young women. N. Engl. J. Med., 284, 878.

Herbst, A. L., D. C. Poskanzer, and S. J. Robboy (1975). Prenatal exposure to stilbestrol: a prospective comparison of exposed female offspring with unexposed controls. New Engl. J. Med., 292, 334-339.

Herbst, A. L., M. M. Hubby, R. R. Blough, and F. Azizi (1980). A comparison of pregnancy experience in DES-exposed and DES-unexposed daughters. J. of Reprod. Med., 24, 62-69.

Jones, L. A., and R. Pacillas-Verjan (1979). Transplantability and sex steroid hormone responsiveness of cervicovaginal tumors derived from female BALB/cCrgl mice neonatally treated with ovarian steroids. Cancer Res., 39, 2591-2594.

Kawashima, S., T. Mori, T. Kimura, Y. Arai, and Y. Nishizuka (1980). Effects of estrogen treatment on persistent hyperplastic lesions of the vagina in neonatally estrogenized mice. Endocrinol. Japon., 27, 533-539.

Lang, R. (1977). Heritable translocation test and dominant-lethal assay in male mice with methyl methanesulfonate. Mutation Research, 48, 75-88.

Lucier, G. W., B. R. Sonawane, O. S. McDaniel, and G. E. R. Hook (1975). Postnatal stimulation of hepatic microsomal enzymes following administration of TCDD to pregnant rats. Chem. -Biol. Interactions., 11, 15-26.

Lucier, G. W., J. A. McLachlan, and G. J. Davis (1978). Transplacental toxicology of the polychlorinated and polybrominated biphenyls. In, D. D. Mahlum, M. R. Sikou, P. C. Hackett, F. D. Andres (Ed.) Developmental Toxicology of Energy-Related Pollutants., Technical Information Center, U. S. Department of Energy. pp. 188-203.

Lucier, G. W., and O. S. McDaniel (1979). Developmental toxicology of the halogenated aromatics: effects on enzyme development. Annals New York Academy of Sciences., 77, 449-457.

Luster, M. I., R. E. Faith, and C. A. Kimmel (1978). Depression of humoral immunity in rats following chronic developmental lead exposure. J. Environ. Path. and Toxicol., 1, 397-402.

Luster, M. I., R. E. Faith, J. A. McLachlan, and G. C. Clark (1979). Effect of in utero exposure to diethylstilbestrol on the immune response in mice. Toxicol. Appl. Pharmacol., 47, 287-293.

Luster, M. I., G. A. Boorman, M. W. Harris, J. A. Moore (1980). Laboratoy studies on polybrominated biphenyl-induced immune alterations following low-level chronic or pre/postnatal exposure. Int. J. Immunopharmacol., 2, 69-80.

MacKenzie, K. M., G. W. Lucier, and J. A. McLachlan (1979). Infertility in mice exposed prenatally to benzo-a-pyrene (BP). Teratology, 19:37A.

Matsunaga, E., and K. Shiota (1979). Threatened abortion hormone therapy and malformed embryos. Teratology, 20, 469-480.

McCormack, S. A., and J. H. Clark (1979). Clomid administration to the pregnant rat causes abnormalities of the reproductive tract in offspring and mothers. Science, 204, 629-631.

McLachlan, J. A. (1977). Prenatal exposure to diethylstilbestrol in mice: toxicological studies. J. Toxicol. Environ. Health, 2, 527-537.

McLachlan, J. A. (Ed.) (1980). Estrogens in the Environment., Elsevier North Holland, New York.

McLachlan, J. A., R. R. Newbold, and B. Bullock (1975). Reproductive Tract lesions in male mice exposed prenatally to diethylstilbestrol. Science, 190, 991-992.

McLachlan, J. A., R. R. Newbold, and B. C. Bullock (1980). Long-term effects on the female mouse genital tract associated with prenatal exposure to diethylstilbestrol. Cancer Research, 40, 3988-3999.

McLachlan, J. A., R. R. Newbold, K. S. Korach, J. C. Lamb, IV, and Y. Suzuki: Transplacental toxicology: prenatal factors influencing postnatal fertility. In, C. A. Kimmel, and J. Buelke-Sam (Ed.), Developmental Toxicity, Raven Press, New York, (in press).

Nelson, J. A., R. F. Struck, and R. James (1978). Estrogenic activities of chlorinated hydrocarbons. J. Toxicol. Environ. Health, 4, 325-340.

Peters, H., and M. Crone (1967). DNA synthesis in oocytes of mammals. Arch. Anat. Micro. Morph. Exp., 56, 160-170.

Reinisch, J. M. (1981). Prenatal exposure to synthetic progestins increases potential for aggression in humans. Science, 211, 1171-1173.

Salomon, D. S., and R. M. Pratt (1979). Involvement of glucocorticoids in the development of the secondary palate. Differentiation, 13, 141-154.

Shapiro, B., A. S. Goldman, and A. W. Root (1974). Prenatal interference with the onset of puberty, vaginal cyclicity and subsequent pregnancy in the female rat. Proc. Soc. Exper. Biol. and Medicine, 145, 334-339.

Shepard, T. H. (1973). Catalog of Teratogenic Agents. Johns Hopkins University Press, Baltimore, Maryland.

Sotomayer, R. E., and R. B. Cumming (1975). Induction of translocations by cyclophosphamide in different germ cell stages of male mice: cytological characterization and transmission. Mutation Research, 27, 375-388.

Vos, J. G., and J. A. Moore (1974). Suppression of cellular immunity in rats and mice by maternal treatment with 2, 3, 7, 8-tetrachlorodibenzo-p-dioxin. Int. Arch. Allergy Appl. Immunol., 47, 777-789.

Vos, J. G., M. J. van Logten, J. G. Kreeftenberg, P. A. Steerenberg, and W. Kruizinga (1979). Effect of hexachlorobenzene on the immune system of rats following combined pre- and postnatal exposure. Drug Chem. Toxicol., 2, 61-76.

Zuckerman, S. S., (Ed.) (1962). The Ovary, Vol. I. Academic Press, New York and London.

WORKSHOP
Alcohol Intoxication and Withdrawal

Moderators: K. Kuriyama, R. G. Thurman

Alcohol Intoxication and Withdrawal:
Introductory Remarks

K. Kuriyama* and R. G. Thurman**

*Dept. of Pharmacology, Kyoto Prefectural University of Medicine,
Kyoto, Japan
**Dept. of Pharmacology, University of North Carolina, Chapel Hill,
N.C., USA

HISTORICAL COMMENTS

Alcohol produced and imbibed from at least the six century has been surrounded by wonder and regulation. Alcoholic beverages have played a central role in all cultures to date. On the other hand, alcoholism is a worldwide social and medical problem, and the accumulation of basic and clinical knowledge to prevent and/or to cure this disease is urgently needed by our modern society. In the past, few pharmacologists have been interested in alcohol research, however,in recent years a growing number of basic scientists including pharmacologists have been attracted to the subject.

BACKGROUND ON ALCOHOL RESEARCH

Pharmacology of alcohol covers a multitude of scientific disciplines ranging from basic biochemistry of the liver and biophysics of cellular membranes to electrophysiology of the central nervous system. Behavioral, psychological and social consequences of alcoholism, prophylactic and therapeutic aspects of alcoholism, and medico-legal aspects of acute alcohol intoxication should be also included in the topics on alcohol research. Presently our information in these area is rather incomplete.

ETHANOL METABOLISM

The metabolism of ethanol has been reviewed repeatedly. The metabolic and nutritional aspects, however, are impossible to separate from other effects of alcohol on the organism. It seems necessary for a coherent discussion to include also these aspects of the physiology of alcohol.
Elimination of ethanol from the organism is almost entirely due to its oxidation mainly in the liver. The first step in alcohol breakdown, ethanol to acetaldehyde, is catalyzed predominantly by the enzyme alcohol dehydrogenase (ADH) which was the first NAD^+-dependent enzyme ever purified from yeast by Negelein and Wulff (1937). Isoenzymes of ADH have been found in man (von Wartburg et al., 1965), rhesus monkey (Papenberg et al., 1965), and rat (Koen and Shaw, 1966).
In addition to ADH, several alternative pathways of ethanol metabolism have

been reported. An NADPH-dependent oxidase catalyzing the oxidation of ethanol
to acetaldehyde has been reported to exist in microsomes obtained by frac-
tionation of livers. Lester and Benson (1969) estimate that the enzyme
account for less than 10 % of the hepatic oxidation of ethanol. Keilin and
Hartree (1936) also demonstrated that catalase can catalyze the oxidation of
ethanol to acetaldehyde. However, peroxide formation in tissues is too slow to
permit very much oxidation of ethanol by catalase. Therefore none of these alternative pathways are considered to be of great significance quantitatively.
The second step in alcohol breakdown, acetaldehyde to actate, is catalyzed by
the NAD^+-dependent aldehyde dehydrogenase. The aldehyde dehydrogenase from
human liver has a very low K_m for acetaldehyde and a very high reaction rate
which explains, in part, why acetaldehyde is not accumulated during the oxidation of ethanol.
Further metabolism of acetate formed from ethanol in the citric acid cycle
occurs mainly extrahepatically. In this process, part of the carbon from
ethanol will be incorporated into amino acids, carbohydrates, C_4 compounds
and lipids.
The rate-limiting step in the break-down of ethanol is the conversion to
acetaldehyde by ADH. Under most conditions, this reaction is regulated by
the supply of the cofactor NAD^+. The reoxidation of NADH appears,in turn,to
be limited by the regulation of energy metabolism. Glucose, fructose and
other monosaccharides, as well as pyruvate, succinate, proteins and amino
acids have all been used in attempts to increase the rate of elimination of
ethanol.

METABOLIC CHANGES INDUCED BY ETHANOL: METABOLIC TOLERANCE

The effects of ethanol on the over-all energy metabolism have been studied intensivel
by various investigators. Ethanol increases the oxygen consumption, alters NAD^+
redox state and inhibits the citric acid cycle in the liver. One of the most
important metabolic changes which occurs during oxidation of ethanol is that
the NAD^+/NADH ratio decreases in the liver and kidneys. Since a great number
of metabolic reactions are inhibited by the change in the redox state of the
cell, it seems important to obtain quantitative data on this aspect of the
effect of ethanol.
Fatty infiltration of the liver has been known as a complication of alcoholism for a long time. It is generally considered that the accumulation of
triglycerides in the liver following continuous ethanol administration is due
to an increase in α-glycerophosphate and peripheral lipolysis coupled with
the inhibition of β-oxidation of acyl CoA compounds by the elevated NADH
redox state.
Little is known about the effect of ethanol on protein and nucleotide metab-
olisms. Although it has been reported that ethanol may decrease the turnover
of protein in the liver, it seems likely that small and moderate dose of
ethanol may have little effect on nitrogen balance.
Metabolic tolerance to ethanol has been known for a long time. This is
defined as the ability of the liver to increase the rate of ethanol elimination following either acute (Yuki and Thurman, 1980) or chronic (Thurman et
al., 1976) treatment of ethanol. This phenomenon involves an accleration
of the rate of reoxidation of NADH due to the effect of ethanol on ATPase
activities in the liver including a decrease in glycolysis (Yuki and
Thurman, 1980) and an increase in Na^+- plus K^+-activated ATPase activity
(Bernstein et al.,1973).

CELLULAR BASIS OF THE ACTION OF ETHANOL ON THE NERVOUS
SYSTEM: CENTRAL NERVOUS SYSTEM TOLERANCE

Presumably the euphoric effect of ethanol on the central nervous system is
the main basis for the widespread use of alcoholic beverages. Since any explanation of the effect of ethanol will involve the molecular mechanism by
which ethanol changes the function of individual nerve cells, intensive studies
have been conducted on this topic in last decade or so. Many electrophysiological, neurochemical and neuropharmacological data have been accumulated on
the cellular basis of ethanol action on the nervous system. Ethanol usually
diminishes the resting potential of nerve and muscle fibers, apparently by
increasing permeability of the membranes to sodium ions. Decrease of the
resting membrane potential to a level which depresses the excitability also
progressively diminishes the action potential until blockage finally ensues.
With respect to transmitter substance, many data concerning synthesis, release, action, and removal are available. Among various transmitters tested,
changes in acetylcholine and biogenic amines seem most closely related to
the central actions of ethanol. For example, ethanol enhances the action of
acetylcholine and of related depolarizing drugs. Ethanol also interacts in
a complex way with calcium, generally antagonizing its effects. This
antagonism is of considerable interest since calcium ions are very important
as stabilizers of the membrane structure and as generators of the action
potential.
Ethanol has also clearly been shown to produce tolerance to many biological
processes (e.g., drop in temperature, sleeping time, etc.). One important
aspect of the mechanism of tolerance to ethanol recently proposed is that
ethanol molecules, by their tendency to assume particular orientation at
lipid-water interphases, may influence charge distribution and interfere
with conformational changes essential for normal membrane function. For
example, ethanol interacts with membraneous cholesterol and subsequently
alters the fluidity of neuronal membranes (Goldstein, this session). The
alteration in fluidity due to ethanol may be attributable, at least in part,
to the central action of ethanol. Also withdrawal of ethanol in ethanol
dependent subjects induces rapid and significant increase in cerebral β-
adrenergic receptor binding as well as an activation of cerebral cyclic AMP
generating system. When animals which have inhaled ethanol for 10 days were
withdrawn, a statistically significant increase in [³H]-dihydroalprenolol
(DHA) binding to brain particulate fractions occurred in 8 hrs (Kuriyama et
al., 1981). Since the activity of cyclic AMP-dependent protein kinase in
synaptic membrane fractions from the brain also increased in these animals,
the following hypothesis is proposed: During ethanol withdrawal, an abrupt
increase in β-adrenergic receptor responsiveness may lead to the increase of
intracellular cyclic AMP and subsequently activate the cyclic AMP dependent
protein kinase in synapses. The resulting increase in phosphorylated protein
in synapses may play an important role in the occurrence and/or maintenance
of the abstinence syndrome, possibly by changing the functional state of
synaptic membrane.
The above two examples may give some suggestions on the future direction for
the studies on molecular neuropharmacology of ethanol.

CONCLUSION

In this workshop we have attempted to present and to discuss recent advances
and future prospects in this rapidly growing research area in pharmacology.
Due to the shortage of time, we have limited ourselves to the effect of
ethanol on the liver and brain.
The present state of this research field seems like a typical, classical
Japanese painting: The aim and figure are quite clear, but are very vague in

details. To clarify the details, obviously continuous and systematic funda-
mented research efforts on the pharmacology of alcohol should be intensified.

REFERENCES

Bernstein, J., Videla, L. and Israel, Y. (1973) Biochem.J., 134, 515-522.
Koen, A.L. and Sham, C.R. (1966) Biochem.Biophys.Acta., 128, 48-54.
Kuriyama, K., Muramatsu, M., Aiso, M. and Ueno, E. (1981) Neuropharmacol.,
20, 659-666.
Lester, D. and Benson, G.D. (1969) Fed.Proc., 28, No.2, 546.
Negelein, E. and Wulff, H.J. (1937) Biochem.Z., 293, 351-389.
Papenberg, J., Wartburg, J-P,von and Aebi, H. (1965) Biochem.Z., 342, 95-
107.
Thurman, R.G., McKenna, W.R. and McCaffery, T.B. (1975) Mol.Pharmacol.,
12, 156-166.
Von Wartburg, J-P., Papenberg, J. and Aebi, H. (1965) Can.J.Biochem.Physiol.,
43, 889-898.
Yuki, T. and R.G. Thurman (1980) Biochem.J., 186, 119-126.

KEYWORDS

Alcohol intoxication, Alcohol withdrawal, Ethanol metabolism, Metabolic
changes induced by ethanol,Cellular basis of ethanol action, Metabolic
tolerance, CNS tolerance.

The Role of Mitochondrial NADH Reoxidation in the Hepatic Metabolism of Ethanol: Studies with Perfused Livers from Ethanol and CCl4-Treated Rats

T. Yuki*, R. G. Thurman** and K. Kuriyama*

*Dept. of Pharmacol., Kyoto Pref. University of Medicine,
Kamikyo-Ku, Kyoto 602, Japan
**Dept. of Pharmacol., University of North Carolina, Chapel Hill,
N.C. 27514, USA

ABSTRACT

The effect of ethanol and CCl4 treatments on alcohol dehydrogenase (ADH) dependent metabolism of ethanol was assessed employing a non-recirculating hemoglobin-free liver perfusion system. The administration of one large dose of ethanol (5 g/kg) nearly doubled hepatic O_2 and ethanol uptakes within 2.5 hrs. This Swift Increase in Alcohol metabolism (SIAM) may be explained as follows: Ethanol produces a stress reaction which leads to a increase in circulating catecholamine. This in turn activates glycogenolysis leading to decreased ATP synthesis by glycolysis. Ultimately ADP not phosphorylated via the anaerobic pathway activates O_2 uptake. This sequence of events then stimulates ethanol metabolism by providing more NAD^+ for the ADH reaction. In another experimental series, acute and chronic CCl4 treatments decreased hepatic ethanol uptake as well as O_2 consumption approximately 50 % and 70 %, respectively. CCl4 treatment did not significantly alter hepatic ADH activity but changed mitochondrial NADH oxidation in both groups significantly. The present results clearly indicate that the mitochondrial NADH reoxidation system plays a major role determining rates of hepatic metabolism of ethanol.

INTRODUCTION

It is well documented that alcohol dehydrogenase (ADH) plays a major role in hepatic ethanol metabolism, and non-ADH pathways (e.g., catalase; Thurman, Hesse & Scholz, 1974; and microsomal ethanol oxidizing system (MEOS); Lieber & DeCarli, 1970) contributes very little to total ethanol oxidation in vivo. When ethanol is metabolized to acetaldehyde by ADH, the cofactor NAD^+ is reduced to NADH. The reoxidation of NADH is most likely the rate-limiting step in ethanol metabolism in the liver (Theorell & Chance, 1951; Videla, L. et al ., 1973). Recently, we have studied hepatic ethanol metabolism using a non-recirculating hemoglobin-free liver perfusion system (Scholz, Hansen & Thurman, 1973). This system has many advantages over the methods of isolated hepatocytes and liver slices, since various metabolic parameters such as mitochondrial respiration and hormone responses are well preserved. First, we studied the rapid adaptive increase in ethanol metabolism. Many investigators have demonstrated that an enhanced ethanol metabolism is seen in animals (Videla, Bernstein & Israel, 1973) and humans (Mendelson, Stein & Mello, 1965) following chronic exposure to ethanol. This increase involves the

ADH pathway, since it is sensitive to 4-methylpyrazole, an inhibitor of alcohol dehydrogenase. In addition, it has been found that this phenomenon occurs at low ethanol concentration (< 1 mM), where the operation of non-ADH-dependent pathway may be minimal. Furthermore, ethanol treatment increased both oxygen and ethanol uptakes in liver slices (Bernstein, Videla & Israel, 1973) and perfused liver (Thurman, McKenna & McCaffrey, 1976). This increase in oxygen uptake is responsible for the stimulation of ethanol metabolism by enhancing the reoxidation of NADH. Wendell & Thurman (1979) have shown that one single large dose of ethanol (5.0 g/kg) increases the rate of ethanol metabolism approximately 60 % in the rat in vivo within few hours. This observations also have shown that one large dose of ethanol stimulates hepatic oxygen uptake in such a short period of time. The experiments reviewed here were designed to determine the minimal time needed to rapidly increase ethanol metabolism in the perfused liver.

In the second study, CCl₄ was employed to investigate the effect of liver damage on ethanol metabolism. While it is well established that the liver metabolizes approximately 90 % of ethanol, it is not clear whether or not ethanol oxidation is impaired in human (Lieberman, 1963) and animal (Khanna et al., 1971) studies in the presence of liver injury. Most of these studies, however, measured the rate of elimination of ethanol from blood in vivo and estimated the effect of liver injury upon the hepatic metabolism of ethanol. Under these conditions, the possible involvement of various extrahepatic factors such as the distribution of ethanol and the effect of drugs administered concomitantly should be taken into consideration. Therfore, in this study, we have used the perfused liver to examine directly the effect of acute and chroni treatment with CCl₄ on ethanol metabolism.

MATERIALS AND METHODS

Animals

In first study, female albino Sprague-Dawley rats (80-150 g) were allowed free access to laboratory chow and water. Some rats were starved 24 hrs before surgical preparation. Ethanol treated rats were given one single dose of ethanol (5.0 g/kg) 2.5 hrs before surgery. Control rats were intubated with 0.9 % NaCl. Adrenalectomized and hypophysectomized rats were employed for the study at 1 week and 2 weeks after surgery, respectively.

In the second study, fed male Wistar rats (120-200 g) were employed. Rats were divided into 3 groups. Control rats received olive oil in the same volume as the treated animals. For acute CCl₄ treatment, a single dose of 4.16 mmoles of CCl₄/kg was given i.p. as a 20 % v/v solution in olive oil 24 hours before perfusion. For chronic treatment, rats received 2.08 mmoles/kg CCl₄ twice weekly for 8 to 12 weeks.

Non-Recirculating Hemoglobin-Free Liver Perfusion

The perfusion technique has been described elsewhere (Scholz, Hansen & Thurman, 1973). The perfusion fluid was Krebs-Henseleit bicarbonate buffer, pH 7.4, saturated with O_2/CO_2 (19/1). The perfusate flowed past an oxygen electrode before it was discarded to determine the oxygen concentration polarographically. Metabolic rates were calculated from the influent minus effluent concentration differences, the flow rate and the liver wet weight.

Biochemical determinations

Samples of the effluent perfusate were collected every 2 min. for determination of glucose, lactate, pyruvate, β-hydroxybutyrate and acetoacetate by standard enzymatic procedures (Bergmeyer, 1963). Alcohol dehydrogenase (ADH) activity was determined in the 105,000 x g supernatant fraction as described Crow et al., (1977). Catalase activity was measured in the liver homogenate according to Lück (Bergmeyer, 1963). The microsomal ethanol oxidizing system

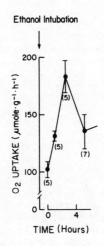

Fig. 1. Effect of ethanol administration in vivo on
         oxygen consumption by perfused liver.

(MEOS) activity was assayed using the 105,000 x g pellet by the method of
Lieber & DeCarli (1968). The activity of mitochondrial NADH oxidation was
measured on isolated pure mitochondria by the method of Rawat & Kuriyama
(1972). Plasma catecholamine concentrations in portal venous blood was
determined by radioenzymatic techniques (Peuler & Johnson, 1977). Protein
content was determined by the method of Lowry et al.(1951). Statistical
comparisons were performed using Student's t-test.

RESULTS & DISCUSSION

Swift Increase in Alcohol Metabolism (SIAM)
To determine the minimal time necessary for ethanol to increase hepatic oxygen
uptake, rats were given ethanol (5.0 g/kg) via gastric intubation. Basal rates
of oxygen uptake by the ethanol-free perfused livers were between 100-110
μmoles/g/h and were unchanged by gastric intubation with saline. The oxygen
uptake increased swiftly and nearly doubled 2.5 hrs after ethanol treatment
(Swift Increase in Alcohol Metabolism; SIAM)(Yuki & Thurman, 1980). The
respiration subsequently declined nearly to basal values at 5 hrs.(Fig. 1.).
This increase in respiration was blocked approx. 75-80 % by KCN (2 mM), an
inhibitor of mitochondrial respiration under these conditions, the rate of
ethanol uptake was also nearly doubled [control (8), 68 ± 8 μmoles/g/h:
ethanol-treated (7), 137 ± 14 (P < 0.01)] and was inhibited approximately 80 %
by 4-methylpyrazole, an inhibitor of ADH. These data suggest that ADH and
mitochondrial respiration are involved in the mechanismof this phenomenon.
However, acute ethanol treatment did not affect the activities of ADH, MEOS
or catalase. The livers from animals treated with ethanol were characterized
by low glycogen contents and rates of glycolysis of only 30 % of control values.
Since glycolysis is an ATP-producing reaction, the inhibition of glycolysis
is equivalent to the stimulation of an ATPase and supply more ADP for mitochondrial respiration. Because the activation of oxygen uptake was rapid
(2-3 hr), the involvement of hormonal factors may be involved. This hypothesis

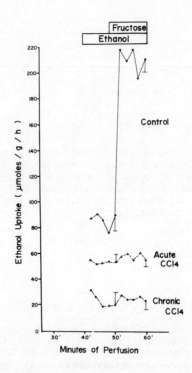

Fig. 2. Ethanol (1.5 mM) and Fructose (4. mM) stimulated
rates of ethanol uptake in perfused livers from
normal and CCl₄-treated rats.
Each point represents the mean ± S.E.M. for 4-5
animals.

is supported by the observation that epinephrine (2 mg/kg) injected into the
rat partially mimicked the observed increase in O₂ uptake due to ethanol. In
addition, the increase in hepatic respiration was blocked by phenoxybenzamine
(40 mg/kg), an α-blocker, and propronolol (40 mg/kg), a β-blocker, as well as
by adrenalectomy and hypophysectomy. Finally, plasma levels of both epinephrine
and norepinephrine were elevated by ethanol treatment approximately 80 % above
the control level indicating that the rapid increase in hepatic oxygen uptake
may be triggered, at least in part, via ethanol-mediated release of catecholamines.
One possible explanation for the consequence of metabolic events responsible
for the SIAM as follows; hormone secretion stimulated by ethanol leads to a
depletion of glycogen, which in turn causes glycolysis to decline. Since
glycolysis is an ATP-producing reaction, ADP not phosphorylated via glycolysis
enters the mitochondria and is phosphorylated by the electron transport chain.
As a consequence of these events, NADH is reoxidized at a faster rate thereby
providing more NAD⁺ for the reaction of ADH with ethanol.

Ethanol Metabolism in Carbon Tetrachloride-Treated Rats
Carbon tetrachloride is actively metabolized in liver to the CCl₃ radical

(Recknagel, 1967). This production of radicals has been shown to diminish a number of membrane bound enzyme fractions (Christie and Judah, 1954) and to enhance the peroxidation of lipids (Slater, 1969). Previously, Khanna et al. showed that acute treatment with CCl_4 abolished cytochrome P-450 mediated ethanol oxidation without affecting the rate of ethanol elimination in vivo. This study strongly suggests that microsomal ethanol oxidation does not play a major role in the elimination of ethanol in vivo. On the other hand, it is possible that CCl_3 generation could also damage mitochondrial membranes and diminish the rate of NADH reoxidation.

Acute and chronic CCl_4 treatments decreased ethanol uptake by the perfused liver by approximately 50 % and 75 % respectively (Fig. 2). The addition of fructose (4 mM), agent which increases the supply of NAD and accelerates ethanol oxidation by increasing reoxidation of NADH (Scholz & Nohl, 1976), doubled the rate of ethanol uptake in livers from control rats. In contrast, no such increase in the hepatic uptake of ethanol was seen in livers from CCl_4-treated animals (Fig. 2). The activity of ADH was unaltered by CCl_4 treatment, while catalase and MEOS activities were reduced significantly. The ratios of lactate/pyruvate and β-hydrobutyrate/acetoacetate reflect the cytosolic and mitochondrial NADH/NAD redox states, respectively (Bücher, 1970). Following acute CCl_4 treatment, the lactate/pyruvate ratio was unchanged, whereas chronic CCl_4 treatment tended to increase this ratio. In contrast, the β-hydroxybutyrate/acetoacetate ratio was increased approximately 3-4 fold following both acute and chronic treatment with CCl_4. In addition, mitochondria isolated from the livers of animals treated with CCl_4 for 24 hrs oxidized NADH at rates of about 65 % of control. Moreover, chronic CCl_4 treatment reduced mitochondrial NADH oxidation by approximately 70 %. Both acute and chronic CCl_4 treatments inhibited hepatic oxygen uptake 16 % and 51 %, respectively. Ethanol (1.5 mM) infusion and the addition of fructose (4 mM) stimulated oxygen uptake in livers from control rat but not in livers from CCl_4-treated rats.

The generation of CCl_3 radical from CCl_4 most likely damages the mitochondrial membrane as evidenced by decreased O_2 uptake by the perfused liver and diminished NADH oxidation by isolated mitochondria. Further, the failure of fructose to stimulate O_2 uptake following CCl_4 treatment suggests that ADP regulation of oxidative phosphorylation has been lost. Thus, these data are consistent with the hypothesis that the decrease in ethanol metabolism observed in this study by CCl_4 treatment is due primarily to a decrease in the rate of NADH reoxidation for the ADH reaction. Under the conditions of this study, non-ADH pathways were minimized by employing 1.5 mM ethanol, a value one order of magnitude below the concentration of ethanol for activation of ethanol by non-ADH pathways.

KEY WORDS

SIAM; glycolysis; Oxygen uptake; ethanol metabolism; Liver perfusion; CCl_4-treated liver; mitochondrial NADH oxidation.

REFERENCES

Bernstein, J., L. Videla and Y. Israel (1973). Biochem.J., 134, 515-522.
Bergmeyer, H.U. (1963); Methods of enzymatic analysis. Academic press, New York, Weinham/Bergstr; Verlag Chemie. GMBH
Bücher, T. (1970). In Sund, H. (eds) Pyridine Nucleotide Dependent Dehydro- genases. New York, Springer. pp.439-461.
Christie, G.S. and Judah, J.D. (1954). Proc.Roy.Soc., Ser.B. 142, 241-257.
Crow, K.E., N. Cornell, R.L. Veech (1977). Alcoholizm Clin.Exp.Res., 1, 43-47.
Khanna, J.M., H. Kalant, G.G. Lin and G.O. Bustos (1971). Biochem.Pharmacol., 20, 3269-3279.

232   T. Yuki, R. G. Thurman and K. Kuriyama

Lieber, C.S. and L.M. DeCarli (1968). Science, 162, 917-918.
Lieber, C.S. and L.M. DeCarli (1970). J.Biol.Chem., 245, 2505-2512.
Lieberman, F.L. (1963). Gastroenterology, 44, 261-266.
Lowry, O.H., N.J. Rosebrough, A.L. Farr, and R.J. Randall (1951). J.biol.
    Chem., 193, 265-275.
Mendelson, J., S. Stein and N. Mello (1965). Metabolism, 14, 1255-1266.
Peuler, J.D. and G.A. Johnson (1977). Life Sci., 21, 625-636.
Rawat, A.K. and K. Kuriyama (1972). Arch.Biochem.Biophys., 152, 44-52.
Recknagel, R.O., S. Malamed (1958). J.Biol.Chem., 232, 705-713.
Recknagel, R.O. (1967). Pharmacol.Rev., 19, 145-208, 1967.
Scholz, R., W. Hansen, and R.G. Thurman (1973). Eur.J.Biochem., 38, 68-73.
Scholz, R. and H. Nohl (1976). Eur.J.Biochem., 63, 449-458.
Slater, T.F. (1969). In Bajusz, E. and Jasmin, G. (eds) Methods and
    Achievements in Experimental Pathology, Karger, Basel pp.30.
Theorell, H. and B. Chance (1951). Acta Chem.Scand., 5, 1127-1144.
Thurman, R.G., S. Hesse, and R. Scholz (1974). In R.G. Thurman, T. Yonetani,
    J.R. Williamson and B. Chance (eds), Alcohol and Aldehyde Metabolizing
    Systems, Academic Press. New York pp.257-270.
Videla, L., J. Berstein, and Y. Israel (1973). Biochem.J., 134, 507-514.
Wendell, G.D. and R.G. Thurman (1979). Biochem.Pharmacol., 28, 273-279.
Yuki, T. and R.G. Thurman (1980). Biochem.J., 186, 119-126.

Ethanol and Membrane Cholesterol

D. B. Goldstein, J. H. Chin, C. K. Daniels, L. M. Parsons and R. C. Lyon

Department of Pharmacology, Stanford University School of
Medicine, Stanford, California 94305, USA

ABSTRACT

Ethanol is among the drugs whose potencies can be predicted from their lipid
solubilities. Physical chemical methods reveal what it does in this hydrophobic
environment; it disorders the membrane bilayer. Order parameters are reduced by
ethanol and by other alcohols, in proportion to their in vivo potency. When mice are
chronically treated with ethanol, their cell membranes become tolerant to the
disordering effects of ethanol, and these tolerant membranes contain more cholesterol than controls. Studies with model membranes made of egg lecithin and
cholesterol showed that the sterol makes membranes more ordered, and it also
blocks the disordering effect of ethanol. Furthermore, ethanol facilitates the
transfer of cholesterol between membranes. We speculate that changes in membrane cholesterol, mediated by ethanol itself, may contribute to ethanol tolerance.

KEYWORDS

Ethanol; cholesterol; membrane; lipid; tolerance; erythrocytes; EPR.

During the past several years, our laboratory has studied chronic effects of ethyl
alcohol in mice. We are interested in the molecular mechanism of functional
tolerance and physical dependence. Our general hypothesis is that functional
tolerance and physical dependence represent adaptive mechanisms, whereby the
organism offsets the initial drug effects. Having done so, it has become maladapted
for a drug-free state, with the result that abnormalities occur on withdrawal of the
drug. This general notion applies to any addicting drug. Investigators seeking the
adaptive mechanisms have focussed on proteins, since most drugs act by binding to
proteins. Ethanol, however, may have a different mode of primary action for which
lipids are more important than proteins. We know from early work (Meyer, 1901;
Seeman, 1972) that ethanol is among the drugs whose potency can be predicted from
their lipid solubility, so we assume that this drug has its primary site of action in a
hydrophobic region of the cell. There are several such regions among the lipids and
protein surfaces, but perhaps the most likely is the lipid bilayer of the cell

membrane. It is this site that we have been examining.

The techniques of physical chemistry have recently been used to show that anesthetic drugs disorder lipid bilayers. They disrupt the packing of phospholipids, allowing spin label probes to report more motion (Trudell and co-workers, 1973; Paterson and co-workers, 1972). The electron paramagnetic resonance (EPR) and nuclear magnetic resonance evidence (Metcalfe and co-workers, 1968) along with calorimetric and fluorescence studies in model membranes (Lee, 1976; Jain and Wu, 1977) suggests that the drugs act by their mere presence in membranes, loosening the bonds between adjacent lipid or protein molecules. We used a sensitive EPR technique to show that low concentrations of ethanol disorder mouse brain and erythrocyte membranes (Chin and Goldstein, 1977a). The effect is significant at ordinary intoxicating concentrations of ethanol, below the lethal range, and it is dose-related; at high ethanol concentrations or when more lipid-soluble alcohols are used, the disordering effect is much larger (Lyon and co-workers, in press). The potency of aliphatic alcohols increases with chain length, in parallel with their increase in lipid solubility and hypnotic potency in vivo. Thus there are excellent correlations between membrane disordering, lipid solubility, and anesthetic potency for this series of compounds.

Next, we inquire how cells respond to the continuous presence of a disordering substance in their membranes. Do they adapt in some way, perhaps analogously to 'homeoviscous adaptation' in bacteria (Sinensky, 1974), modifying their membrane lipids so as to offset the change in their environment? We looked first to see whether membranes from mice that had been chronically treated with ethanol had changed their response to ethanol in vitro (Chin and Goldstein, 1977b). We treated mice for eight or nine days with ethanol in a liquid diet, using controls pair-fed an isocaloric sucrose-containing diet. Their synaptosomal plasma membranes and erythrocyte membranes, washed free of ethanol, and spin-labeled with 5-doxyl-stearic acid, had normal order parameters in vitro. With this probe, which monitors motion fairly near the surface of the membrane, there was no indication that the membranes had become more ordered in response to ethanol. However, when ethanol was added back in vitro, the membranes were found to be resistant to the disordering effect of the drug. In other words, the membranes were tolerant.

We then considered what kind of a biochemical change could have made this physical difference in the membranes. Any of the lipids might have changed. Indeed, a change had already been shown in the fatty acid composition of brain membrane phospholipids in mice that had been treated chronically with ethanol (Littleton and John, 1977). We chose to look at cholesterol, which is probably the most important determinant of membrane fluidity in mammalian plasma membranes. We found that the membranes of the tolerant mice contained slightly but significantly more cholesterol than those of normal mice (Chin and co-workers, 1978). This was true in red cells, where there might be a trivial explanation if serum cholesterol had changed, and it was also true in synaptosomal plasma membranes, where it may be more meaningful. Others have replicated this finding (Johnson and co-workers, 1979).

Recently, we looked at the problem in two more ways, asking reciprocal questions: How does cholesterol influence the sensitivity of membranes to ethanol? And how might ethanol cause a change in membrane cholesterol? To study the former, we used model membranes of egg lecithin with different proportions of cholesterol, and studied their order parameters with two spin labels, 5- and 12-doxylstearic acid (Chin and Goldstein, 1981). The probes sample different depths in the membrane and they reveal the well-known fact that membranes are more fluid at their core than near the surface. Ethanol is not a very lipid-soluble compound; its hydroxyl group might be expected to hold it near the aqueous interface. We thought there might be no effect of ethanol at the regions monitored by the 12-doxylstearic acid label. Unexpectedly we found that there was more disruption with the 12- than with the 5-position label. In other experiments we used synaptosomal plasma membranes labeled with 5-, 12-, or 16-doxylstearic acid and again found larger effects of ethanol at deeper locations. Ethanol clearly has a stronger effect halfway down the acyl chains than at the surface. We used this same model system to study the ordering effects of cholesterol. Addition of cholesterol increased the order parameter; the effect was greater with the 12-doxyl than with the 5-doxyl label. This is also a bit surprising, since the rigid sterol nucleus of the cholesterol extends down only to about the ninth carbon along the chain (Huang, 1977). It now appears that the magnitude of changes in order parameters with different labels tells us little about the location of the drug; it does tell us that the drug effect is strongly felt in the deep regions of the bilayer.

The model system allows us to examine whether cholesterol affects the sensitivity of membranes to ethanol. Addition of cholesterol to phosphatidylcholine liposomes decreased their sensitivity to ethanol. Cholesterol progressively blocked the ethanol effect. This is qualitatively consistent with the in vivo observation that cholesterol was increased in ethanol-tolerant membranes. However, the quantitative agreement is not as good. When we used model membranes that contained high concentrations of cholesterol such as exist in plasma membranes (40 mol % or more), addition of 10% more sterol had little or no effect on the order parameter or the sensitivity to ethanol. We do not know whether model membranes differ from biomembranes in this respect.

Finally, we are looking at the mechanism by which chronic ethanol exposure causes the membrane cholesterol to increase. Is there a physiologic feedback mechanism that monitors the membrane fluidity and activates transfer systems? Perhaps there is, but we started with a simpler hypothesis. Perhaps the mere presence of ethanol in membranes might allow them to take up more cholesterol; we might see this in vitro in the absence of physiologic controls. We incubated red cells with various cholesterol donors, labeled with tritiated cholesterol, and followed the movement of cholesterol. As is well known, cholesterol exchanges readily among plasma lipoproteins and erythrocytes. We could follow the process to equilibrium. When the donors contained high levels of cholesterol, as in cholesterol-enriched plasma or in high-cholesterol model membranes, there was a net transfer of sterol into the red cells; low-cholesterol donors did not cause a net transfer but the exchange could be followed with the radioactive label. Halftimes for this process varied with the cholesterol donor. Whole plasma, HDL, and model membranes with low cholesterol content (equimolar with phospholipid) transferred cholesterol rapidly, with half-times of an hour or two, whereas cholesterol-enriched plasma, LDL, and high-cholesterol vesicles (cholesterol:phospholipid molar ratio of 1.6) were much slower. In each system, addition of ethanol accelerated the transfer (Daniels and Goldstein, 1980). There was little or no effect on the amount of tritiated cholesterol in the recipient membrane at equilibrium, but the exchange or transfer process was speeded by ethanol. The magnitude of the ethanol effect was similar for all the donors. The effect was concentration-related, and a concentration of 0.35 M accelerated the process by about 30-40%.

This in vitro system contains no lecithin:cholesterol acyl transferase activity (since the plasma has been heated), so there is no esterification of the cholesterol. In several other ways it differs from the situation in vivo. Our system comes to equilibrium; by contrast, steady state conditions must prevail in vivo where the cholesterol can travel from membrane to membrane. Thus it is not surprising that we do not reproduce in vitro the net increase in cell membrane cholesterol seen in vivo in mice chronically treated with ethanol. Nevertheless, membranes disordered by ethanol may transfer cholesterol faster than normal and this must have important consequences for many organs.

In summary, it seems likely that chronic exposure to ethanol evokes changes in many different lipids and protein surfaces. If we focus on cholesterol for the moment, we can put together a coherent body of data. Cholesterol may determine not only cell membrane fluidity but also the membrane's sensitivity to ethanol. Ethanol's effects may be offset by an increase in cell membrane cholesterol. And ethanol itself, apparently by a purely physical mechanism, may facilitate entry of cholesterol into membranes. This may be a novel mechanism of tolerance.

ACKNOWLEDGEMENT

The work of our laboratory is supported in part by USPHS grants AA01066, DA00322, and a research salary award to Dora B. Goldstein, DA00048.

REFERENCES

Chin, J.H. and D.B. Goldstein (1977a). Effects of low concentrations of ethanol on the fluidity of spin-labeled erythrocyte and brain membranes. Mol. Pharmacol., 13, 435-441.

Chin, J.H. and D.B. Goldstein (1977b). Drug tolerance in biomembranes: A spin label study of the effects of ethanol. Science, 196, 684-685.

Chin, J.H. and D.B. Goldstein (1981). Membrane-disordering action of ethanol: Variation with membrane cholesterol content and depth of the spin label probe. Mol. Pharmacol., 19, 425-431.

Chin, J.H., L.M. Parsons, and D.B. Goldstein (1978). Increased cholesterol content of erythrocyte and brain membranes in ethanol-tolerant mice. Biochim. Biophys. Acta, 513, 358-363.

Daniels, C.K. and D.B. Goldstein (1980). Ethanol facilitates cholesterol uptake by erythrocytes in vitro. Fed. Proc., 39, 744.

Huang, C.H. (1977). A structural model for the cholesterol-phosphatidylcholine complexes in bilayer membranes. Lipid, 12, 348-356.

Jain, M.K. and M.N. Wu (1977). Effect of small molecules on the dipalmitoyl lecithin liposomal bilayer: III Phase transition in lipid bilayer. J. Membrane Biol., 34, 157-201.

Johnson, D.A., N.M. Lee, R. Cooke, and H.H. Loh (1979). Ethanol-induced fluidization of brain lipid bilayers: Required presence of cholesterol in membranes for the expression of tolerance. Mol. Pharmacol., 15, 739-746.

Lee, A.G. (1976). Interactions between anesthetics and lipid mixtures. Normal alcohols. Biochemistry, 15, 2448-2454.

Littleton, J.M. and G. John (1977). Synaptosomal membrane lipids of mice during continuous exposure to ethanol. J. Pharm. Pharmacol., 29, 579-580.

Lyon, R.C., J.A. McComb, J. Schreurs, and D.B. Goldstein (in press). A relationship between alcohol intoxication and the disordering of brain membranes by a series of short-chain alcohols. J. Pharmacol. Exp. Ther.

Metcalfe, J.C., P. Seeman, and A.S.V. Burgen (1968). The proton relaxation of benzyl alcohol in erythrocyte membranes. Mol. Pharmacol., 4, 87-95.

Meyer, H. (1901). Zur Theorie der Alkoholnarkose. 3. Mittheilung: Der Einfluss wechselnder Temperatur auf Wirkungsstarke und Theilungscoefficient der Narcotica. Naunyn-Schmiedebergs Arch. Exp. Pathol. Pharmakol., 46, 338-346.

Paterson, S.J., K.W. Butler, P. Huang, J. Labelle, I.C.P. Smith, and H. Schneider (1972). The effects of alcohols on lipid bilayers: A spin label study. Biochim. Biophys. Acta, 266, 597-602.

Seeman, P. (1972). The membrane actions of anesthetics and tranquilizers. Pharmacol. Rev., 24, 583-655.

Sinensky, M. (1974). Homeoviscous adaptation - a homeostatic process that regulates the viscosity of membrane lipids in Escherichia coli. Proc. Nat. Acad. Sci., 71, 522-525.
Trudell, J.R., W.L. Hubbell, and E.N. Cohen (1973). The effect of two inhalation anesthetics on the order of spin-labeled phospholipid vesicles. Biochim. Biophys. Acta, 291, 321-327.

Susceptibility to Ethanol of Neurons in Lateral Vestibular, Spinal Trigeminal and Lateral Geniculate Nuclei

M. Sasa*, Y. Ikeda*, S. Fujimoto*, J. Ito**, I. Matsuoka**
and S. Takaori*

*Dept. of Pharmacol., Faculty of Medicine, Kyoto University,
Kyoto 606, Japan
**Dept. of Otorhinolaryn., Faculty of Medicine, Kyoto University,
Kyoto 606, Japan

ABSTRACT

An electrophysiological study was performed to determine the susceptibility to ethanol of neurons in the lateral vestibular nucleus (LVN), spinal trigeminal nucleus (STN) and lateral geniculate body (LGB) using cats and rats. The LVN neurons were classified into monosynaptic, polysynaptic I and polysynaptic II neurons, the STN neurons into relay neuron, type-A and type-B interneurons, and the LGB neurons into principal cell (P-cell) and interneuron (I-cell). Ethanol, i.v. administered, inhibited spike generation most effectively in the LVN monosynaptic and polysynaptic II neurons, and slightly in the STN type-B interneuron, LVN polysynaptic I neuron and LGB I-cell with little effects on the STN relay neuron and LGB P-cell. Iontophoretic application of ethanol more effectively inhibited spike generation upon vestibular nerve stimulation of the LVN monosynaptic neuron than of the polysynaptic I neuron, and blocked glutamate- and acetylcholine-induced spikes of the monosynaptic neuron. These results indicate that the LVN monosynaptic neuron is most sensitive to ethanol, suggesting that ethanol inhibits transmitter release from preterminal and/or the membrane excitability of monosynaptic neuron.

KEYWORDS

Ethanol; lateral vestibular nucleus neuron; spinal trigeminal nucleus neuron; lateral geniculate body neuron; electrophysiology; iontophoresis.

INTRODUCTION

The acute effects of ethanol on neurons in the central nervous system are not uniform, and regional and dose-response differences have been reported. For example, ethanol inhibits the locus coeruleus neuron (Pohorecky and Brick, 1977) but excites Renshaw cells (Meyer-Lohmann and co-workers, 1972). However, different effects of ethanol on cerebellar Purkinje cells have been obtained by two other groups. Rogers and co-workers (1980) and Siggins and Bloom (1980) reported an increase in climbing fiber bursts with ethanol, while Sinclair and Lo (1981) observed a decrease in the bursts with an increase in spontaneous firing of Purkinje cells. The effects of ethanol on hippocampal pyramidal cells seem to be much more complex than on Purkinje cells, because it has been reported that ethanol applied by micropressure excited half of the pyramidal cells tested and inhibited the other half of the cells, or the drug applied on hippocampal slice by perfusion produced no change, depolarization or hyperpolarization of the pyramidal cells (Siggins and Bloom, 1980). The present studies were done in an attempt to determine the susceptibility to ethanol of neurons in primary nuclei in afferent transmission and to elucidate the mechanism underlying the action of ethanol using microiontophoretic technique.

METHODS

Single neuron activities were extracellularly recorded from the LVN and rostral part of the STN in cats using a glass-insulated silver wire microelectrode, and from the LGB in rats using a glass microelectrode filled with 2 M sodium acetate. These animals were anesthetized with α-chloralose, immobilized with gallamine and artificially respired. The LVN neurons were classified by stimulating orthodromically the vestibular nerve located in the labyrinth and antidromically the vestibulospinal tract, the STN neurons by stimulating the intracranial trigeminal nerve and contralateral medial lemniscus, and the LGB neuron by optic chiasma and visual cortex stimulation. The positions of the recording and stimulating electrodes were marked by passing a direct current through the electrode and histologically verified. Ethanol (25 %, w/v) dissolved in saline was administered i.v. in cumulative doses which were increased logarithmically at 10-min intervals. The responses of neurons were recorded 5 and 10 min after each injection. In several animals, femoral blood pressure was monitored using a pressure transducer and blood concentration of ethanol was determined using a gas chromatograph. The effects of microiontophoretically applied ethanol were examined in the LVN neuron using a seven-barreled micropipette filled with 10 % ethanol, 2 M monosodium glutamate and 0.5 M acetylcholine chloride and attached along a glass-insulated silver wire microelectrode (Sasa and coworkers, 1979). The distance of tips between the recording microelectrode and micropipette was within 20 μm. Poststimulus latency histogram obtained from 40-50 successive responses was constructed using a computer (ATAC-350) and the spontaneous firing rate was continuously recorded on a rate meter. Statistical significances were determined by Student's t-test.

RESULTS

Intravenous Administration of Ethanol

According to the responses to orthodromic vestibular nerve stimulation and antidromic vestibulospinal tract stimulation, the LVN neurons were classified into three groups: monosynaptic, polysynaptic I and polysynaptic II neurons, as shown in Fig. 1 (Ikeda, Sasa and Takaori, 1980). The monosynaptic neuron, which was first described by Shimazu and Precht (1965) and Precht and Shimazu (1965), fired spike on a monosynaptic component of the field potential upon orthodromic stimulation with a mean latency of 1.3 ± 0.1 msec (n=7) and upon antidromic stimulation with a mean spike latency of 1.1 ± 0.1 msec. The antidromic spike consistently followed high frequency stimuli to the vestibulospinal tract up to 200 Hz. The polysynaptic I neuron responded to vestibular nerve stimulation with a mean spike latency of 2.8 ± 0.2 msec (n=7), but the spike latency was not consistent. The polysynaptic II neuron fired spikes upon orthodromic stimulation with the spike latency much longer than the two types of neurons mentioned above (mean latency: 20.1 ± 3.8 msec, n=7). Ethanol given i.v. to the animals dose-dependently inhibited the orthodromic spike generation of the LVN monosynaptic and polysynaptic II neurons, with little

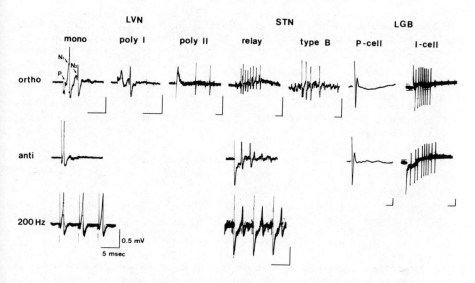

Fig. 1. Typical examples of spikes in LVN, STN and LGB neurons.
P, N_1 and N_2: pre-, mono- and polysynaptic components
of the field potential upon vestibular nerve stimulation. 200Hz: high frequency stimuli of 200 Hz.

effect on the polysynaptic I neuron and without affecting the antidromic spike
of the monosynaptic neuron (TABLE 1). A significant inhibition was observed
in 3 out of 7 monosynaptic and 2 out of 7 polysynaptic II neurons with a dose
as low as 0.2 g/kg of ethanol. When 0.4 g/kg of ethanol was administered, the
mean spike number of the orthodromic spikes in the monosynaptic and polysynaptic II neurons were significantly reduced to 1.3 $\pm$ 0.2 and 1.5 $\pm$ 0.2 from
2.1 $\pm$ 0.2 and 3.2 $\pm$ 0.7, respectively. Spike generation of the polysynaptic I
neuron was, however, significantly inhibited only by a maximum dose of ethanol
tested (1.6 g/kg). The STN neurons were classified into three types as previously reported (Sasa and co-workers, 1974, 1977): relay neuron, type-A and
type-B interneurons (Fig. 1). Briefly, the relay neuron was activated by
orthodromic trigeminal nerve stimulation and antidromic medial lemniscus
stimulation with the mean latencies of 3.0 $\pm$ 0.3 and 1.2 $\pm$ 0.2 msec (n=6),
respectively. The antidromic spike followed high frequency stimuli to the
medial lemniscus up to 200 Hz. The type-A interneuron responded to orthodromic stimulation, and transsynaptically to antidromic stimulation. The
type-B interneuron fired spikes upon orthodromic stimulation with a long
latency (mean latency: 8.9 $\pm$ 1.2 msec, n=7). When the effects of ethanol were
examined on the relay neuron and type-B interneuron, it was found that ethanol
up to 1.6 g/kg rarely affected orthodromic or antidromic spike generation of
the relay neuron and that only a maximum dose of 1.6 g/kg significantly inhibited the orthodromic spike of type-B interneuron (P<0.05, TABLE 1). The LGB
neurons were classified into principal cell (P-cell) and interneuron (I-cell)
as described by Burke and Safton (1966). As shown in Fig. 1, the P-cell fired
a single spike upon orthodromic optic chiasma stimulation and antidromic visual
cortex stimulation. The orthodromic and antidromic spike latencies were 3.5 $\pm$
0.3 and 3.1 $\pm$ 0.4 msec (n=5), respectively. In contrast, the I-cell repeti-
tively fired upon both orthodromic and antidromic stimulation with the means
of the first spike latencies of 9.5 $\pm$ 1.7 and 4.2 $\pm$ 0.6 msec (n=7), respectively. The orthodromic and antidromic spike generation of P-cells remained

TABLE 1   Effects of Ethanol i.v. Administered on Neurons in Lateral Vestibular
Nucleus, Spinal Trigeminal Nucleus and Lateral Geniculate Body

	Ethanol (g/kg)				
	0	0.2	0.4	0.8	1.6
Lateral vestibular nucleus					
Monosynaptic neuron (n=7)	2.1+0.2#	1.6+0.2	1.3+0.2*	1.2+0.2**	0.9+0.2**
Polysynaptic I neuron (n=7)	0.9+0.1	0.9+0.1	0.9+0.1	0.8+0.1	0.5+0.2
Polysynaptic II neuron (n=7)	3.2+0.7	2.2+0.4	1.5+0.2*	0.8+0.2**	0.1+0.1**
Spinal trigeminal nucleus					
Relay neuron (n=6)	4.0+1.0	4.2+1.1	4.1+1.1	4.2+1.4	3.9+1.3
Type-B interneuron (n=7)	4.5+0.9	4.4+1.0	3.9+0.9	3.8+1.1	0.7+0.4**
Lateral geniculate body					
P-cell (n=5)	0.9+0.1	0.8+0.2	0.8+0.1	0.7+0.1	0.9+0.1
I-cell (n=7)	9.3+1.1	8.6+1.7	8.5+1.6	7.7+1.8	5.5+1.6*

* $P<0.05$, ** $P<0.01$.   #: Mean orthodromic spike number + S.E.

unaffected with ethanol up to 1.6 g/kg (TABLE 1). The orthodromic spikes of
I-cells were not significantly affected with ethanol up to 0.8 g/kg and
inhibited only with 1.6 g/kg, but spikes produced by cortical stimulation
remained unaltered with the drug up to 1.6 g/kg. The systemic blood pressure
monitored on cats was not significantly altered during or after ethanol injection up to 1.6 g/kg. The ethanol concentrations in blood were 0.53 +0.07,
0.87 +0.18, 1.95 + 0.36 and 4.47 + 0.51 mg/ml (n=4-5) 5 min after ethanol
injection in cumulative doses of 0.2, 0.4, 0.8 and 1.6 g/kg, respectively.

Iontophoretic Administration of Ethanol

The effects of iontophoretic application of ethanol were examined on the LVN
monosynaptic and polysynaptic I neurons. A typical example of monosynaptic
neuron is shown in Fig. 2. Orthodromic spike generation of the monosynaptic
neuron was dose-dependently inhibited with 100 and 200 nA of ethanol. The
polysynaptic I neuron was less sensitive to ethanol iontophoretically applied
than the monosynaptic neuron. A significant inhibition of the orthodromic
spike with 100 and 200 nA of ethanol was obtained in 17 (50 %) and 24 (71 %)
out of 34 monosynaptic neurons, and in 3 (25 %) and 5 (42 %) out of 12 polysynaptic I neurons, respectively. To determine whether ethanol affects the
synaptic transmission or membrane excitability of monosynaptic neuron, the
effects of ethanol were examined on spike firing induced by glutamate and
acetylcholine. As represented in Fig. 3, iontophoretic ethanol of 100 and
200 nA dose-dependently inhibited spikes produced by both glutamate and
acetylcholine.

DISCUSSION

The LVN monosynaptic and polysynaptic II neurons were most sensitive to ethano
but the LVN polysynaptic I neuron, STN type-B interneuron and LGB I-cell were
inhibited by only the highest dose tested (1.6 g/kg). The STN relay neuron an
LGB P-cell were resistant to ethanol. These results indicate that the effects
of ethanol on the central neurons show regional differences even in the primar
relay nuclei and neurons specified in the same nucleus. The LVN neurons have
been classified into kinetic and tonic neurons by Shimazu and Precht (1965).

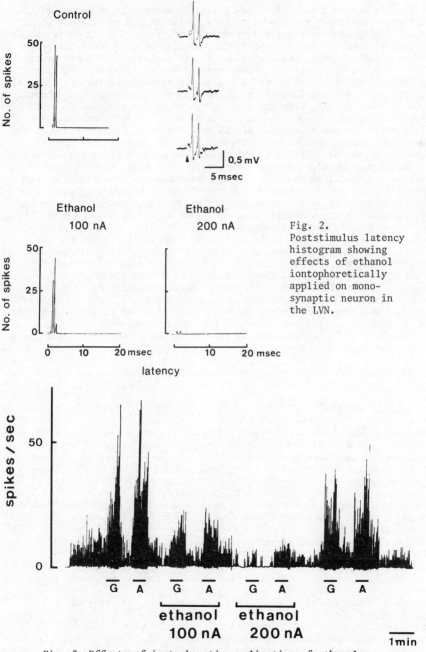

Fig. 2. Poststimulus latency histogram showing effects of ethanol iontophoretically applied on monosynaptic neuron in the LVN.

Fig. 3. Effects of iontophoretic application of ethanol on glutamate- and acetylcholine-induced spike firing of monosynaptic neuron in the LVN. G: glutamate 75 nA, A: acetylcholine 100 nA.

The kinetic neuron fired spikes on N_1 wave (monosynaptic component of the field potential) upon vestibular nerve stimulation and revealed an absent or a sporadically irregular pattern of spontaneous firing, which increased steeply in response to horizontal rotation with constant angular acceleration and decreased with constant angular velocity. In contrast, the tonic neuron fired spikes on N_2 wave (polysynaptic component of the field potential) upon vestibular nerve stimulation and showed a regular spontaneous firing, which initially increased with rotation, maintaining a constant value during the remainder of the rotation. Judging from characteristics of spikes produced by vestibular nerve stimulation and spontaneous firing pattern, the LVN monosynaptic and polysynaptic I neurons recorded herein are considered to correspond to the kinetic and tonic neurons, respectively. The LVN monosynaptic neuron was affected by ethanol of 0.4 g/kg, which brought about a blood ethanol concentration of 0.87 mg/ml. At this level, vestibular signs such as equilibrium disorder and nystagmus have been observed in humans with a low tolerance to ethanol (Ashan, 1958; Wallgren and Barry, 1970). Therefore, ingestion of a moderate dose of ethanol impairs the LVN monosynaptic neuron, thereby suggesting that the monosynaptic neuron may play a primary role in controlling body balance against sudden changes of the body, although the role of polysynaptic II neuron remains to be determined. An inhibition of the LVN polysynaptic I neuron was produced by increasing the blood ethanol concentration to 4.47 mg/ml, which is a toxic dose to humans. Therefore, the polysynaptic I neuron may be involved in the maintenance of standing posture. The spike generation of the LVN monosynaptic neuron upon vestibular nerve stimulation was also inhibited by iontophoretically applied ethanol. The low susceptibility of polysynaptic I neuron to ethanol was observed in the iontophoretic study. Therefore, differences of susceptibility of neurons to ethanol are considered to be due to transmitter substances and/or the membrane characteristics. Iontophoretic application of ethanol blocked glutamate- and acetylcholine-induced spike firing, suggesting ethanol inhibits synaptic transmission and/or membrane excitability of the monosynaptic neuron.

REFERENCES

Ashan, G. (1958). Acta Otolaryngol., Suppl. 140, 69-78.
Burke, W., and A.J. Safton (1966). J. Physiol. (London), 187, 201-212.
Ikeda, Y., M. Sasa, and S. Takaori (1980). Japan. J. Pharmacol., 30, 665-675.
Meyer-Lohmann, J., R. Hagenah, C. Hellweg, and R. Benecke (1972). Naunyn-Schmiedeberg's Arch. Pharmacol., 272, 131-142.
Pohorecky, L.A., and J. Brick (1977). Brain Res., 131, 174-179.
Precht, W.,and H. Shimazu (1965). J. Neurophysiol., 28, 1014-1028.
Rogers, J., G.B. Siggins, J.A. Schulman, and F.E. Bloom (1980). Brain Res., 196, 183-198.
Sasa, M., S. Fujimoto, S. Igarashi, K. Munekiyo, and S. Takaori (1979). J. Pharmacol. exp. Ther., 210, 311-315.
Sasa, M., S. Igarashi, and S. Takaori (1977). Brain Res., 125, 369-375.
Sasa, M., K. Munekiyo, H. Ikeda, and S. Takaori (1974). Brain Res., 80, 443-460.
Shimazu, H., and W. Precht (1965). J. Neurophysiol., 28, 991-1013.
Siggins, G.R., and F.E. Bloom (1980). Pharmacol. Biochem. Behav., 13, Suppl. 1, 203-211.
Sinclair, J.G., and G.F. Lo (1981). Brain Res., 204, 465-471.
Wallgren, H., and H. Barry, III (1970). Action of Alcohol, Vol. I. Biochemical, Physiological and Psychological Aspects, Elsevier Publ. Co., Amsterdam, pp. 1-400.

Dissociation of Components of Ethanol Intoxication and Tolerance

C. J. P. Eriksson*, R. A. Deitrich**, M. Rusi*, K. Clay**
and D. A. Petersen***

*Research Laboratories of the State Alcohol Monopoly (Alko),
Box 350, SF-00101 Helsinki 10, Finland
**Department of Pharmacology, University of Colorado, Denver,
Colorado, USA
***School of Pharmacy, University of Colorado, Boulder, Colorado,
USA

ABSTRACT

The present investigation represents an effort to study if ethanol intoxication and tolerance should be dissociated into differentially regulated
components. The degree of ethanol-mediated hypothermia in individual mice
of a genetically heterogenous line was not significantly correlated to the
period of time the animals were void of the loss of righting reflex (sleep
time). Brain homovanillic acid concentration (determined 3 days after the
ethanol treatment) correlated with sleep time ($r = 0.358$, n=33, $p < 0.05$)
but not with hypothermia ($r = -0.009$). Ethanol-induced sleep time was
assessed in rat lines genetically selected for high (ANT) and low (AT)
sensitivity to ethanol as determined by the tilting-plane motor performance test. No sleep-time line differences were found. In experiment 3,
ANT and AT rats were treated for 5 consecutive days with ethanol. No
significant tolerance differences developed between the two lines as
measured by tilting-plane performance.

In summary, it appears that ethanol intoxication can be dissociated into
several different components, which may be regulated by genetically separate mechanisms. It seems possible that the primary mechanisms regulating
initial intoxication are genetically distinct from those determining
acquired tolerance.

KEYWORDS

Ethanol, intoxication, tolerance, genetic factors, hypothermia, righting
reflex, motor performance, homovanillic acid.

INTRODUCTION

The etiology of ethanol intoxication and tolerance involves the following
basic questions: 1. Are ethanol-induced impairments of motor performance,
hypothermia, narcosis, and other components of intoxication, determined by
one common regulatory mechanism? 2. Are the mechanisms regulating initial

245

intoxication and acquired tolerance common or separate? These questions
have been approached by pharmacological manipulation of ethanol intoxication. Inhibition of acquired tolerance but no effect on initial impairment of motor performance by p-chlorophenylalanine (Frankel and co-
workers, 1975), and hypothermia and sleep time by 6-hydroxydopamine
(Ritzmann and Tabakoff, 1976), has been observed. Intoxication has been
dissociated by Kiianmaa (1980), who observed reduction in hypothermia,
increased impairment of motor performance and no effect on narcosis by
ethanol after intra-cerebral treatment with 6-hydroxydopamine.

The relationships between different components of intoxication or tolerance can also be investigated by assessing the individual correlations
between the various parameters within a genetically heterogenous population. This approach was recently employed by Erwin, McClearn and Kuse
(1980), who did not find a significant association between initial ethanol
sensitivity and acquisition of acute tolerance. The individual correlation technique was used in the present study (experiment 1) to determine
the relationship between ethanol-induced hypothermia, narcosis, and the
possible dopaminergic influence on each of these parameters.

Comparisons of inbred strains have been more commonly used than individual
correlations. the idea has been that any difference found after ethanol
treatment in two, or more, inbred strains must be due to genetic factors.
This kind of study has recently been reviewed by Belknap (1980) and
following conclusions were obtained: BALB mice are consistently more
sensitive to ethanol (loss of righting reflex and hypothermia) than C57 or
DBA mice. Results regarding the different intoxication and tolerance
parameters in C57 compared with the DBA strain are inconsistent.
Outbred animal lines genetically selected for a specific components of
intoxication or tolerance may prove to be a powerful tool applicable to
dissociating these phenomena. Ethanol-induced hypothermia was found to be
more severe in mice selected for ethanol sensitivity, measured by duration
of loss of righting reflex (LS = long sleep) than in less sensitive short
sleep (SS) mice (Moore and Kakihana, 1978; Tabakoff and others, 1980).
Similarly, ethanol sensitive rats, selected for greater motor impairment
by ethanol (MA), were also more sensitive, when loss of righting reflex
was used as index of sensitivity, than the LA (least affected) line (Riley
and co-workers, 1977). The relationship between initial sensitivity and
acquired tolerance has been more diffuse. Bass and Lester (1980) reported
no difference between the MA and LA lines in regards to acquisition of
tolerance, whereas Tabakoff and others (1980) observed that animals which
were less sensitive (SS) also developed tolerance more quickly.

Rats genetically selected for more (ANT) and less (AT) ethanol-induced
impairment of motor performance (Rusi, Eriksson and Mäki, 1977) were used
in the present study. In experiments 2 and 3, duration of loss of righting reflex and development of acquired tolerance with regards to the
impairment of motor performance on the tilting plane were investigated.

PROCEDURES AND RESULTS

Experiment 1: Individual Correlations between Sleep Time, Hypothermia and
Brain Homovanillic Acid

Male mice (age: 50-59 days, n=98) of the genetically heterogenous population (HS/IBG), obtained from the Institute for Behavioral Genetics,
University of Colorado, Boulder, Colorado, were employed. In the morning

of day 1 of the experiments, animals were injected with 4 g ethanol per kg
b.wt. (given as 20 %, w/v, in distilled water). After the mice lost the
righting reflex (within 3 min), they were placed on their backs in V-
shaped plastic troughs and the time (sleep time) until regaining righting
reflex (critera: able to right themselves twice within 30 sec) was
recorded. Body temperature was determined before, and 30 and 60 min
after, ethanol administration by inserting the lubricated termiston probe
2.5 cm into the rectum. Half of the animals (ethanol group) were again
injected with ethanol on day 4 of the experiments (4 g/kg). One hour
after the ethanol administration, the treated and control mice were killed
by cervical dislocation and the brains excised (within 1 min). Each brain
was divided at the mid line and one half was used for the determination of
homovanillic acid (HVA) in the following manner. To the brain sample was
added deuterated HVA (D_5-HVA) as internal standard and 50 μl of 3 N HCl.
The brains were immediately homogenized in 0.5 ml saline and quickly
frozen until extracted. After thawing, brain proteins were precipitated
by addition of 3 ml ethanol and centrifugation. The ethanol was removed
by rotary evaporator and 0.5 ml 0.01 N HCl was added to the residue.
Ether, 3 x 3 ml was used to extract HVA. After removal of ether with a
stream of nitrogen, HVA was converted to its trimethylsilyl derivative and
gas chromatography-mass spectrometry in the selected ion monitoring mode
was used to measure the ratio D_0-HVA/D_5-HVA.

ORIGINAL:

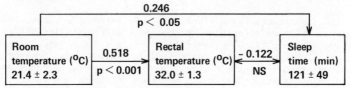

CORRECTED FOR ROOM TEMPERATURE:

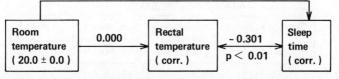

Fig. 1. Relation between hypothermia and duration of loss of righting
        reflex. Rectal temperature was measured 60 min after i.p.
        injection of ethanol (4 g/kg) in 98 HS male mice. Values are
        means ± SD and correlation coefficients (above the arrows).

Figure 1 summarizes the day 1 results. No significant correlation was
observed between sleep time and hypothermia under conduction of the experiment. However, the rectal temperature correlated positively to the
ambient temperature, which ranged between 18.5 and 25.6°C. Since room
temperature also correlated positively to sleep time it was realized that
the effects associated with room temperature could "hide" a true negative
correlation between hypothermia and sleep time. Therefore, both rectal
temperature and sleep-time values were "normalized" according to Hays
(1963), holding room temperature fixed, which lead to a significant

partial correlation between these two intoxication parameters (Fig. 1). A significantly (p < 0.001) higher brain concentration of HVA was found in the ethanol group (D_0-HVA/D_5-HVA:1.76±SD of 0.80, n = 32) compared with the controls (1.06±0.53, n = 33). HVA correlated in the control group significantly to the sleep time (r = 0.358, p < 0.05) but no correlation was found to the rectal temperature of day 1 (r = -0.009). No relationship was found between HVA and hypothermia or sleep time within the ethanol group.

Experiment 2: Sleep Times in Rats Selected for Motor Performance

Male and female rats (age: 3 - 4 months; generation: F_{12}), selectively bred for a high (ANT = alcohol nontolerant) and a low (AT = alcohol tolerant) degree of motor impairment by ethanol (Rusi, Eriksson and Mäki, 1977), from the Research Laboratories of the State Alcohol Monopoly (Alko), Finland, were employed. Motor impairment was determined by the tilting-plane test as described previously (Rusi, Eriksson and Mäki, 1977). About two weeks after the tilting-plane tests, part of the animals were tested for ethanol-induced duration of loss of righting reflex. Sleep times were determined as for the HS mice except that the rats were placed directly with their backs on a plain surface. Ethanol (4 g/kg) was given as 15 % (w/v) in saline. Tail-blood samples were taken immediately after both behavioral tests and the ethanol concentration was determined by head-space gas chromatography.

Table 1 summarizes the behavioral results. In spite of a marked line difference in impaired motor performance, no significant line difference was observed in sleep time. A sex difference (p < 0.05), with male AT rats "sleeping" longer than the corresponding females, was, however, found. Blood ethanol determinations revealed no line differences during the tilting-plane tests. Similarly, no line difference was found in ethanol concentration at the time the animals regained the righting reflex.

TABLE 1. Ethanol-Induced Narcosis and Impairment of Motor Performance
in AT and ANT Rats*

Animals	Sleep time (min)	Blood ethanol (mM)	Decrease in sliding angle (in degrees)	Blood ethanol (mM)
ANT ♂	334±48 (18)	68.5±12.6	21±10 (43)	49.1±8.0
AT ♂	311±43 (14)	71.5±10.0	9± 6 (29)**	49.4±7.0
ANT ♀	300±64 (9)	64.5± 5.9	22± 6 (29)	48.9±7.0
AT ♀	264±65 (11)	69.9± 5.5	9± 5 (17)**	47.6±4.6

*Animals of generation F_{12} were injected with an i.p. dose of ethanol:
4 g/kg (sleep time) and 2 g/kg (tilting-plane test). Values are means ±SD (N).
**Line comparisons: p < 0.001 (Student's t-test)

Experiment 3: Acquired Tolerance in ANT and AT rats

The procedure of this experiment involved two steps. In the preliminary step of the investigation males and females (age: 3.3 - 3.5 months) AT and

ANT rats (second litters of the same parents as for experiment 2) were
tested for their tilting-plane performance at ethanol doses ranging
between 1.0 and 2.5 g/kg. Ethanol was given i.p. as 12 % (w/v) in saline.
The aim of this dose-response test was to determine the dose for each
group of rats which would give the same amount of intoxication. The doses
were found to be the following (for 12 degrees decrease in sliding angle):
1.3 (male ANT); 1.4 (female ANT); 1.9 (female AT); 2.0 (male AT). Three
weeks after these preliminary tests, animals were subjected to a second
set of experiments, in which they were tested for their tilting-plane
performance for 5 consecutive days at the previously obtained ethanol
doses. In addition to these test doses, animals received an ethanol intubation after the tests, so that their total daily ethanol intake was
5 g/kg.

Table 2 lists the results for the males. No significant line differences
were found at any of the days. However, the substantial variation of the
test values could have covered a small line difference, which now was
observed only as a tendency for more acquired tolerance at days 2 and 3 in
the AT compared with the ANT rats. The female rats displayed significant
($p < 0.005$) line differences on day 1, with the initial motor-impairment
values being 19.4 ± 5.5 (ANT, n = 14) and 12.3 ± 6.4 degress (AT, n = 14).
However, no line difference was found in acquired tolerance as determined
in percent of performance impairment on day 1.

TABLE 2. Development of Tolerance in ANT and AT Rats*

Animals (and numbers)	Decrease in sliding angle (in degress)				
	Days of treatment				
	1	2	3	4	5
ANT (13)	10.3 ± 5.4	8.8 ± 6.3	9.3 ± 6.4	6.3 ± 3.9	4.6 ± 3.4
AT (12)	9.9 ± 8.1	5.4 ± 2.5	5.3 ± 5.8	6.2 ± 4.4	6.8 ± 4.2

*Male animals (F_{12}) were injected each day with an i.p. dose of ethanol:
1.3 g/kg (ANT) and 2.0 g/kg (AT) for the tilting-plane test, and
orally: 3.7 g/kg (ANT) and 3.0 g/kg (AT) after the tests. Values are
means ±SD.

DISCUSSION

It is attractive to hypothetize that ethanol-induced impairment of motor
performance, hypothermia, narcosis, and other components of intoxication,
primarily involves a common central effect of ethanol. Membrane fluidization, which has been associated with the anesthetic effect of ethanol
(Seeman, 1972), could be such an effect. If a single common mechanism is
the main determinant of the different components of ethanol intoxication
it follows that there should also be a common genetic factor involved.
Therefore, in a genetically heterogenous population the effect of ethanol
on each of the components of intoxication should be essentially the same,
at least the magnitudes of the different intoxication parameters should
correlate with each other. Moreover, animals genetically selected for one
of these paramters should also become selected for the other components
regulated by the same genetic factor(s). As mentioned in the introduction
section, most of the current data is in favor of a common mechanism for
ethanol-induced hypothermia and narcosis. However, the results of the
present study (experiment 1) demonstrate that, although there may be

common factors, the main factors regulating hypothermia and narcosis seem to be separate. The correlation between brain HVA and sleep time, but not hypothermia, further supports this notion. Similarly, Pohorecky and Rizek (1981) point out the necessity to consider a dissociation of ethanol-induced hypothermia and impairment of motor performance. Ethanol-induced impairment of motor performance and narcosis has also been suggested to involve common genetic mechanisms (Riley and co-workers, 1977). This notion is not supported by the results of experiment 2 of the present study, in which no sleep-time differences were found between the ANT and AT strains. It is suggested that the main regulators of ethanol-induced narcosis is genetically different from those regulating impairment of motor performance.

With regard to ethanol-induced narcosis, Ritzmann and Tabakoff (1976) have reported that intra-cerebroventricular injection of 6-hydroxydopamine had no effect on initial sensitivity to ethanol but prevented development of acquired sleep-time tolerance in C57 mice. However, by comparing the acquired sleep-time tolerance in LS and SS mice, Tabakoff and others (1980) observed faster development of acquired tolerance in the SS mice. With regard to ethanol-induced impairment of motor performance, Bass and Lester (1980) found no relationship between initial sensitivity and acquired tolerance in their MA and LA rat lines. The results of the present study (experiment 3) support the notion of independent genetic influence upon initial ethanol sensitivity as opposed to acquired ethanol tolerance. It is, however, emphasized that common regulatory factors, perhaps being of minor importance for the overall regulation of initial intoxication and acquired tolerance, cannot be excluded based on the results of the present study.

ACKNOWLEDGEMENTS

Part of this study is supported by Alcohol Research Center Grant AA 03527. Thanks are due to Dr. Rodney Baker for his technical assistance.

REFERENCES

Bass, M.B., and D. Lester (1980). Tolerance to ethanol-induced impairment of water escape in rats bred for ethanol sensitivity. Psychopharmacology, 71, 153-158.
Belknap, J.K. (1980). Genetic factors in the effects of alcohol: neurosensitivity, functional tolerance and physical dependence. In H. Rigter and J.C. Crabbe, Jr. (Eds), Alcohol Tolerance and Dependence. Elsevier/North- Holland Biomedical Press, New York. Chap. 7, pp. 157-180.
Erwin, V.G., G.E. McClearn, and A.R. Kuse (1980). Interrelationships of alcohol consumption, actions of alcohol, and biochemical traits. Pharmac. Biochem. Behav., 13, Suppl. 1, 297-302.
Frankel, D., J.M. Khanna, A.E. LeBlanc, and H. Kalant (1975). Effect of p-chlorophenylalanine on the acquisition of tolerance to ethanol and pentobarbital. Psychopharmacologia (Berl.), 44, 247-252.
Hays, W.L. (1963) Statistics, Holt, Rinehart and Winston, London, pp. 574-576.
Kiianmaa, K. (1980). Alcohol intake and ethanol intoxication in the rat: effect of a 6-OHDA-induced lesion of the ascending noradrenaline pathways. European J. Pharmacol., 64, 9-19.
McClearn, G.E., and S.M. Anderson (1979). Genetics and ethanol tolerance. Drug Alcohol Depend., 4, 61-76.

Moore, J.A., and R. Kakihana (1978). Ethanol-induced hypothermia in mice: influence of genotype on development of tolerance. Life Sci., 23, 2331- 2338.

Pohorecky, L.A., and A.E. Rizek (1981). Biochemical and behavioral effects of acute ethanol in rats at different environmental temperatures. Psychopharmacology, 72, 205-209.

Riley, E.P., E.D. Worsham, D. Lester, and E.X. Freed (1977). Selected breeding of rats for differences in reactivity to alcohol. An approach to an animal model of alcoholism. II. Behavioral measures. J. Stud. Alc., 38, 1705-1717.

Ritzmann, R.F., and B. Tabakoff (1976). Dissociation of alcohol tolerance and dependence. Nature, 263, 418-420.

Rusi, M., K. Eriksson, and J. Mäki (1977). Genetic differences in the susceptibility to acute ethanol intoxication in selected rat strains. In M.M. Gross (Ed.), Alcohol Intoxication and Withdrawal, Vol. IIIa, Plenum Press, New York. pp. 97-109.

Seeman, P. (1972). The membrane actions of anesthetics and tranquilizers. Pharmacol Rev., 24, 583-655.

Tabakoff, B., R.F. Ritzmann, T.S. Raju, and R.A. Deitrich (1980). Characterization of acute and chronic tolerance in mice selected for inherent differences in sensitivity to ethanol. Alcoholism, 4, 70-73.

WORKSHOP

Models of Experimental Peptic Ulcers and Therapeutic Agents

Moderators: S. Okabe, Y. Osumi

Models of Experimental Peptic Ulcers and Therapeutic Agents

S. Okabe* and Y. Osumi**

*Department of Applied Pharmacology, Kyoto College of Pharmacy,
Kyoto, Japan
**Department of Pharmaology, Faculty of Medicine, Kochi Medical
School, Nankoku, Kochi, Japan

The factors related to the genesis of peptic ulceration in humans are even
today poorly understood. Despite the numerous animal models of acute and
chronic peptic ulceration, these approaches leave much to be desired when
attempts are made to extrapolate the findings into clinical significance.
Only on the basis of an appropriate model can effective and safe chemical
compounds be prepared for clinical treatment.
It is our wish that this Workshop will provide the opportunity for a frank
interchange of ideas and open discussions that will be fruitful for the
production of compounds that will benefit those with gastric and duodenal
disorders.

KEYWORDS

Ulcer models, anti-ulcer agents, screening, peptic ulcer

Possible Roles of Central Catecholamines in Regulation of Gastric Functions

Y. Osumi

Department of Pharmacology, Kochi Medical School, Nankoku, Kochi 781-51, Japan

ABSTRACT

In the present study, possible roles of central noradrenaline (NA) in formation of gastric ulcer induced by water-immersion stress, and in regulation of gastric functions such as acid secretion and mucosal blood flow were investigated in rats. We suggested that; (1) An increased mobilization of NA in the brain might promote the formation of stress-induced gastric ulcer, (2) Central noradrenergic inhibitory mechanisms originating from the locus coeruleus seem to be involved in regulation of gastric functions, probably at the level of the brain stem ala cinerea, and (3) When there is an elevation in gastric acid secretion but with no parallel increase in mucosal blood flow, gastric ulceration may occur under condition of stress.

KEY WORDS

Gastric ulceration; stress; acid secretion; mucosal blood flow; noradrenaline; dopamine; brain.

INTRODUCTION

Since a wide variety of stress experienced by humans results in gastric ulceration, stress-induced gastric ulcers in laboratory animals can serve as a models for assessing the pathogenesis and pharmacological basis of anti-ulcer agents. As there is still a paucity in information concerning central neurogenic mechanisms in regulation of gastric functions, the possible roles of central NA in formation of stress-induced gastric ulcer and in regulation of gastric functions such as acid secretion and mucosal blood flow, and finally a relation of acid secretion to mucosal blood flow was investigated in rats.

CENTRAL NA ON STRESS-INDUCED GASTRIC ULCER

It has been well documented that a wide variety of stress in experimental animals results in reduction of NA content in the brain. After the administration of ᴅ-methyl-p-tyrosine, an inhibitor of NA synthesis at the step of tyrosine hydroxylase, NA contents in the hypothalamus, lower brain stem, and cerebral cortex decreased progressively. Water-immersion stress, by the method of Takagi and Okabe (1968), accelerated the decrease in NA contents in the brain after the administration of ᴅ-methyl-p-tyrosine. This accelerated decrease by the stress is attributed to the increased activity of NA containing neurons with a subsequent release of this amine exceeding the rate of neuronal resynthesis. Based on this working hypothesis, effects of fusaric acid, a potent dopamine β-hydroxylase inhibitor, and tetrabenazine, a central monoamine depletor, on formation of stress-induced gastric ulceration were examined (Osumi and co-workers, 1973).

Water-immersion stress for 3 hrs decreased NA contents in the brain to approximately 70 % of control(0.33 + 0.02 µg/g, n=8). Treatment of non-stressed normal animals with 100 mg/kg of fusaric acid decreased NA content in the brain to approximately 52 % of control within 3 hrs. Combined treatment of the rats with the same dose of fusaric acid plus water-immersion stress did not accelerate the decrease of NA to any great extent, as compared to rats treated with this substance alone. Dopamine content in the brain was not modified either by water-immersion stress and/or administration of fusaric acid. These biochemical data indicate that mobilization of NA in the brain by the stress was completely blocked by the pretreatment of animals with fusaric acid. In these fusaric acid pretreated animals, the ulcerative changes in the stomach were all but completely abolished. Mean ulcer index of animals treated with fusaric acid was 0.5 ± 0.3 (n=8) as compared with that of controls, 3.3 + 0.2 (n=12). Such a protective effect of fusaric acid was also obtained by the intracerebroventricular administration of this substance 0.5 mg/animal. On the other hand, treatment of animals with tetrabenazine accelerated the mobilization of catecholamines in the brain and rather exacerbated the formation of gastric ulcerative changes, as induced by water-immersion stress (ulcer index; 4.4 + 0.4, n=8). These results suggested that an increased mobilization of NA in the brain might promote the formation of stress-induced gastric ulcer. Furthermore, it is reasonable to assume that NA in the brain may affect physiological gastric functions such as acid secretion and mucosal blood flow.

CENTRAL MONOAMINES IN REGULATION OF GASTRIC ACID SECRETION AND MUCOSAL BLOOD FLOW

Much attention has been focused on the central regulation in gastric functions, and stimulation of certain regions of the brain promotes an alteration in these functions. Whether or not central monoaminergic mechanism directly affect such functions apparently has not been determined.

In this series of experiment, fasted rats of Wistar strain were
used under urethane anesthesia. A cannula was inserted into the
stomach via an incision in the duodenum and the animal was
placed in the stereotaxic instrument. Gastric solution (glycine
: mannitol = 1:5 [v/v], pH 3.5, 300 mosM, 38°C) was infused into
the stomach at the beginning of each 15-min collection period.
Gastric mucosal blood flow was measured by the aminopyrine
clearance technique develoed by Jacobson and co-workers (1966).
Precise experimental procedures and results has been presented
elesewhere (Osumi and co-workers, 1977, 1981).

Mean basal gastric acid output and mucosal blood flow was 3.1 $\pm$
0.2 µEq/15 min and 1.4 $\pm$ 0.1 ml/15 min, respectively. Intra-
ventricularly administered NA 10 µg decreased both gastric acid
output and mucosal blood flow to some 60 % in the first 15 min,
after which there was a return toward the respective basal
value. The same dose of other test substances such as dopamine,
and serotonin did not significantly affect these gastric parameters. Therefore, gastric inhibition by centrally applied NA
is fairly specific, as compared to the other central neuro-
transmitter candidates used.

Effect of NA on the electrical stimulation-induced increase
in gastric functions was then examined. In a preliminary
experiment, repetitive stimulation of the lateral hypothalamic
area at 10 cycles/sec, 0.5 mA, 2 msec for 10 min using a bipolar
stainless electrode induced a consistent and reproducible
increase in acid output and mucosal blood flow. Percent
increases in gastric acid output and mucosal blood flow 15 min
after the stimulation were 473 (p $<$ 0.05, n=5) and 193 (p $<$ 0.01,
n=5), respectively. Since these lateral hypothalamic area-in-
duced increases were abolished by a small dose of atropine
intravenously administered, the increases in acid secretion and
mucosal blood flow can be explained by the activation of the
efferent descending motor pathways to the brain stem vagal
nuclei, originating from the lateral hypothalamic area. The
administration of NA 10 µg into the lateral ventricle 5 min
prior to the second stimulation all but completely blocked the
stimulation-induced increases in these gastric parameters.
Seventy-five min after the second stimulation, gastric acid output and mucosal blood flow responded well to the third stimulation. As the lateral hypothalamic area and the brain stem
vagal nuclei have a large number of NA terminals, the inhibitory
effect of intraventricular NA is probably mediated by adrenergic
receptors located in these regions. These possibilities were
confirmed in other experiments in which a minute amount of NA
was microinjected into both the lateral hypothalamic area and
the brain stem vagal nuclei. Whether or not electrical stimulation of the central neuron system would inhibit gastric functions, as was the case with NA exogenously applied was then
determined.

The distribution of catecholamine-containing nerve cell bodies
and terminals in the central nervous system has been reported
by many investigators (Andèn and co-workers, 1966; Ungerstedt,
1971; Olson and Fuxe, 1972). The locus coeruleus, located in
the dorsolateral tegmentum in the pons, is the largest nucleus
composed of cell bodies which contain NA. Unilateral electrical

stimulation of the locus coeruleus decreased both gastric acid output and mucosal blood flow to around 60 % of the respective basal level. From these results, we concluded that central noradrenergic inhibitory mechanisms originating from the locus coeruleus seem to be involved in regulation of gastric functions, probably at the level of the brain stem ala cinerea. Noradrenergic inhibitory mechanism within the lateral hypothalamic area might also be involved in regulation of gastric functions (Okuma and co-workers, 1980). Its precise neural mechanism is under investigation.

RELATION OF MUCOSAL BLOOD FLOW TO GASTRIC ACID SECRETION

As for the relation of mucosal blood flow to gastric acid secretion, many workers reported a close relationship in animals treated with secretory substances such as histamine and gastrin (Jacobson and co-workers, 1966; Harper and co-workers, 1968; Reed and Sanders, 1971; Main and Whittle, 1973). An increase in acid secretion, regardless of the stimulus is considered to induce a secondary increase in mucosal blood flow. Such a close parallelism was also obtained by stimulation of the central nervous system (Osumi and co-workers, 1977). The coefficient r was 0.896. On the other hand, it is interesting to note that this parallelism was not observed under conditions of stress.

In this series of experiment, gastric cannulation was performed under light ether anesthesia. Precise experimental procedures and results has been presented elesewhere (Kitagawa and co-workers, 1979). Acid output and mucosal blood flow at 3 hr after the discontinuation of ether exposure were 16.5 ± 2.3 μEq/15 min and 4.9 ± 0.6 ml/15 min, respectively. By water-immersion stress, acid output remarkably and significantly increased (465%) immediately after the onset of this stress, yet the mucosal blood flow did not show any corresponding increase. A small amount of atropine 10 μg/kg was given subcutaneously prior to the stress loading. By this pretreatment, the increase in acid output induced by the stress was completely abolished and mucosal blood flow decreased. Such a result was also obtained in vagotomized rats. The increase in acid output corresponded well to the formation of the ulcerative changes. The coefficient r was 0.849. These results suggest that when there is an elevation in gastric acid secretion, but with no parallel increase in mucosal blood flow, gastric ulceration may occur under conditions of stress.

REFERENCES

Andén, N. E., A. Dahlström, K. Fuxe, K. Larsson, L. Olson, and U. Ungerstedt (1966). Ascending monoamine neurons to the telencephalon and diencephalon. Acta physiol. Scand., 67, 313-326.

Harper, A. A., J. B. Reed, and J. R. Smy (1968). Gastric blood
flow in anesthetized cats. J. Physiol. 194, 795-807.
Jacobson, E. D., R. H. Linford, and M. I. Grossman (1966).
Gastric secretion in relation to mucosal blood flow by a
clearance technique. J. Clin. Invest., 45, 1-13.
Kitagawa, H., M. Fujiwara, and Y. Osumi (1979). Effects of
water-immersion stress on gastric secretion and mucosal
blood flow in rats. Gastroenterology, 77, 298-302.
Main, I. H. M., and B. J. R. Whittle (1973). Gastric mucosal
blood flow during pentagastrin and histamine-stimulated
acid secretion in the rats. Br. J. Pharmacol. 49, 534-542.
Okuma, Y., M. Nagata, and Y. Osumi (1980). Effects of acetylcholine and noradrenaline applied into the lateral hypothalamic area on gastric functions in rats. Japan. J.
Pharmacol., 30(Suppl.) 220p.
Olson, L., and K. Fuxe (1972). Further mapping out of central
noradrenaline system. Projections of the "subcoeruleus"
area, Brain Res., 43, 289-295.
Osumi, Y., S. Takaori, and M. Fujiwara (1973). Preventive
effect of fusaric acid, a dopamine β-hydroxylase inhibitor,
on the gastric ulceration induced by water-immersion
stress in rats. Japan. J. Pharmacol. 23, 904-906.
Osumi, Y., S. Aibara, K. Sakae, and M. Fujiwara (1977). Central
noradrenergic inhibition of gastric mucosal blood flow and
acid secretion in rats. Life Sciences, 20, 1407-1416.
Osumi, Y., T. Ishikawa, Y. Okuma, Y. Nagasaka, and M. Fujiwara
(1981). Inhibition of gastric functions by stimulation of
the rat locus coeruleus. Eur. J. Pharmacol. (in press).
Reed, J. D., and D. J. Sanders (1971). Splanchnic nerve stimulation of gastric acid secretion and mucosal blood flow
in anesthetized cats. J. Physiol. 219, 555-570.
Takagi, K., and S. Okabe (1968). The effect of drugs on the
production and recovery process of the stress ulcer. Japan.
J. Pharmacol. 18, 9-18.

Duodenal Ulcer and Dopamine: New Elements in Pathogenesis and Therapy

S. Szabo, G. T. Gallagher, A. Blyzniuk, E. A. Maull and A. W. Sandrock

Department of Pathology, Brigham and Women's Hospital,
Harvard Medical School, Boston, Mass. 02115, USA

ABSTRACT

This review demonstrates the usefulness of cysteamine- or propionitrile-
induced duodenal ulcers in the rat for pharmacologic and pathophysiologic
studies. The animal models were used to elucidate the involvement of dopamine which may represent a new element in both the pathogenesis and therapy
of duodenal ulceration. Dopamine agonists (e.g., bromocriptine or lergotrile), either as a pre- or post-treatment, decreased the intensity of the
acute and chronic duodenal ulcers and diminished the output of gastric acid
in animals given cysteamine or propionitrile. We also demonstrated the existence of specific dopamine binding sites in gastric and duodenal mucosa and
muscularis propria. The chemically induced duodenal ulceration was associated with changes in the sensitivity and number of these dopamine receptors.

KEYWORDS

Duodenal ulcer; Animal models; Dopamine, Ergot alkaloids; Dopamine receptors;
Gastric secretion.

INTRODUCTION

Although duodenal ulcer disease is more frequent in most countries than
gastric ulcer, until recently easily reproducible animal models have been
available only for gastric erosions and ulcers (Wormsley, 1976; Szabo and
co-workers). A few years ago we described that injection of propionitrile
(Szabo and Selye, 1972) or cysteamine (Selye and Szabo, 1973; Szabo, 1978),
produces a rapidly developing acute duodenal ulcer in the rat. Subsequent
structure-activity studies revealed that the duodenal ulcerogenic effect may
be a unique property of certain short chain alkyl chemicals which bear on
one or both ends nucleophilic radicals like -CN, -SH, -NH$_2$, -Cl (Szabo and
Reynolds, 1975; Szabo and co-workers). The structure-activity studies also
suggested the involvement of putative neurotransmitters (e.g., histamine,
dopamine, serotonin, GABA) in the mediation or modulation of duodenal ulcer
disease.

These acute, but especially chronic (Szabo, 1978) experimental duodenal ulcers resemble the human duodenal ulcer disease in both structural (e.g., localization of the ulcer on the anterior and posterior wall of the duodenum, light microscopic appearance of the lesions) and functional criteria (e.g., role of gastric acid, effectiveness of antacids, anticholinergics, vagotomy, histamine H_2 antagonists) (Szabo, 1980, 1978; Szabo and co-workers, 1979; Robert, 1975). Thus, the cysteamine- or propionitrile-induced duodenal ulcers in the rat are suitable models to study the pathogenesis of acute and chronic ulcer disease as well as to test antiulcer drugs for therapeutic effect.

MATERIALS AND METHODS

Female Sprague-Dawley rats (150-200g) had, unless otherwise stated, unlimited access to Purina lab chow and tap water. Each group contained 3-4 rats and every experiment was repeated at least twice and the results were pooled.

In the acute ulcerogenic studies, groups of animals were pretreated with the dopamine agonist bromocriptine or lergotrile (1mg/100g p.o. once daily, for 1 week) before the administration of either cysteamine (28mg/100g p.o. x3, on 1st day) or propionitrile (s.c. x3 daily, 6mg/100g on 1st, 8mg/100g on 2nd, and 10mg/100g on 3rd day). Survivors were killed on the 3rd day after cysteamine or on the 4th day after propionitrile. In chronic studies, rats were given cysteamine (as above) to induce ulcers, then on the 2nd day they were placed on drinking water containing 0.01% cysteamine. On the 2nd day, certain groups of animals were also given 1mg/100g of bromocriptine or lergotrile, p.o. once daily for 1 or 3 weeks, when the survivors were killed. At autopsy, samples of duodenum and stomach were fixed in 10% formalin and processed for light microscopic examination.

In the secretory studies, a stainless steel gastric fistula was implanted according to the method of Hotz and co-workers (1975). One week later, following an overnight fast rats received a single dose (0.2 or 1mg/100g) of bromocriptine or lergotrile and, 30 min later, cysteamine (15mg/100g s.c.) or propionitrile (2mg/100g s.c.). The rats were then placed in mildy restraining cages, and gastric and duodenal/pancreatic secretions were collected through separate tubes under mild vacuum (-7cm H_2O) at hourly intervals for 7 hr. Acid and base were titrated to pH 7.0 in samples of gastric and duodenal/pancreatic juice.

In the biochemical experiments, slight modifications of labelled ligand (^{3}H-dopamine and ^{3}H-haloperidol) binding assays (Burt and co-workers, 1976; List and co-workers, 1980) were used. Groups of rats received a single dose of cysteamine or propionitrile (see above) and they were killed by decapitation 1, 4 or 8 hr later. The mucosa and muscularis propria of the duodenum and glandular stomach were rapidly dissected over ice and immersed into 25 volumes of ice-cold 15mM TES buffer. Following homogenization and centrifugation, the tissues were resuspended (25 vol) 3 times. Membrane suspensions containing ^{3}H-dopamine were incubated in the presence or absence of cold dopamine. After incubation for 30 min at 22°C, aliquots were vacuum filtered through Whatman GF/B filter along with three 4 ml washes of TES buffer. Cold dopamine (10 µM) was used to define specific ^{3}H-dopamine binding (about 60-80% specific binding)

RESULTS AND DISCUSSION

The acute ulcerogenic studies confirmed the rapid production of duodenal ulcers on the anterior and/or posterior wall of the proximal duodenum in rats given cysteamine or propionitrile. Perforation of the anterior ulcers occurred about 24-48 hr after the initiation of treatment with duodenal ulcerogens. The posterior ulcers usually penetrated into the pancreas. Inflammatory cells infiltrated the ulcer crater in rats killed or dead on the 3rd or 4th day.

The cysteamine-induced acute duodenal ulcers were virtually abolished by bromocriptine or lergotrile in a dose- and time-response manner: a single high dose
of either dopamine agonist was slightly active, while a daily treatment with
small quantities almost completely prevented the cysteamine-induced duodenal
ulcer (Fig. 1,2). These studies which were described in detail earlier (Szabo,
1979) also revealed that the dopamine antagonists haloperidol or pimozide
aggravated the experimental duodenal ulcers. New results presented in Table 1
now demonstrate that the intensity of propionitrile-induced acute duodenal
ulcers was also decreased by about 50% after pretreatment with bromocriptine
or lergotrile.

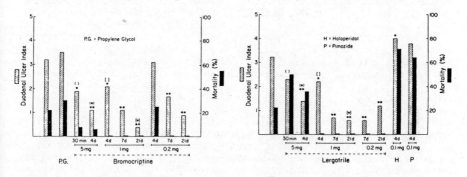

Fig. 1,2.   Effect of bromocriptine (Fig. 1 - left) and lergotrile,
            haloperidol or pimozide on duodenal ulcer produced by
            cysteamine in the rat. (Reprinted from Szabo, 1979).

$$^{*} p<0.05; \quad ^{**} p<0.005$$

TABLE 1 Effect of Bromocriptine or Lergotrile on
Propionitrile-Induced Duodenal Ulcers in the Rat

Group	Pretreatment[#]	Duodenal ulcer		Mortality
		Incidence (Pos./Tot.)	Intensity (Scale:0-3)	(%)
1.	None	16/17	1.2±0.2	88
2.	Bromocriptine	5/9*	0.6±0.3*	100
3.	Lergotrile	6/9	0.6±0.2*	75

[#]In addition, rats of all groups were given propionitrile 30 min after the administration of dopamine
agonists.

$$^{*} = p<0.05$$

The dopamine agonists seem to exert an antiduodenal ulcerogenic effect not
only as pretreatment but also as a post-treatment. It can be seen (Table 2)
that the intensity of cysteamine-produced chronic duodenal ulcers was diminished in rats which started to receive bromocriptine or lergotrile after the
acute duodenal ulcers were formed. After one week of therapy, only the

intensity of duodenal ulcers was reduced, while after three both the incidence and intensity were decreased (Table 2). These results imply an accelerated healing in animals bearing chronic duodenal ulcers and treated with
these ergot alkaloids.

TABLE 2 The Effect of Post-treatment with Lergotrile or
Bromocriptine on the Cysteamine-induced Chronic Duodenal Ulcer
in the Rat

Group	Pretreatment[#]	Duration of Experiment	Duodenal ulcer Incidence (Pos./Tot.)	Intensity (Scale:0-3)	Mortality (%)
1.	Water	7-21 days	38/45	2.0+0.4	47
2.	Lergotrile	7 days	19/25	1.0+0.1*	20
3.	Bromocriptine	7 days	19/25	1.1+0.2*	20
4.	Lergotrile	21 days	9/20*	0.6+0.2*	45
5.	Bromocriptine	21 days	8/21*	1.1+0.2*	33

[#]In addition, rats of all groups received cysteamine.

* = p<0.005

The secretory studies with duodenal ulcerogens alone confirmed our previous
findings with this method (Gallagher and co-workers , 1980). Bromocriptine
or lergotrile, given as a single dose or as a daily pretreatment for one week,
decreased the cysteamine- or propionitrile-induced gastric acid output. The
inhibition was especially prominent during the first 3 hr of collections, but
the total 7 hr gastric acid output was also diminished after a single dose of
the drugs (Table 3).

TABLE 3 Effect of Lergotrile or Bromocriptine on Propionitrile-Induced
Gastric and Pancreatic/Duodenal Secretions in Conscious Rats with
Chronic Gastric Fistula

Group	Pretreatment[#]	Acid output (µEq+SEM) Initial 3hr	Total 7hr	Base output (µEq+SEM) Initial 3hr
1.	None	630+92	920+62	145+13*
2.	Lergotrile (0.2mg, once)	104+57***	398+86**	74+24
3.	Bromocriptine (0.2mg, once)	69+32***	405+85**	148+46
4.	Lergotrile (0.2mg, once daily for 1 week)	264+72*	814+129	142+19
5.	Bromocriptine (0.2mg, once daily for 1 week)	103+49***	818+221	135+30

[#] In addition, rats of all groups were given propionitrile 30 min after
the administration of dopamine agonists.

* = p<0.05;   ** = p<0.01;   *** = p<0.001

TABLE 4 Effect of Cysteamine or Propionitrile on Specific ^{3}H-Dopamine
Binding to Duodenal and Gastric Membranes in the Rat

Tissues	^{3}H-dopamine (pmol/mg protein)						
	Control	1 hr		4 hr		8 hr	
		Cyst.	Prop.	Cyst.	Prop.	Cyst.	Prop.
Du. mucosa	2.9±0.2	2.5±0.9	2.7±1.4	4.9±0.7*	5.9±1.0*	2.8±0.3	4.5±1.1
" musc.	7.7±0.8	2.7±0.5**	2.1±0.6**	7.2±0.7	6.1±0.2	12.4±2.5	20.1±6.7
Gs. mucosa	2.4±0.2	2.0±0.5	2.6±0.9	4.4±0.5**	5.3±0.8*	2.6±0.8	1.9±0.3
" musc.	7.7±0.7	3.3±0.8**	8.7±0.3	4.6±0.4	5.9±0.1	6.7±1.5	9.4±2.5

* = $p<0.01$; ** = $p<0.001$

Surprisingly, the antisecretory effects of a single dose and that of a daily
pretreatment for a week of dopamine agonists were either similar or the one
treatment was better, although in the ulcerogenic studies one or three weeks
of treatment was significantly superior to one dose (Fig. 1,2). Thus, inhibition of gastric acid output cannot completely account for the anti duodenal ulcerogenic effect of these ergot alkaloids. Duodenal/pancreatic base
output cannot explain that either, since, unexpectedly, the values for base
output were also decreased in rats given bromocriptine or lergotrile (Table
3). All these actions of dopamine agonists were more prominent at 1 mg than
at 0.2mg dose. Results not presented here also indicate that these two
drugs also reduced the duodenal/pancreatic output of trypsin and amylase.
These enzymes might represent additional ulcerogenic factors, the activity of
which could be diminished by bromocriptine or lergotrile. New experiments
are in progress in our laboratory to gain further insight into these possibilities.

The biochemical experiments on the characterization of dopamine receptors in
the gut showed a saturable specific binding site in both gastric and duodenal
mucosa and muscularis propria. These results, which were presented in detail
elsewhere (Sandrock, 1981) also demonstrated that the muscle layer of the gut
contains about twice as many specific dopamine sites as the mucosa. Since
we also found a dopamine-sensitive adenylate cyclase in the duodenal mucosa
(Nafradi and Szabo, 1981), these binding sites might be called D_1-receptors.
Duodenal mucosa, known to contain relatively large concentration of dopamine,
proved sensitive to treatment with cysteamine or propionitrile (Szabo et al.,
1978).

Administration of cysteamine or propionitrile in 1 hr resulted in a 2-3 fold
decrease in dopamine binding in duodenal muscularis propria, and in 4 hr in
about a doubling of dopamine binding sites in duodenal and gastric mucosa
(Table 4). These differences seem to disappear 8 hr after the administration
of duodenal ulcerogens (Table 4).

The timing of changes in dopamine binding sites in the stomach and duodenum
correlates well with other biochemical and functional changes related to
the development of duodenal ulcer. Namely, the motility changes and the
delayed gastric emptying are maximal at 30 min - 1 hr after cysteamine or
propionitrile (Lichtenberger et al., 1977), while the gastric acid output
seems to peak around 3-4 hr (Ishii et al., 1976; Szabo et al., 1977; Gallagher

et al., 1980). A dopamine-sensitive early alteration in duodenal motility
has been implicated (Browers and Tytgat, 1980; Malagedala, 1980; Lam, 1980)
in the mechanism of anti duodenal ulcerogenic action of dopamine agonists
(Szabo, 1979). Thus, the biochemical and functional status of dopamine receptors in the stomach and duodenum and its relationship to the pathogenesis
of duodenal ulcer deserves further investigations.

ACKNOWLEDGEMENTS

We greatly appreciate the excellent secretarial help of Ms. Joanne Pirie
in the preparation of this manuscript. These studies were supported in part
by grants AM25229 and ES01876 from the National Institutes of Health.
S. Szabo is a Research Career Development Awardee (AM00600). A.W. Sandrock
was a Summer Research Student Awardee of the American Gastroenterological
Association.

REFERENCES

Brouwers, J.R.B.J., and G.N. Tytgat (1980). Gastroenterology, 79, 184-185.
Burt, D.R., I. Creese and S.H. Snyder (1976). Mol. Pharmacol., 12, 800-812.
Gallagher, G.T. and S. Szabo (1980). Fed. Proc. 39, 326.
Hotz, J., M. Zwicker, H. Minne and R. Ziegler (1975). Pflugers Arch., 353,
171-189.
Ishii, Y., Y. Fujii, and M. Homma (1976). Eur. J. Pharmacol., 36, 331-336.
Lam, S.K. (1980). Gastroenterology, 79, 185.
Lichtenberger, L.M., S. Szabo and E.S. Reynolds (1977). Gastroenterology,
73, 1072-1076.
List, S., M. Titeler, and P. Seeman (1980). Biochem. Pharmacol., 29, 1621-1622.
Malagelada, J.-R. (1980). Gastroenterology, 79, 185.
Nafradi, J. and S. Szabo (1981). Fed. Proc., 40, 709.
Robert, A., J.E. Nezamis, C. Lancaster, and J.N. Badalamenti, (1974).
Digestion, 11, 199-214.
Robert, A., J.E. Nezamis and E. Lancaster, (1975). Toxicol. Appl. Pharmacol.,
31, 201-207.
Sandrock, A.W. and S. Szabo (1981). Gastroenterology, 80, 1362.
Selye, H. and S. Szabo, (1973). Nature, 244, 458-459.
Szabo, S., (1978). Amer. J. Pathol., 93, 273-276.
Szabo, S., (1979). Lancet, 2, 880-882.
Szabo, S., (1980). Amer. J. Pathol., 101, Suppl., S78-S86.
Szabo, S., L.R. Haith, Jr., and E.S. Reynolds, (1979). Amer. J. Dig. Dis.
(Dig. Dis. Sci.), 24, 471-477.
Szabo, S., H.C. Horner, and K.A. Bailey, (1978). Proc. 7th Int. Congr.
Pharmacol, Paris, 33.
Szabo, S., H.C. Horner and G.T. Gallagher, (in press) In: Drugs and Peptic
Ulcer, Pfeiffer, C.J. (ed), CRC Press.
Szabo, S. and E.S. Reynolds, (1975). Environm. Health Perspect., 11, 135-140.
Szabo, S., E.S. Reynolds, L.M. Lichtenberger, L.R. Haith, Jr. and V.J. Dzau,
(1977). Res. Commun. Chem Pathol. Pharmacol., 16, 311-323.
Szabo, S. and H. Selye, (1972). Arch. Pathol., 93, 389-390.
Wormsley, K.G., (1976). Duodenal Ulcer, Horrobin, D.E. (ed), Eden Press,
Montreal, Canada, 1-100.

Defensive Mechanism in Peptic Ulcer and Assessment of Anti-ulcer Agents

K. Ohe, T. Shirakawa, Y. Yokoya, H. Matsumoto, T. Fujiwara,
Y. Okada, M. Onda, M. Inoue and A. Miyoshi

First Department of Internal Medicine, Hiroshima University
School of Medicine, Hiroshima, Japan

ABSTRACT

Defensive mechanism of gastric mucosa was studied. (1) In guinea pig gastric mucosa in vitro, reduction in ATP content occurred preceeding the back diffusion of mucosal acid induced by aspirin or taurocholate. (2) The hydrogen ion permeability increases before the increase in activated pepsin in rat gastric mucosa with aspirin-induced ulceration. (3) Increase in the hydrogen ion permeability was specific for the presence of erosions and intestinal metaplasia in gastric ulcer patients. (4) Anti-ulcer agents showed different patterns in inhibiting the events leading to aspirin-induced ulceration in rats. From these findings, it has been concluded that the increase in hydrogen ion permeability is the consequence of cellular damage in the gastric mucosa and to cause erosions which forms the background for ulceration.

KEYWORDS

Defensive mechanism; H^+ permeability; energy metabolism; gastric mucosa; aspirin; taurocholate; erosion; ulcer; intestinal metaplasia; anti-ulcer agents.

INTRODUCTION

According to Shay's hypothesis (1961), peptic ulcer is formed on the imbalance between aggressive factors and mucosal defensive factors. Therefore, when the defensive mechanism of gastric mucosa is impaired, gastric ulcers occur even if the acid secretion is subnormal. This aspect of ulcerogenesis is of particular interest since many cases of gastric ulcer with hypoacidity are found in Japan because of a high incidence of atrophic gastritis.

INCREASE IN THE HYDROGEN ION PERMEABILITY OF THE GASTRIC MUCOSA AS THE RESULT OF CELLULAR DAMAGE

Method. Guinea pig gastric mucosa was perfused in vitro with a glucose-Ringer solutions continuously titrated to pH 4 and 7.4 at the mucosal and serosal side, respectively (Ohe, Hayashi, Shirakawa and others,1980). The content of high-energy compounds was determined by fluorometric enzyme method (Williamson and Corkey, 1969) in the mucosa removed from the apparatus at an appropriate time.

Results and discussion. After addition of aspirin to 2 mM or taurocholate to 3 mM in the mucosal solution, the potential difference (PD) decreased in approximately equal rate, and the ATP content in the gastric mucosa decreased rapidly to show a significant reduction when the PD was 1/2 (Fig. 1, upper panel). However, the alkalinization of the serosal solution continued for a while until it started to be acidified so that titration with alkali instead of acid was necessary. The acidification became significant when the PD was zero (Fig. 1, lower panel). This finding indicates that the hydrogen ions diffuse from the mucosal to serosal solution through the gastric mucosa which has become permeable as the result of cellular damage.

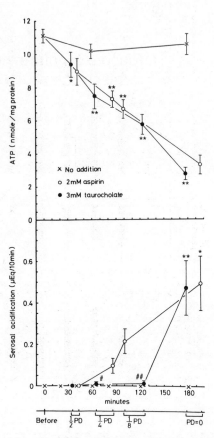

Fig. 1.   Effect of 2 mM aspirin and 3 mM taurocholate on ATP content (upper panel) and serosal acidification (lower panel). Statistically significant difference from the value before addition is shown by *($p \leq 0.05$) or by ** ($p \leq 0.01$).

INCREASE IN HYDROGEN ION PERMEABILITY OF GASTRIC MUCOSA IN ASPIRIN-INDUCED ULCERATION IN RATS

Method.   The aspirin suspension (1 ml of 50 mg/ml) was instilled into the stomach of male Wistar rats through a plastic tube fixed at the pyloric ring.   After an appropriate time, the suspension was replaced by 5 ml of the test solution (100 mM HCl-15 mM NaCl-78 mM mannitol-40 mg/l phenol red), an aliquot was taken (sample 1), and the remaining test solution was left for 30 minutes (sample 2).   The net fluxes of sodium and hydrogen ions were calculated from their concentrations in the samples 1 and 2, according to the formula reported by Skillman, Gould, Chung and others (1974).   The ratio of activated to total pepsinogen was calculated from the acid-protease activities in alkali-treated (pH 8.2 for 20 minutes at 37°C) and untreated homogenates of the gastric mucosa (Ohe, Yokoya, Kitaura and others, 1980).

Results and discussion.   A significant increase in sodium ion net flux and a significant decrease in hydrogen ion net flux were seen immediately after instillation of aspirin (Fig. 1, second and third panels from the top), but the number of ulcers increased significantly after 2 hours (Fig. 3, top penel). A significant but transient increase in the ratio of activated to total pepsinogen in the gastric mucosa was observed 30 minutes after instillation of aspirin, which is between the significant decrease in hydrogen ion net flux and the significant increase in the number of ulcers (Fig. 2, bottom panel).

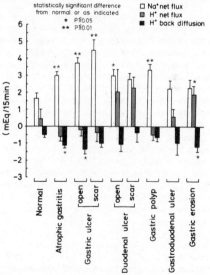

Histological examination revealed a layer of regenerated cells formed at the surface of the gastric mucosa at this time point and comes off thereafter leaving erosions. These findins indicate that the increase in hydrogen ion permeability of gastric mucosa preceeds the peptic process toward ulceration.

INCREASE IN HYDROGEN ION PERMEABILITY OF THE GASTRIC MUCOSA IN VARIOUS MUCOSAL LESIONS IN PATIENTS WITH GASTRIC ULCER

Increase in Hydrogen Ion Permeability in the Gastric Mucosa with Erosions

Method. (1) Using a gastric tube, 200 ml of the above test solution was instilled and left for 15 minutes in the stomach of the patients without pretreatment with gastric secretion inhibitor (Ohe, Shirakawa, Yokoya and others, 1980). The net fluxes of sodium and hydrogen ions and the hydrogen ion back diffusion (H^+ net flux plus neutralized H^+ minus secreted H^+) were calculated according to the formulations by Skillman, Gould, Chung and others, 1974), based on Hollander's two-component hypothesis (Hollander, 1954).

(2) After treating the patients with 400 mg of cimetidine (oral) and 0.5 mg atropine sulfate (intramuscular), the pylorus was blocked by a baloon under the direct vision with a gastrofiberscope (Olympus, GIF-Q), and 100 ml of the above test solution was instilled and left in the stomach for 15 minutes. The net flux of sodium and hydrogen ions were calculated simply by subtracting the amount of ions at the beginning of 15 minutes from the amount at the end, because the above modifications eliminated the necessity of calculating the pyloric loss and the hydrogen ion back diffusion, which includes impractical assumptions.

• (p≤0.05), •• (p≤0.01): Significant difference from zero-time or as indicated

Fig. 2. Number of ulcers, the net flux of sodium and hydrogen ions and the ratio of activated to total pepsinogen in gastric mucosa during the course of aspirin-induced ulceration.

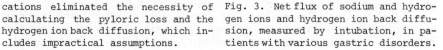

Fig. 3. Net flux of sodium and hydrogen ions and hydrogen ion back diffusion, measured by intubation, in patients with various gastric disorders.

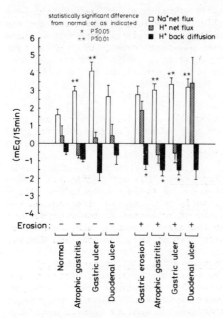

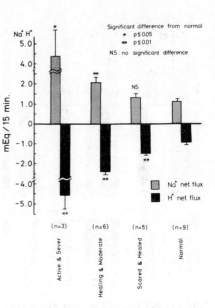

Fig. 4. Net flux of sodium and hydrogen ions and hydrogen ion back diffusion, measured by intubation, in patients classified according to the presence of erosions.

Fig. 5. Net flux of sodium and hydrogen ions, measured after inhibiting the gastric secretion and blocking the pylorus by endoscopy, in gastric ulcer patients classified according to the stage of ulcer (active, healing and scar) and the severity of erosions (severe, moderate and healed).

Results and discussion. In patients not treated with gastric secretion inhibitor and tested using a gastric tube, a significant increase in hydrogen ion back diffusion was specific for atrophic gastritis, open gastric ulcer and gastric erosions whereas the increase in sodium ion net flux seemed to be non-specific (Fig. 3). However, in patients with atrophic gastritis and those with gastric ulcer, the increase in hydrogen ion back diffusion was found to be specific for the presence of erosions (Fig. 4). Further, when tested in gastric ulcer patients treated with cimetidine plus atropine after blocking the pylorus by endoscopy, the hydrogen ion net flux was significantly decreased in parallel with the severity of erosions (Fig. 5). Particularly, the fact that the patients with gastric ulcer in scar stage without detectable erosion showed a significantly lower hydrogen ion net flux than normal subjects indicated the increased hydrogen ion permeability of gastric mucosa even after the ulcer and accompanied erosions healed. The sodium ion net flux was also increased, but in patients with the ulcer in scar stage without erosion there was no difference from normal subjects. From the above findings, it has been speculated that the hydrogen ion permeability of the gastric mucosa increases to cause the gastric erosions which form the background for ulceration.

Increase in the Hydrogen Ion Permeability in the Gastric Mucosa with Intestinal Metaplasia

In the gastric mucosa with diffuse intestinal metaplasia, tested by endoscopy, the hydrogen ion net flux was significantly higher than in the fundic and py-

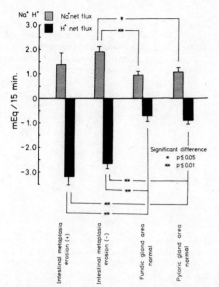

Fig. 6. Net flux of sodium and hydrogen ions in the gastric mucosa with intestinal metaplasia in comparison with those in normal fundic and pyloric gland area.

loric gland area of normal subjects (Fig. 6), indicating that the intestinal metaplasia also increases the hydrogen ion permeability of the gastric mucosa.

ASSESSMENT OF ANTI-ULCER AGENTS

Using the above experimental model of aspirin-induced gastric ulceration in rats, a few anti-ulcer agents were tested (TABLE 1).

Cimetidine. The intraperitoneal injection of 50 mg/kg of cimetidine significantly inhibited the increase in the ratio of activated to total pepsinogen in the gastric mucosa and the ulceration without affecting the ion fluxes.

Carbenoxolone and prostaglandin-E_2. The intragastric administration of 160 mg/kg of carbenoxolone and the subcutaneous injection of 600 μg/kg of prostaglandin-E_2 inhibited significantly the increase in sodium ion net flux and the decrease in hydrogen ion net flux as well as the ulcer formation in rats pretreated with atropine (1 mg/kg) to inhibit the acid secretion.

Cetraxate. The intragastric administration of 300 mg/kg of cetraxate inhibited the increase in the ratio of activated to total pepsinogen in the gastric mucosa and the ulceration without affecting the ion fluxes, being pro-

TABLE 1. Protective Effect of Anti-Ulcer Agents against Aspirin-Induced Gastric Mucosal Damage

	Inhibition of the increase in[1]			
Anti-ulcer agent	Na^+ net flux	H^+ net flux[2]	Mucosal pepsin (%)[3]	Number of ulcers
Cimeticine	−	−	+	+
Carbenoxolone	+	+	NT	+
Prostaglandin-E_2	+	+	NT	+
Cetraxate	−	−	+	+
Zolimidine	−	+	NT	+
Geranyl-geranylacetone	−	+	NT	+
Pirenzepine	+	+	NT	+

[1]Significant inhibition by the agent in comparison with the control without the agent.
[2]The negative increase in the H^+ net flux.
[3]The ratio of activated to total pepsinogen in the gastric mucosa.
NT: not tested.

274   K. Ohe *et al.*

bably due to its anti-plasmin activity.

Zolimidine and geranyl-geranylacetone. The intragastric administrayion of either 300 mg/kg of zolimidine or 200 mg/kg of geranyl-geranylacetone inhibited the decrease in hydrogen ion net flux and the ulcer formation without inhibiting the increase in sodium ion net flux in atropine-treated rats.

Pirenzepine. The intraperitoneal injection of 100 mg/kg of pirenzepine inhibited the increase in sodium ion net flux, the decrease in hydrogen ion net flux and ulcer formation in rats treated with YM-11170 (5 mg/kg), a new H_2-receptor antagonist.

The above anti-ulcer agents showed different patterns in inhibiting the events leading to ulcer formation, probably indicating the complexity of the process to form ulcers by impairment of defensive mechanism.

CONCLUSIONS

1) From the results of experimental and clinical studies on hydrogen ion permeability of gastric mucosa, the following chain of events were proposed as the process leading to ulcer formation caused by the impairment of defensive mechanism; e. g., cellular damage - increase in hydrogen ion permeability - erosions - peptic process - ulcer. The intestinal metaplasia may also cause the increase in hydrogen ion permeability in gastric ulcer patients.

2) Different anti-ulcer agents showed different patterns in inhibiting the events leading to ulceration induced by aspirin. To find out the reason for these differences, further investigations are required in relation to the validity of the above proposal on the mechanism of ulcer formation.

REFERENCES

Hollander, F (1954). Two-component mucous barrier. Its activity in protecting the gastroduodenal mucosa against peptic ulceration. A. M. A. Arch. Int. Med., 93, 107-120.
Ohe, K., K. Hayashi, T. Shirakawa, K. Yamada, T. Kawasaki and A. Miyoshi (1980). Aspirin- and taurocholate-induced metabolic damage in mammalian gastric mucosa in vitro. Am. J. Physiol., 239, G457-G462.
Ohe, K., T. Shirakawa, H. Yokoya, M. Onda, A. Noguchi, S. Uraki, M. Inoue and A. Miyoshi (1980). Studies on the hydrogen ion back diffusion in patients with gastric ulcer. Hiroshima J. Med. Sci., 29, 1-5.
Ohe, K., H. Yokoya, T. Kitaura, T. Kunita and A. Miyoshi (1980). Increase in pepsin content in gastric mucosa during the course of aspirin- and taurocholate-induced gastric ulceration in rats. Digest. Dis. Sci., 25, 849-856.
Shay, H. (1961). Etiology of peptic ulcer. Am. J. Digest. Dis., 6, 29-49.
Skillman, J. J., S. A. Gould, R. S. K. Chung and W. Silen (1974). The gastric mucosal barrier: clinical and experimental studies in critically ill and normal man, and in rabbit. Ann. Surg., 172, 564-584.
Williamson, J. R. and B. E. Corkey (1969). Assay of intermediates of citric acid cycle and related compounds by fluorometric enzyme methods. In S. Fleischer and L. Packer (Ed.), Methods in Enzymology, Vol. 13, Academic Press, New York. pp. 434-513.

Differential Role of Histamine in Duodenal versus Gastric Experimental Ulcer

C. J. Pfeiffer

Laboratory of Investigative Gastroenterology, Memorial University of
Newfoundland, Faculty of Medicine, St. John's, Nfld., Canada

ABSTRACT

Although exogenous histamine is clearly established as a potent gastric acid
stimulator, vasoactive agent, and ulcer-inducing chemical, the role of endogenous histamine in ulcer pathogenesis remains unclear. The present report reviews this topic, and presents recent data on the guinea pig treated
with histamine and a specific H_2 agonist in light of gastric and duodenal
ulcer and other tissue responses. The predominance of H_2 receptor activity
in duodenal ulcer etiology and H_1 receptor stimulation in experimental gastric ulcer pathogenesis is suggested.

KEYWORDS

Histamine; guinea pig; ulcer; stomach; duodenum; H_1-H_2 receptors.

INTRODUCTION

Exogenous histamine is an established inducer of experimental ulcer; due to
its effects on both acid-peptic secretion and its actions on the vascular
system, and due to the multifactorial basis of ulcer in general, its mechanisms of ulcer induction are probably multiple. Further, spontaneous ulcer
formation in humans may depend upon some action of endogenous histamine,
known to be present in high quantities in the gastric mucosa, but this phenomenon remains obscure. Although hydrochloric acid is required for ulcer
development and H_2 blocking agents inhibit both ulcer formation and acid
secretion, it is still not known if endogenous histamine is a necessary link
in the acid secretory mechanism, and if released histamine is a primary or
secondary event in the early pathogenesis of gastric or duodenal mucosal
erosion. Furthermore, the specific cellular sources of the total pool of
endogenous, mucosal histamine are still debated; only some of the histamine-
containing cells have been clearly identified. Recent development of rather
specific H_1 and H_2 agonists and antagonists have made possible the more detailed exploration of these problems, and some of this information is reviewed in the present communication.

275

EXOGENOUS HISTAMINE AND ULCER INDUCTION

Since 1920 it has been known that histamine is a powerful gastric stimulant, and since 1942 that exogenous histamine is ulcerogenic in animals. Gastric ulcers have been induced by histamine in guinea pigs (Halpern and Martin, 1946), rats (Moreno and Brodie, 1962), mice (Schayer, 1959), and monkeys, dogs, cats, and rabbits (Hay and co-workers, 1942). Because exogenous histamine is rapidly metabolized, slow release preparations or multiple injections are frequently required. In histamine resistant species such as the rat, large doses are required for ulcer induction but in highly sensitive species such as the guinea pig, single low doses are ulcerogenic to the stomach. An interesting finding on site sensitivity for ulcer induction in the guinea pig has been reported by Eagleton and Watt (1967, 1971) and confirmed by Cho and Pfeiffer (1981); i.e., single i.p. doses of histamine induced gastric ulceration but repeated i.m. doses induced duodenal ulceration.

ENDOGENOUS HISTAMINE AND ULCER INDUCTION

The important question of whether endogenous histamine is a primary or secondary factor in ulcer pathogenesis is not yet proven. Such a relationship would likely depend upon site of ulcer formation, species, and whether the ulceration is spontaneous, is related to a particular drug or chemical, whether there is a particular stress-related or microvascular perfusion change, etc. In animal models the prototype of endogenous histamine releasers, Compound 48/80, is ulcerogenic in the rat. Furthermore, in experimental ulcer models there is considerable evidence for gastric histamine release. Gastric mucosal tissue histamine is depleted during reserpine, glucocorticoid, insulin, indomethacin, aspirin, fluphenamic acid, acetic acid, and serotonin induced ulceration, or after electrical stress. Enhanced histamine synsthesis, as reflected by an elevation in histidine decarboxylase activity, also occurs after the above drug administrations, as well as during restraint ulceration in the rat. Mast cell degranulation is associated with release of 5-HT and other amines as well as histamine, and this phenomenon occurs after treatment with such ulcerogenic drugs as reserpine and glucocorticoids. An increase in gastric juice histamine content has also been reported after the rat gastric mucosa has been damaged by the irritants, acetic or salicylic acid (Johnson, 1967). As reviewed by Schwartz (1971), to demonstrate that endogenous histamine is involved in ulcer production it is necessary to prove that histamine itself is ulcerogenic, that it is present locally, and that it is released during the pathogenesis of the lesions. These criteria have been satisfied but they do not prove a primary role for histamine in ulcer pathogenesis. Further information has been provided by experiments of Rees and co-workers (1977) in which H_1 and H_2 antagonists were studied in relation to gastric mucosal barrier disruption induced in the canine pouch in response to sodium taurocholate. Only when these two classes of histamine antagonists were used in combination, was bile salt damage reduced, suggesting that mucosal histamine did play an etiologic role in adverse mucosal ionic flux changes. Later data (Rees and co-workers, 1978) suggested that this endogenous histamine was derived from a nonmast cell pool in the gastric mucosa.

Accordingly, both mast cell and nonmast cell endogenous pools may contribute to the histamine released during gastric mucosal damage. Disodium cromoglycate, which inhibits the liberation of mediators of anaphylaxis, has been postulated to act by stabilizing the mast cell membrane. It inhibits promethazine-induced gastric ulcers in the guinea pig in a dose-dependent fashion (Sadeghi and co-workers, 1976). Also it has been reported by Ogle and Lau (1979) that disodium chromoglycate pretreatment inhibited reserpine-induced gastric ulcers in the rat, and that mucosal mast cell degranulation was concurrently prevented. The ulcer-preventive agent, zinc sulfate, also inhibited mast cell degranulation (Cho and Ogle, 1977), but acts as well by stabilizing lysosomal membranes (Pfeiffer and co-workers, 1980). Further evidence supporting the active role of endogenous histamine in experimental ulcer development is the finding of Ritchie and co-workers (1967) that there was a fall in incidence of stress ulcers in the rat stomach when the level of tissue histamine was reduced by inhibiting histidine decarboxylase activity.

In the course of gastric damage induced in rats by instillation of ethanol (25, 50, or 98%), the gastric content of histamine was increased. However, if exogenous histamine was provided and absorbed in this preparation, gastric lesion scores were not enhanced, and 16,16-dimethyl prostaglandin E_2 was found to reduce endogenous histamine release, as well as lesion formation (Aures and co-workers, 1980). Also, in rats the gastric mucosal barrier disruption caused by exposure to 40mM acetylsalicylic acid was inhibited by H_2 blocking agents but not by mepyramine, an H_1 antagonist (Bommelaer and Guth, 1979).

The relationship of endogenous histamine with human peptic ulcer has recently been studied. Prospective analyses of men with duodenal ulcer revealed that the mucosal histamine content was lower by 30 percent in ulcer patients than in control subjects, and it was suggested that histamine release was increased during duodenal ulcer pathogenesis (Troidl and co-workers, 1976). Histamine methyltransferase activity was found to be reduced in the gastric mucosa of duodenal ulcer patients, and this may partially explain the elevated hydrochloric acid secretion commonly observed in association with duodenal ulcer (Barth and co-workers, 1977). Although too rare to explain typical peptic ulcer disease, isolated case reports have also shown that hyperhistaminemia associated with chronic myelogenous leukemia can result in severe gastrointestinal ulceration (Hirasuna and co-workers, 1979).

MECHANISMS OF ACTION OF HISTAMINE IN ULCER PATHOGENESIS

To the extent that histamine is involved in ulcer pathogenesis, its modes of action are probably numerous. For simplicity they can be characterized as acid-peptic secretory effects, vascular effects, and other effects. The acid-secretory stimulation is well established, and was suggested above for human duodenal ulcer disease. Okabe and co-workers (1981) have reported that histamine-induced gastric and duodenal ulcers in the dog appear to be induced mainly by gastric hypersecretion. We have reported that the experimental duodenal but not gastric ulceration in the guinea pig was associated with enhanced gastric acid-peptic secretion (Cho and Pfeiffer, 1981). Further, the duodenal ulcer model in the rat, induced by the combination of histamine plus carbachol appears to depend upon gastric hypersecretion (Robert and co-workers, 1972). However, the histamine derivative, imidazole, exerts antisecretory effects in the isolated gastric mucosa (Goto and Watanabe, 1978) in common with other inhibitory histamine analogs.

An etiologic role for localized mucosal circulatory insufficiency has long been hypothesized in peptic ulcer (Pfeiffer and Sethbhakdi, 1971) particularly for human stress ulceration and experimental stress ulceration. Furthermore, enhanced mucosal flow has been shown to exert cytoprotective

effects in experimental erosive gastritis (Moody and co-workers, 1978).
Histamine induces gastric mucosal vasodilatation, plasma leakage and hemo-
concentration, and eventually circulatory stasis and anoxia in the gastric
mucosa. In angiograms of rats and dogs studied after histamine treatment,
the vasopressor drugs that protected against ulcers and vascular plethora
did not reduce the histamine-induced acid secretion (Kowalewaki, 1975).
It has recently been shown that independent H_1 and H_2 receptors, both sub-
serving vasodilatation, are present in rat gastric submucosal arterioles,
and that the H_1 influence was predominant in the antrum (Guth and co-workers
1978, 1980) or in the whole stomach, as reported recently in Japan. In the
dog Heidenhain gastric pouch the mucosal vasculature appeared to be more
sensitive to histamine than the parietal cell and less sensitive to H_2
blocking agents (Knight, 1979).

We have reported that the selective H_2 agonist, dimaprit, induces duodenal
ulceration, and to a far lesser degree, gastric ulceration, in the guinea
pig. An H_1 antagonist, diphenhydramine, inhibited histamine-induced gastric
ulceration in the guinea pig, but cimetidine (H_2 blocker) was particularly
effective in inhibiting histamine and dimaprit-induced duodenal ulcers.

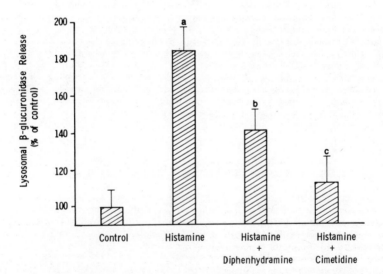

Fig. 1.
Histamine-treated group. Each value is the mean of
five determinations. Vertical bars stand for S.E.M.

Because of these findings, the increased gastric secretion observed in the
guinea pigs with duodenal ulcer (mentioned above), the same observation in
humans with duodenal ulcer, and the reported H_1 and H_2 vascular responses
in the gastroduodenal mucosa, it is suggested that there is predominance of
H_2 receptor activity in duodenal ulcer, and H_1 activity in gastric ulcer,
and that the former is mediated mainly through vascular mechanisms and the

latter through gastric secretory mechanisms. There is, nonetheless, over-lap in these functions. Our observation that the guinea pig gastric ulcers were localized to the antrum further supports this concept, as H_1-responsive arterioles were more prevalent in the antrum than in the corpus.

The effect of histamine on other membrane systems possibly associated with ulcer pathogenesis (Pfeiffer and co-workers, 1980), i.e., lysosomal mem-branes, has also been demonstrated. As shown in (Fig. 1), in vitro studies with isolated hepatic lysosomes indicated release of β-glucuronidase in-duced by histamine, a phenomenon inhibited by both H_1 and H_2 blocking agents. Both of these agents alone were also stabilizers of non-histamine treated lysosomes, whereas excitation specifically of H_2 receptor sites in this system did not labilize the membranes as did excitation of both H_1 and H_2 receptors (by histamine; Fig. 2). In lysosomes isolated from the gastric mucosa of histamine treated guinea pigs, an H_1 blocking agent reduced the release of β-glucuronidase caused by histamine in the stomach, but did not

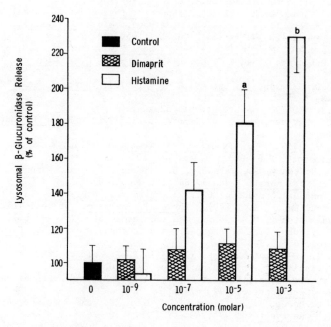

Fig. 2. Lysosomal membrane alterations in isolated
         hepatic lysosomes.

alter duodenal lysosomal permeability. Cimetidine similarly affected the gastric but not duodenal acid hydrolase release in the mucosa.

The above mechanisms may account for part of the actions of histamine in ulcer pathogenesis, and histamine is only one factor in this complex dia-thesis. Other actions of histamine less well understood may include its stimulation of adenylate cyclase activity and cyclic AMP production, mainly in conjunction of H_2 receptor sites.

ACKNOWLEDGMENT

The author is most appreciative of Dr. C.H. Cho, who collaborated in obtaining the data presented in Figs. 1 and 2.

REFERENCES

Aures, D., Guth, P.H., Paulsen, J., and Grossman, M.I. (1980). Gastro-
    enterol. 78, 1133 (abst.).
Barth, H., Troidl, H., Lorenz, W., Rohde, H., and Glass, R. (1977). Agents
    and Actions 7, 75-79.
Bommelaer, G., and Guth, P.H. (1979). Gastroenterol. 77, 303-308.
Cho, C.H., and Ogle, C.W. (1977). Europ. J. Pharmacol. 43, 315-322.
Cho, C.H., and C.J. Pfeiffer (1981). Digest. Dis. and Sci. 26, 306-311.
Eagleton, G.B., and J. Watt (1967). J. Pathol. Bacteriol. 93, 694-696,
    1967.
Eagleton, G.B., and J. Watt (1971). In C.J. Pfeiffer (Ed.), Peptic Ulcer,
    J.B. Lippincott, Philadelphia, Chap. 4, pp. 34-44.
Goto, Y. and Watanabe, K. (1978). Japan. J. Pharmacol. 28, 185-195.
Guth, P.H., Moler, T.L., and Smith, E. (1980). Microvas. Res. 19, 320-328.
Guth, P.H., and Smith, E. (1978). Gut 19, 1059-1063.
Halpern, B., and J. Martin (1946). C.R. Soc. Biol. (Paris), 140, 830-832.
Hay, L.J., R.L. Varco, and C.F. Code (1942). Surg. Gynec. Obstet. 75,
    178-182.
Hirasuna, J.D., Shelub, I., and Bolt, R.J. (1979). West. J. Med. 131,
    140-143.
Johnson, L.R. (1967). Gastroenterol. 52, 8-15.
Knight, S.E., McIsaac, R.L., and Rennie, C.D. (1979). Brit. J. Pharmacol.
    66, 458.
Kowalewski, K. (1975). in Experimental Ulcer, Gheorghiu, T. et al (Ed.).
    G. Witzstrock, Pub. Baden-Baden, pp. 105-112.
Moody, F.G., McGreevy, J., Zalewsky, C., Cheung, L.Y., and Simons, M.
    (1978). Acta physiol. scand. Special Suppl. 35-43.
Moreno, O., and D.A. Brodie (1962). J. Pharmacol. exp. Ther. 135, 259-264.
Ogle, C.W., and Lau, H.K. (1979). Europ. J. Pharmacol. 55, 411-415.
Okabe, S. and Ohtsuki, H. (1981). Gastroenterol. 80, 1242 (abst.).
Pfeiffer, C.J., Cho, C.H., Cheema, A., and Saltman, D. (1980). Europ. J.
    Pharmacol. 61, 347-353.
Pfeiffer, C.J. and Sethbhakdi, S. (1971) in Peptic Ulcer, Pfeiffer, C.J.
    (Ed.), Lippincott, Philadelphia, pp. 207-220.
Rees, W.D.W., Rhodes, J., Wheeler, M.H., Meek, E.M., and Newcombe, R.G.,
    (1977). Gastroenterol. 72, 67-71.
Rees, W.D.W., Rhodes, J., Williams, B.C., Owen, E., and Newcombe, R.G.
    (1978). Gastroenterol. 74, 492-492.
Ritchie, W.P., Breen, J.J., Grigg, D.I., and Wangensteen, O.H. (1967). Gut
    8, 32-35.
Robert, A., Nezamis, J.E., Dale, J.E., and Stowe, D.F. (1972). Digestion
    6, 35-45.
Sadeghi, D., Zarrindast, M.R., and Ghaffarpur, F.A. (1976). Toxicol. Appl.
    Pharmacol. 35, 179-181.
Schayer, R.W. (1959). Physiol. Rev. 39, 116-126.
Schwartz, J.C. (1971). In C.J. Pfeiffer, (Ed.). Peptic Ulcer, J.B.
    Lippincott, Philadelphia, Chap. 20, pp. 190-198.
Troidl, H., Lorenz, W., Rohde, H., Häfner, G., and Ronszhimer, M. (1976).
    Klin. Wschr. 54, 947-956.

Can the Mechanisms of Aspirin-induced Gastric Mucosal Injury be Identified?

G. L. Kauffman, Jr

Center for Ulcer Research and Education, and Surgical Service,
Wadsworth V. A. Medical Center, Los Angeles, California 90064,
USA

ABSTRACT

In combination with luminal acidification, gastric mucosal injury occurs with oral and parenteral aspirin administration. The magnitude of rat gastric bleeding and cat antral ulceration is the same regardless of the route of aspirin administration. Although oral and parenteral aspirin administration profoundly depress rat fundic and antral prostaglandin synthesis, certain parameters with which gastric mucosal integrity has been associated are affected in different ways by each mode of aspirin administration. Non-stimulated canine gastric mucosal blood flow, as measured by mucosal aminopyrine clearance, increases 30% when aspirin is topically applied to the gastric mucosa and is reduced about 30% when aspirin is given intravenously. Topical aspirin produces gastric bleeding in dog which is associated with a significant reduction in transmucosal potential difference and change in net H^+ and Na^+ flux whereas, in cat, intravenous aspirin also produces gastric bleeding and ulceration but is not associated with any change in these mucosal permeability parameters. Topical aspirin produces a small increase in gastric acid secretion yet, intravenous aspirin significantly reduces histamine-stimulated gastric acid secretion in dog. Parenteral aspirin reduces luminal fluid soluble glycoprotein output as well as reducing glycoprotein biosynthesis, indicating a reduction in gastric mucus formation. When placed on the nutrient side of amphibian gastric mucosa in vitro, aspirin reduces bicarbonate secretion from the surface epithelial cells. Although the effect of topical aspirin on these two functions has not been studied, these observations do suggest that reduction of the bicarbonate-rich unstirred layer of gastric gel mucus may play a role in aspirin-induced gastric mucosal injury. In summary, the mechanisms of aspirin-induced gastric mucosal injury are multiple and may be related to inhibition of gastric mucus and bicarbonate production.

KEYWORDS

Aspirin, prostaglandins, gastric mucosal injury, gastric acid secretion, gastric blood flow, gastric mucosal barrier

INTRODUCTION

Topical and parenteral aspirin administration produce the same degree of gastric mucosal injury. If the assumption is made that the mechanism of topical and parenteral aspirin-induced injury is the same, then the effect of topical and parenteral aspirin administration on the parameter through which aspirin might work should also be identical. Based on the work of a variety of investigators, a comparison has been made between the effect of topical and parenteral aspirin administration on gastric mucosal blood flow, the "gastric mucosal barrier", and gastric acid secretion in an attempt to identify the mechanism of aspirin-induced gastric mucosal injury.

MUCOSAL INJURY INDUCED BY ASPIRIN

The degree of gross gastric mucosal injury produced by the topical application of aspirin in acid is the same as that produced by parenteral aspirin with either stimulated gastric acid secretion or exogenous luminal acid. Brodie and Chase (1967) found that the dose-response for gastric irritation, measured as percent of rats with intragastric hemorrhage, following administration of oral or intraperitoneal aspirin was similar. Hansen, Aures and Grossman (1980) reported that in cats receiving histamine, aspirin (40 mg·kg^{-1}) administered as a bolus either intravenously or intragastrically within 4 hours developed antral ulcers. The mean area of ulceration and plasma and mucosal salicylate concentrations at the end of the study were not significantly different in the two groups. These observations indicate that experimentally, topical aspirin produces the same degree of gastric mucosal injury as does parenteral aspirin.

EFFECT OF ASPIRIN ON MUCOSAL PROSTAGLANDIN FORMATION

Vane (1971) showed that aspirin inhibits endogenous prostaglandin biosynthesis. A comparison of the effect of oral and intragastric aspirin on the ability of the gastric mucosa to generate prostacyclin and PGE$_2$ has been made by Konturek et al (1981). They found that aspirin given intravenously or intragastrically to rats, in doses producing gastric mucosal lesions, produced a dose-dependent decrease in the mucosal generation of prostacyclin and PGE$_2$. These observations do not shed additional light on the mechanism of aspirin-induced injury but do suggest that reduction in tissue prostaglandin synthesis may play a role.

EFFECT OF ASPIRIN ON GASTRIC MUCOSAL BLOOD FLOW

Augur (1970) found that gastric mucosal blood flow, as measured by the aminopyrine clearance technique, in canine Heidenhain pouches increased about 30% during and following irrigation with 20 mM aspirin in 100 mN HCl. Yet, aspirin, 100 mg·kg^{-1}, given intravenously to dogs has been reported by Kauffman, Aures, and Grossman (1980) to significantly reduce by 30% Heidenhain pouch mucosal blood flow also as measured also by the aminopyrine clearance technique. Although maintenance of adequate mucosal blood flow may be an important mechanism in mucosal protection, it seems unlikely, based on these studies, that the mechanism of aspirin induced mucosal injury is related to a change in this parameter.

EFFECT OF ASPIRIN ON THE "GASTRIC MUCOSAL BARRIER"

Under normal conditions, the gastric epithelium can maintain a large H^+ gradient, the mucosal pH being 7.4 and that of the luminal fluid at times 2 or lower. Davenport (1965) showed that with exogenous 100 mN HCl in a canine Heidenhain pouch, the loss of H^+ from the fluid was around 200 $\mu mol \cdot 30$ min^{-1}, and the gain in fluid Na^+ and K^+ was around 250 $\mu mol \cdot 30$ min^{-1} and 10 $\mu mol \cdot 30$ min^{-1} respectively. Instilling 20 mM aspirin in 100 mN HCl in the pouch resulted in a significant change in net cationic flux with the H^+ loss being around 800 $\mu mol \cdot 30 min^{-1}$, Na^+ gain 1000 $\mu mol \cdot 30$ min^{-1} and K^+ gain 55 $\mu mol \cdot 30$ min. Also Bugat et al (1976) reported that in cats prepared with gastric pouches, the topical application of 20 mM aspirin in 100 mN HCl caused a net H^+ loss of 450 $\mu mol \cdot 30$ min^{-1}, and net gain of Na^+ of 500 $\mu mol \cdot 30$ min^{-1} and transmucosal potential difference of -25 mv yet in the same model, administration of intravenous aspirin, 100 $mg \cdot kg^{-1} \cdot day^{-1}$ for 7 days, was not associated with significant change in these permeability characteristics. The net H^+ loss was 40 $\mu mol \cdot 30$ min^{-1}, net Na^+ gain 130 $\mu mol \cdot 30$ min^{-1} and transmucosal potential difference -50 mv. Although the "gastric mucosal barrier has been considered to be important in the maintenance of mucosal integrity, these different effects of topical versus parenteral aspirin administration suggest that the mechanism of aspirin-induced gastric mucosal injury is not related to change in "mucosal barrier" characteristics.

EFFECT OF ASPIRIN ON GASTRIC ACID SECRETION

Topical aspirin appears to affect acid secretion in a different way than intravenous administration. Davenport (1969) demonstrated that the net loss of H^+ from a canine Heidenhain pouch during irrigation with 5 and 10 mM aspirin in 100 mN HCl was slightly less than with 100 mN HCl alone and with 20 mM aspirin in 100 mN HCl slightly less than with 100 mN HCl alone. These observations suggest that topical aspirin (5 mM and 10 mM) minimally stimulates acid secretion. As has been suggested by Davenport (1966) this is likely due to liberation of histamine into the interstitial fluid. In contrast to this topical aspirin effect, Kauffman and Grossman (1981) have reported that in the canine Heidenhain pouch and gastric fistula, intravenous aspirin, 100 mg kg^{-1}, given as a bolus significantly inhibits submaximal histamine-stimulated acid secretion 24% and 28% respectively. It is not known whether this inhibitory response is secondary to a primary effect of aspirin on the parietal cell or reduced mucosal blood flow. Again, different effects of aspirin, as a function of route of administration have been observed for gastric acid secretion, which suggests that the mechanism by aspirin-induced gastric mucosal injury is not related to that parameter.

EFFECT OF ASPIRIN ON GASTRIC MUCUS AND BICARBONATE SECRETION

The effect of aspirin on gastric mucus synthesis and secretion has not been studied quite as extensively comparing the topical versus parenteral routes as have the aforementioned parameters. Most of the studies are comparable to the parenteral route of administration since aspirin was given either parenterally or studied in an in vitro preparation with aspirin being placed in the nutrient solution. Menguy and Masters (1965) observed that in rats, parenteral administration of aspirin caused a decrease in gastric mucosal content of mucus measured by periodic acid schiff staining and direct measurement of mucosal hexosamine and fucose content. They also found that oral administration of aspirin in dogs with denervated antral pouches resulted in lower mucus volume with reducted carbohydrate concentration. Rainsford (1977) reported that oral aspirin administered to rats at a dose of 200 mg·kg^{-1} caused a marked inhibition of $^{35}SO_4$= incorporation into gastric glycoproteins. Kent and Allen (1968) found that in the presence of 15 mM salicylate the incorporation of D-[U-^{14}C] glucose was significantly reduced in human gastric mucosal tissue. These observations suggest that the synthesis and secretion of gastric mucus is reduced by parenteral aspirin.

Gastric bicarbonate secretion, which is thought to be a product of the surface epithelial cell, has also been shown by Garner (1977) to be significantly reduced in Necturus and Rana temporaria fundic mucosa in vitro by 3mM aspirin. No information on the effect of topical aspirin on gastric bicarbonate secretion is available.

The potential role of an unstirred layer of gastric gel mucus which is rich in bicarbonate in mucosal protection was first hypothesized by Heatley (1959). More recently, the concept has been expanded by Allen and Garner (1980) but many questions about the true physiologic significance of gastric gel mucus and bicarbonate secretion remain unanswered.

CONCLUSION

In an attempt to identify the mechanism of aspirin-induced gastric mucosal injury, topical and parenteral aspirin producing nearly equal damage, the effect of topical versus parenteral aspirin on gastric mucosal blood flow, the gastric "mucosal barrier" and gastric acid secretion has been reviewed. Topical aspirin stimulates an increase in mucosal blood flow, changes the "mucosal barrier" characteristics and stimulates acid secretion. Parenteral aspirin reduces mucosal blood flow, has no effect on the gastric "mucosal barrier" and reduces stimulated acid secretion. From these data, no conclusion can be drawn regarding a mechanism of aspirin action. Parenteral aspirin does reduce the synthesis and secretion of gastric mucus and bicarbonate. Presently it can be concluded that the mechanisms of aspirin-induced gastric mucosal injury are multiple and may be in part related to inhibition of gastric mucus and bicarbonate production.

ACKNOWLEDGEMENT

This work was supported by grants AM17328 and AM27465 from the National Institutes of Health. The author expresses appreciation to Anita Boesman for typing the manuscript.

REFERENCES

Allen, A., and Garner, A. (1980). Gut, 21, 249-262.
Augur, N. (1970). Gastroenterology, 58, 311-320.
Brodie, D. A., and Chase, B. J. (1967). Gastroenterology, 53, 604-610.
Bugat, R., Thompson, M. R., Aures, D., and Grossman, M. I. (1976).
   Gastroenterology, 71, 754-759.
Davenport, H. W. (1965). Gastroenterology, 49, 189-196.
Davenport, H. W. (1966). Gastroenterology, 50, 487-499.

Davenport, H. W. (1969). Gastroenterology, 56, 439-449.
Garner, A. (1977). Acta Physiol. Scand., 99, 281-291.
Hansen, D., Aures, D., and Grossman, M. I. (1980). Proc. Soc. Expt. Biol. and Med., 164, 589-592.
Heatley, N. (1959). Gastroenterology, 37, 313-318.
Kauffman, G. L. Jr., Aures, D., and Grossman, M. I. (1980). Am. J. Physiol., 238, G131-G134.
Kauffman, G. L. Jr., and Grossman, M. I. (1981). Gastroenterology, 80, 1189.
Kent, P. W., and Allen, A. (1968). Biochem. J., 106, 645-658.
Konturek, S. J., Piastucki, I., Brzozowski, T., Radecki, T., Dembinska-Kiec, A., Zmuda, A., and Grejglewski (1981). Gastroenterology, 80, 4-9.
Menguy, R., and Masters, Y. F. (1965). Surg. Gyn. and Obstet., 120, 92-98.
Rainsford, K. D. (1978). Biochem. Pharmacol., 27, 877-885.
Vane, J. R. (1971). Nature New Biol., 231, 232-235.

Screening of Anti-Ulcer Agents Using Experimental Ulcer Models

S. Okabe

Department of Applied Pharmacology, Kyoto College of Pharmacy,
Kyoto, Japan

ABSTRACT

Several problems as to the screening methods for anti-ulcer agents are
described.

KEYWORDS

Anti-ulcer agents; screening methods; ulcer models; recurrence; rodents;
large animals.

INTRODUCTION

Peptic ulcer is a frequently encountered clinical entity and presents a
most difficult challenge for the physician since there is a high rate of
recurrence even after the initial healing (Fig. 1). Different types of
drugs are prescribed for patients with various types of ulcers and related
conditions. However, the effects of these compounds are often unsatisfacto-
ry. Thus, the development of more effective and safe drugs is required for
the treatment of ulcers.

SCREENING METHODS

To screen anti-ulcer agents, various animal models have been produced by
surgical procedures, pharmacological agents, and by the induction of stress
(Table 1). Using these acute and chronic ulcer models in a variety of
species, the following three types of screening were used to determine
whether these test compounds are effective to:
1) prevent the development of acutely-induced gastric and duodenal ulcers
   (test compounds are given to animals before the induction of ulcers)
2) accelerate the healing of chronic gastric and duodenal ulcers (test
   compounds are given to animals for 10-21 days after the induction of
   chronic gastric and duodenal ulcers)
3) prevent the recurrence of healed gastric and duodenal ulcers (test
   compounds are given to animals for 30-40 days at the time of

reulceration).
    Concerning acute and chronic gastric ulcers, various methods have
been used. In contrast, duodenal ulcer models are few; i.e., histamine
+ carbachol- or cysteamine-induced ulcers in rats or histamine-induced
ulcers in guinea pigs. Recently, our group found that mepirizole, a
non-steroidal antiinflammatory drug, induces readily discernible ulcers
in the rat duodenum with a high incidence and low mortality (Fig. 2).
Since mepirizole-induced duodenal ulcers are fairly sensitive to anti-
ulcer agents, this ulcer model appears to be useful for assessing newly
prepared anti-ulcer agents. In addition, it was also found that mepirizole-
induced duodenal ulcers persist for longer than 10 days after ulceration.
Thus, this model should be useful to determine whether or not test
compounds accelerate the healing of chronic types of duodenal ulcers.

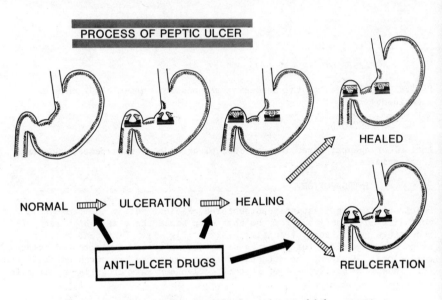

Fig. 1.   Three types of anti-ulcer drugs which prevent
           the development of peptic ulcers, accelerate
           the healing and prevent the reulceration.

TABLE 1. Various types of ulcer models

1. Acute ulcers

Stomach   rats: Shay ulcers, stress ulcers (water-immersion, restraint, cold, exertion, electric shock), drug-induced ulcers (aspirin, indomethacin, phenylbutazone, histamine, reserpine, serotonin)

        guinea pigs: histamine ulcers, aspirin ulcers
        cats: caffeine ulcers, gastrin ulcers
        dogs: aspirin ulcers, indomethacin ulcers, histamine ulcers
        mini pigs: aspirin ulcers

Duodenum rats: histamine-carbachol ulcers, cysteamine ulcers, propionitrile ulcers, mepirizole ulcers
        guinea pigs: histamine ulcers, demaprit ulcers, gastrin ulcers
        cats: gastrin ulcers
        dogs: histamine ulcers
        mini pigs: none

2. Chronic ulcers

Stomach   rats: clamping-cortisone ulcers, acetic acid ulcers, thermal ulcers, thermal-cortisone ulcers
        guinea pigs: none
        cats: acetic acid ulcers
        dogs: acetic acid ulcers, cincophen ulcers, indomethacin ulcers, histamine ulcers
        mini pigs: acetic acid ulcers

Duodenum rats: acetic acid ulcers
        guinea pigs: none
        cats: none
        dogs: acetic acid ulcers
        mini pigs: none

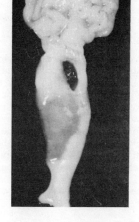

Fig. 2. Mepirizole ulcers in rats

EFFECTS OF ANTI-ULCER AGENTS ON EXPERIMENTAL ULCERS

Most of the clinically prescribed drugs have proven to be effective in inhibiting the development of acute ulcers and/or in accelerating chronic
ulcers, thereby supporting the usefulness of these models. The effects of
several different types of anti-ulcer agents as assessed in our laboratory
are listed in Table 2. However, some compounds now being clinically prescribed have little effect on either acute or chronic ulcers in experimental animals.

TABLE 2. Anti-ulcer agents which showed a significant effect on the following ulcer models

Antacid

    $Al(OH)_3$ (Shay, aspirin, indomethacin, histamine, mepirizole)

Anticholinergics

    Propantheline   (Shay, stress, aspirin, indomethacin, histamine,
                        histamine-carbachol, mepirizole, thermal-cortisone)

    Pirenzepine   (Shay, stress, aspirin, indomethacin, histamine,
                        histamine-carbachol, cysteamine, mepirizole, acetic
                        acid)

Histamine H_2-
blocker

    Cimetidine   (Stress, aspirin, indomethacin, histamine, histamine-
                        carbachol, mepirizole, acetic acid)

Others

    Ulcerlmin   (Shay, stress, aspirin, indomethacin, histamine, acetic
                        acid)

    15- or 16-$DMPGE_2$ (Shay, stress, aspirin, indomethacin, mepirizole, acetic
                        acid)

PREVENTION OF RECURRENCE

Since recurrence of old ulcers is an unavoidable fate of human peptic ulcer
diathesis, drugs which prevent reulceration are in great demand by both
physicians and patients. In fact, the prevention of recurrence of partially
or completely healed ulcers by conventional anti-ulcer agents is difficult.
The effect of drugs on recurrence is given little attention, at least in
laboratory models. This may be due to the difficulty in producing ulcer
models in which the healing and reulceration seen in humans can be repeated (Okabe and co-workers, 1971; Tabata and Okabe, 1981). Empirically
ulcers which develop in laboratory animals heal within a few weeks and do
not reulcerate. The administration of cortisone to rats with healed thermal
ulcers resulted in reulceration of healed lesions (Kahn and co-workers,
1961). However, to my knowledge, the method had not been used for the

screening of anti-ulcer agents. Two ulcer models in rats, i.e., acetic
acid-induced gastric ulcers (Takagi and co-workers, 1969; Okabe and
Pfeiffer, 1972)(Fig. 3) and thermocautery-induced gastric ulcers (Suguro
and co-workers, unpublished) are found to recur spontaneously. Using these
ulcer models, drugs can be prepared which prevent the recurrence of old
ulcers, regardless of the effect on acute and chronic ulcers. Propantheline
bromide which has a potent preventing effect on various types of acute
ulcers, had no preventive effect on reulceration of acetic acid-induced
gastric ulcers in rats(Okabe and Pfeiffer, 1972). There is no known
experimental model of duodenal ulcers in which reulceration either spontaneously or artificially occurs.

ULCER MODELS IN LARGE ANIMALS

Ulcer models which are frequently used in screening anti-ulcer agents are
usually produced in small animals such as rats and guinea pigs. From the
standpoint of morphology and physiology, probably large animals such as
dogs, cats or mini pigs can be used to acquire information which should be
much more realistic than that obtained from small animals, when we consider
the peptic ulcers in humans. For example, the acetic acid ulcer induced in
mini pigs appears to be useful to screen test compounds expected to accelerate the healing of chronic ulcers (Fig. 4). The gastric ulcers induced
by indomethacin in dogs appears to be useful for screening compounds which
are expected to prevent the development of ulceration and to accelerate the
healing of chronic types of ulcers (Fig. 5). Many compounds have little
effect on experimental ulcers in small animals. However, even such drugs
may have positive results in ulcer models produced in larger animals.

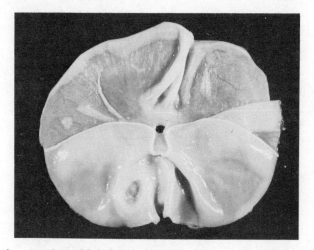

Fig. 3.   Acetic acid-induced gastric ulcer in the rat
          (100 days after ulceration)

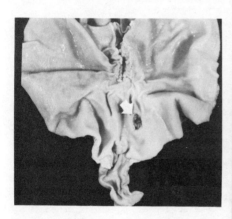 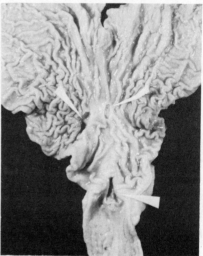

Fig. 4. Acetic acid-induced   Fig. 5. Indomethacin-induced
         gastric ulcer in mini   gastric ulcers in
         pigs (5 days after   dogs (5 days after
         ulceration)   ulceration)

SUMMARY

An extensive screening of various compounds using already established
methods or those now being prepared should result in making available potential drugs for the treatment the peptic ulcers diagnosed clinically
including drugs which prevent the reulceration of healed ulcers.

REFERENCES

Kahn, D. S., M. J. Phillips S. C., Skoryna and co-workers (1961).
   Am. J. Path. 38, 177-187.
Okabe, S., Y. Ishihara and H. Kunimi (1981). Gastroenterology 80, 1241.
Okabe, S. and C. J. Pfeiffer (1972). Amer. J. Dig. Dis. 17, 619-629.
Okabe, S. and C.J. Pfeiffer (1973). Amer. J. Dig. Dis. 18, 746-750.
Okabe, S., R. Saziki and K. Takagi (1971). J. Appl. Physiol. 30, 793-796.
Okabe, S. and K. Tabata (1981). Digestion 21, 179-183.
Tabata, K. and S. Okabe (1980). Dig. Dis. Sci. 25, 439-447.
Takagi, K., R. Saziki and S. Okabe (1969). Japan. J. Pharmacol.19, 418-426.

SYMPOSIUM

Models and Quality Control of Laboratory Animals

Chairmen: G. P. Lewis, T. Nomura

Introduction to Models and Qu
Control of Laboratory Anim

G. P. Lewis

Department of Pharmacology, Royal College of Surgeons of England,
UK

In spite of the public criticism levelled at experimental work on animals
there seems little doubt among the majority of the informed public that there
is a need for the use of animals not only for drug testing and development
but for basic research too. The object of using animals in basic research is
to learn how living tissues work. We justify such use of animals, and we do
need justification, on the grounds that without such an understanding there
would be no rational basis for medical, dental or veterinary practice. It is
clear that our difficulties increase when this basic knowledge is lacking,
and makes even more important the use of a battery of simple test models
referred to as a screen, in drug development.

A compound thought to be interest in such a "primary screen" is subjected to
more detailed study in whole animals recording various physiological functions.
Several species of animal will be used and the choice in each case will
depend on the characteristics of the species or particular strain (1). Thus
cats and monkeys are especially suitable for research on psychotropic or
hypnotic drugs whereas cats and dogs are commonly used in cardiovascular
research or metabolic studies and there are many other examples. We have
two speakers in the Symposium who will be talking about this aspect.
Dr Ohsawa will outline the general principles of characterisation of animal
models and Dr Hiddleston will describe some specific examples.

The majority of animals used in the pharmaceutical industry are rats and mice
and the great advantage of using these rodents is that they can be bred and
kept in very large numbers in a fairly small space. This, of course, does
not mean that the greatest laboratory animal care should not be exercised in
their breeding and maintenance. It is quite clear that the researcher
cannot risk having to repeat laborious and time-consuming work with numerous
animals because of some undetected infection of deficiency. One such factor
in animal care is nutrition, and we have Dr Eva later in the Symposium to
tell us about some of the factors involved.

Until quite recently, all a biologist knew about his animals was more or less
what he could learn from external observation, such as colour, weight and sex.
During the present day, the breeding and care of laboratory animals has become
a science in itself and of course this is one of the main concerns of ICLAS.
Academic and industrial institutions, as well as specialist companies, have

TEM - T

⌐1 farms where they breed standardised species, varieties and
The value of such standardisation is only recently being appreciated
⌐rmacologists in general.

⌐he standardisation process begins with genetic control by inbreeding. Each
strain has its own hereditary attributes which can be exactly specified,
from a characteristics appearance to certain heritable diseases such as
diabetes or proneness to cancer. On the other hand, out-breeding maintains
genetic variability and avoids too close a genetic relationship resulting in
individuals with a broad spectrum of reactions similar to human individuals.
This makes such outbred strains suitable for use in certain pharmacological,
chemotherapeutic, toxicological and teratological work.

Hygiene is of the greatest importance in the breeding of laboratory animals,
which have to be guaranteed free from all pathogenic bacterial and parasitic
infections. The most reliable way of doing this is to have germ-free
animals. The foetus is removed from a pregnant animal by caesarean section
and artificially reared in a sterile incubator. As the animal then has no
natural resistance it can only live in a sterile environment. That necessi-
tates very complicated equipment and organisational measures such as air-
conditioning, the use of very fine air filters, special locks for introducing
sterile food, water, bedding, etc. — in other words, total insulation from
the natural environment. To enable the animal to develop its own resistance,
it can then be fed a specific bacterial flora which provides the gut with a
standard bacterial colonisation. Such animals called "specific pathogen
free" (SPF) are then made available for research as "standardised" laboratory
animals. There is no doubt that great strides have been made in standardising
laboratory animals for drug research in the pharmaceutical industry. But the
ever-increasing difficulty in financing academic institutions is hindering
such development there.

Since not even large research institutions are able to breed all the species
they need, certain animal farms have tended to specialise. In Britain, the
International Index of Laboratory Animals issued periodically by the Medical
Research Council, lists more than 200 pure strains of mice and 100 of rats,
as well as other animals, which are available for research throughout the
world. The list include mice with spontaneously occurring high blood
pressure, obese and diabetic mice, mice which in time will develop leukaemia
or some other forms of cancer, mice which when given special food become
specially subject to coronary heart attack. Another important product of
specialised breeding is the "nude mouse". This strain is important, not
because of the absence of hair, but because having no thymus it shows several
properties found in patients with immunodeficiency diseases, syndromes that
have been particularly difficult to study. In several of these developments,
the Central Institute for Experimental Animals in Tokyo, with Dr Nomura as
its Head, has been in the forefront, and I hope he will tell us about some of
these developments. They are pioneering even deeper by examining not only
new strains but completely new species which might lead to a more effective
use of animals in the future testing of drugs.

One of the important aspects of drug testing and development is safety
evaluation. Catherine de Medici is sometimes credited with being the first
experimental toxicologist at a time when poisoning was developing in Italy.
The aim of the poisoner was to develop a poison which the victims could not
recognise by smell or taste. To counteract this, a bioassay was introduced.
The important person who feared poisonining had someone else to taste the
food first, so that he became the test object (2).

Toxicology is now implicated in the development of a drug right from the beginning of its development and basically never ends. Chronic toxicity studies over periods ranging from several weeks to several months are an essential part of a drug profile, and animal toxicity reports constitute an extremely critical chapter in the dosier prepared for submission to drug regulatory authorities (3).

Over the past twenty years or so the science of toxicology has developed at a remarkable rate, mainly in the toxicology departments of pharmaceutical companies and in special institutes carrying out toxicological studies on contract. On the other hand, academic institutions where young toxicologists can receive appropriate training are very few and far between. And although toxicologists working in the pharmaceutical industry deserve a large amount of the credit for the scientific progress that has been achieved in toxicological research, it is the drug regulations that have become an increasingly important determining factor in the application of the know-how. One of these influences has been the FDA's Good Laboratory Practices, which some have regarded with some trepidation. However, we are lucky enough to have as our final speaker, Dr Lepore of the FDA who will give us an account of GLPs.

There are three areas where there is particular concern because the toxicity may be delayed, difficult to recognise at an early stage and may be the same as natural disease and will therefore be difficult to detect. The first area, teratogenesis, is due to drugs taken during pregnancy. This has already happened with thalidomide. Extensive testing of new drugs in pregnant animals has been mandatory since the thalidomide disaster and since then has increased to include the period before mating, the whole pregnancy, at birth, development of the young and even their reproduction performance. How far such tests, especially when they give positive results only at the highest dose, provide genuine protection for mal still remains uncertain. One important aspect is the species variation and we have Dr Scott to tell us something about that. The second area is mutagenesis, which occurs when drugs cause abnormalities of genetic material of cells so that a permanent change in the hereditary constitution or mutation occurs. At present, many countries, including the WHO, suggest routine tests for mutagenicity in their guidelines for drug evaluation, although both regulatory authorities and drug developers are well aware that our scientific knowledge is not sufficiently advanced to give an assurance of reliable prediction of what will happen in man. The third area of particular concern is carcinogenesis, i.e. malignant tumours which can occur spontaneously or can be induced by drugs and other chemicals or sometimes occur as a result of mutation. Complex and long duration animal tests are in wide use to predict carcinogenicity of chemicals in man but their validity is again open to question.

The reason that these tests are not yet required by law for all drugs in all countries, is that their predictive value for man is uncertain and results may differ from one animal strain to another. For example (4) a new drug, pronethalol, effective against angina pectoris, caused cancer in one genetic strain of mouse but not in another. In the case of bromocriptine (5) the compound was found to give rise to malignant endometrial changes in rats, whereas in women — some of whom received the drug continuously for periods of up to six years — no uterine neoplasia was detectable. Occurrences of this sort provide a nightmare situation for both drug developer and regulatory authority, especially if the drug is to be used long-term in man. Frequently decisions to use or not to use a drug in man must be based finally upon a benefit/risk assessment.

298   G. P. Lewis

The need therefore for fundamental research into the genetic and microbiological backgrounds of the animals themselves and the environment in which
the animals are reared is of paramount importance. Such studies might well
result in a degree of predictability which might prevent regulatory authorities being forced into a position to demand wholesale slaughter of animals
to provide results which are of uncertain value.

REFERENCES

1. Bruhin, H. and Gelzer, J. (1978) Our indispensable substitutes. *Ciba-
    Geigy Journal*.
2. Smyth, D.H. (1978) *Alternatives to Animal Experiments*. London: Scolar
    Press.
3. Gelzer, J. (1978) *Governmental Toxicology Regulations: An Incumbrance
    to Drug Research?* Rome: Consorzio Ricerca Farmaceutica S.p.A.
4. Laurence, D.R. and Black, J.R. (1978) *The Medicine You Take*. Glasgow:
    Fontana Collins.
5. Besser, G.M., Thorner, M.A., Wass, J.A.H., Doniach, I., Canti, G.,
    Curling, M., Grudziniskas, J.G. and Setchell, M.E. (1977) Absence
    of uterine neoplasia in patients on bromocriptine. *Brit. Med. J.*
    2, 868.

Consideration of Provision and Characterization of Animal Models

N. Ohsawa

The 3rd Dept. of Internal Medicine, University of Tokyo Faculty
of Medicine, Tokyo, Japan

ABSTRACT

Useful animal models are indispensable in drug research, in which the extrapolation of animal data to humans is essential. Two approaches of the extrapolation are expected to be useful; simulation of human physiology or pathology
and a comparative approach in which the various species of animals are lined
phylogenetically and compared. The analysis of the present status of laboratory animal science indicates that the development of new experimental animals
and disease models is necessary for the establishment of the principles and
the methods of the extrapolation of animal data to humans. Four methods of
developing new experimental animals are presented. They are 1) from domestic
and wild animals, 2) from mutants, 3) from toxicology and 4) by developmental
engineering.

KEYWORDS

Animal models; drug research; extrapolation; simulation; comparative approach;
developmental engineering.

INTRODUCTION

Experimental animals are indispensable for drug research. In this presentation,
only the general principles and problems in laboratory animal science are discussed and the details of individual problems will be discussed by following
lecturers. Important problems in developing a new drug using experimental
animals are as follows;

TABLE 1 Drug Research using Experimental Animals

1. Discovery of new drug
2. Extrapolation of animal data to humans   1) drug effect
3. Extrapolation of animal data to humans   2) adverse effect

Especially important are the last two problems, which are to predict whether
the new drug would be effective and safe in human trials or clinical trials
from the data obtained by using experimental animals. These are the problems
of the extrapolation of laboratory animal data to humans. The present status
of development of laboratory animals is believed to be far from the ideal.

PRINCIPLES OF EXTRAPOLATION

In order to extrapolate the data from laboratory animals to humans, two principles are analyzed.

TABLE 2   Principles and Approaches of Extrapolation

1.	Simulation
2.	Comparative approach

Simulation

The first approach of extrapolation is to search for the suitable experimental
animals or disease models which simulate human physiology or pathology most
effectively. In this approach, the research starts from the analysis of human
diseases to the discovery of the most suitable animal models (Fig. 1).   The
simulation of human diseases in experimental animals should not simply be
phenomenal but also fundamental. For these purposes, the cooperative research
with clinical investigators is essential.

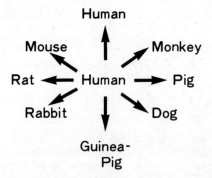

Fig. 1. Simulation procedure.

Since simulation is the partial simulation of humans or human diseases, careful
consideration is needed to extrapolate the experimental results to the analysis
of human diseases. From this standpoint, one of the most excellent models is
in vivo culture systems of normal or pathological human tissues. This can be
achieved by the heterotransplantation of human tissues to nude mice or nude
rats which reveal no rejection reaction due to the congenital thymus deficiency. As an example, animal models for muscular dystrophy research are presented.

TABLE 3   Animal Models for Muscular Dystrophy Research

---

1. Dystrophy mouse

2. Dystrophy chicken

3. Human dystrophied muscles transplanted
   into nude mice or nude rats

Dystrophy mice and chickens are currently used as useful animal models for
muscle dystrophy. Muscular dystrophy of mice and chickens, however, are apparently different from human muscular dystrophy in several fundamental points.
We have recently succeeded in the heterotransplantation of specimens of human
dystrophied muscles to nude mice. The *in vivo* culture system of dystrophied
muscles gives us a unique opportunity to evaluate whether the genetically
inherited and progressive human muscular dystrophy can be influenced by an
environmental factor or factors, including drugs. Another example of *in vivo*
culture systems of human tissues is the human tumor/nude mouse system or human
tumor/nude rat system for the development of anticancer drugs. Human cancer
tissues transplanted into nude mice or nud rats are expected to be more efficient in screening anticancer drugs, than using animal tumors (Fig. 2)
(Rygaard, 1973).

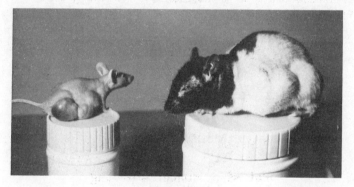

Fig. 2.   Nude mouse and rat bearing a human cancer.

Comparative Approach

The second approach is the comparative approach in which the various species
of animals are lined phylogenetically, such as mouse, rat, guinea-pig, rabbit,
dog, pig, monkey and human. The experimental data obtained from these animals
are compared and extrapolated to humans (Fig. 3).

The method is multispecies method and is evaluated to be useful for drug
research, especially for safety studies, since this approach follows the
phylogenetical processes. The method gives the theoretical basis for the
extrapolation to humans. As an example, the species difference of adrenal
glucocorticoids is shown in Fig. 4. Mouse, rat and rabbit have inactive
steroid 17α-hydroxylase in the adrenal cortex which is essential to synthesize
cortisol instead of corticosterone. Animals which produce corticosterone as
a major adrenal glucocorticoid are quite different in several features from
animals producing cortisol, such as guinea-pig, dog, monkey and human.

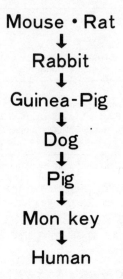

Fig. 3. Comparative approach.

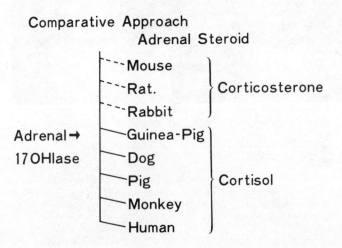

Fig. 4. Comparative approach -adrenal steroid synthesis-

The former group of animals have high sensitivity to adrenal glucocorticoids, tendency to develop hypertension and resistance to infection. Since humans belong to the cortisol producing group, care should be taken when the data of corticosterone producing animals such as rat, mouse and rabbit are extrapolated to humans. The comparative approach is an excellent procedure but is usually difficult to apply, because a complete series of the experimental animals is not easily obtained at present.

DEVELOPMENT OF NEW ANIMAL MODELS

The analysis of the present status of laboratory animal science indicates that the development of new experimental animals and disease models is necessary for the establishment of the principle and the methods of the extrapolation of the laboratory animal data to humans. Several methods of developing new experimental animals are presented in Table 4.

TABLE 4   Development of New Animal Models

1.   from domestic and wild animals
2.   from mutants
3.   from toxicology
4.   by developmental engineering

Development of New Experimental Animals from Domestic and Wild Animals

This is the most traditional way of developing new animal models which includes the discovery of a useful feature through a wild survey and the development of animals with suitable size for experiments. The following are such examples.
Göttingen miniature pig. (Fig. 5). Pigs are evaluated to be extremely useful experimental animals, especially for arteriosclerosis research and immunological studies. The wide application of ordinary pigs, however, has been hampered by their large size. Göttingen miniature pigs are extremely small and proved to be suitable for routine experiments (Beglinger and co-workers, 1975).

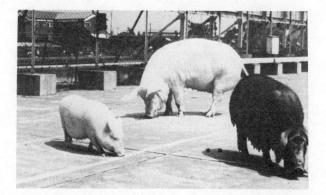

Fig. 5.   Göttingen miniature pig (front left), Omini-pig
          (front right) and ordinary pig (back).

Marmosets. (Fig. 6). Marmoset monkeys are very small primates of the new world, which are easy to handle. The marmosets are useful for the studies of drug safety and some viral diseases. Since macaca monkeys widely used as

experimental primates are now in extremely short supply, marmoset monkeys are
expected to become substitutes for macaca monkeys.

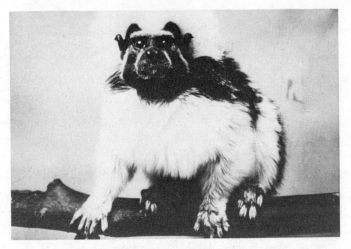

Fig. 6.   Common marmoset.

Pica (*Ochotona rufescens rufescens*) (Fig. 7). The pica is a small, non-
rodent animal of approximately the same size as rats. Since picas have
simillar characteristics to rabbits, they are expected to become a small and
easily handled substitute for rabbits as a non-rodent experimental animal
(Puget, 1973).

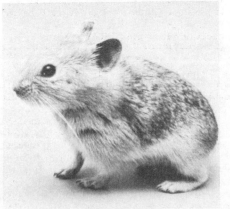

Fig. 7.   Pica.

Development of New Experimental Animals from Mutants

Many mutant animal models including nude mutants are now widely used but still many more new mutants are needed. A careful search for mutants by animal breeders with the collaboration of clinical researchers is expected to be fruitful for the new discovery of various mutant animals.

Development of New Experimental Animals from Toxicology Studies

During toxicology studies, prolonged administration of large quantities of new chemical substances results in the development of various adverse effects in test animals. Some of them might be useful models for human diseases. For instance, oral administration of cyproheptadine, an anti-serotonin substance, causes diabetes in rats (cyproheptadine diabetes rat). This diabetes mellitus is caused by a unique disturbance in insulin secretion from the rat's pancreatic islets and is useful for studies on the mechanism of insulin secretion.

Development of New Experimental Animals by Developmental Engineering

One of the fascinating approaches of developing new experimental animals is the use of the technique of microsurgery of mammalian eggs or embryos to produce artificially developed animals (Table 5).

TABLE 5   Development of New Experimental Animals by
          Developmental Engineering -Microsurgery of
          Mammalian Embryos-

1. Aggregation chimeras
   Intraspecies (mouse ↔ mouse, rat ↔ rat)
   Interspecies
2. Injection chimeras
   mouse embryo ↔ mouse embryonal cell
   mouse embryo ↔ mouse teratoma cell
3. Uniparenteral homozygous diploid animal
4. Parthenotes
5. Nuclear transplantation

Aggregation chimeras. Two embryos of a different mouse or rat were aggregated in vitro and developed to a single blastocyst which was transplanted into the uterus of pseudopregnant foster mothers to obtain congenitally chimeric animals (Fig. 8) (Mclaren, 1976; Mintz, 1971).
Injection chimeras. Mouse embryonal cells or teratoma cells are injected into a mouse blastocyst. Injected cells are organized into the blastocyst and developed in to normal tissues, including gonadal tissues. When teratoma cells are developed into sperms or eggs within the chimeric mouse, normal F1 mice can be obtained. If teratoma cells become mutant cells by irradiation or mutagens and develop in to sperms or eggs in injection chimeras, a mutant-normal F1 hybrid mouse can be obtained. Using these procedures, a new mutant mouse can be induced antificially from mutant cells (Dewey and co-workers, 1977). The technique is expected to be useful in developing new mutant animal models.
Uniparenteral homozygous diploid animals. A mouse embryonal cell is obtained before two pronuclei of sperm and ovum are fused and one pronuclei is removed by a micropipette to form a haploid cell. The cell is treated with cytochalasin B to induce a karyokinesis without cytokinesis which produces a uniparenteral complete homozygous diploid embryonal cell. The embryo is caused to develop into a blastocyst. The blastocyst is transplanted to the uterus of a pseudo-

pregnant foster mother and a uniparenteral homozygous diploid animal is
obtained (Hoppe and Illmensee, 1977). The technique will be extremely useful
in developing completely homozygous diploid animals within a short period.
These microsurgical techniques are expected to open a new field of experimental
animals.

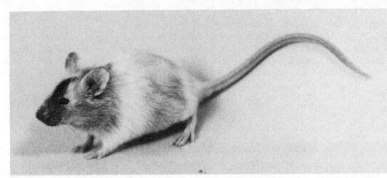

Fig. 8.   Chimeric mouse: BALB/c ↔ C57BL.

CONCLUSION

Laboratory animal science is closely related to biomedical research through
which laboratory animal science will contribute to develop new drugs for
clinical medicine.   Laboratory animal science is also closely related to
basic biology (Fig. 9).

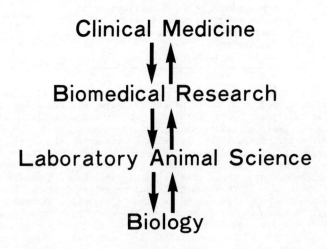

Clinical Medicine

Biomedical Research

Laboratory Animal Science

Biology

Fig. 9.   Relationship between laboratory animal science
and other research fields.

Thus, laboratory animal science is located in the key position between basic

biology and clinical medicine. Therefore, experimental animals are indispensable and should be developed further. These experimental animals should be
well defined genetically, microbiologically and nutritionally, under the GLP.

ACKNOWLEDGEMENT

The help and advice of Dr. T. Nomura and his colleagues of the Central Institute for Experimental Animals are greatly appreciated.

REFERENCES

Beglinger, R., M. Becker, E. Eggenberger, und C. Lombard (1975). Das Göttinger
    Miniaturschwein als Versuchstiere. Res. exp. Med., 165, 251-261.
Dewey, M.J., D.W. Martin, Jr., G.R. Matin, and B. Mintz (1977). Mosaic mice
    with teratocarcinoma-derived mutant cells deficient in hypoxanthine phospho-
    ribosyl transferase. Proc. Natl. Acad. Sci. USA, 74, 5564-5568.
Hoppe, P.C., and K. Illmensee (1977). Microsurgically produced homozygous
    diploid uniparenteral mice. Proc. Natl. Acad. Sci. USA, 74, 5657-5661.
Illmensee, K., and L.C. Stevens (1979). Teratomas and chimeras. Scientific
    American, 86, 87-97.
Mclaren, A. (1976). Mammalian Chimeras. Cambridge University Press, Cambridge.
Mintz, B. (1971). In J.C. Daniel, Jr. (Ed.), Method in Mammalian Embryology.
    W.H. Freeman and Company, San Francisco. pp. 186-214.
Puget, A. (1973). The Afghan pika (Ochotona rufescens rufescens): a new
    laboratory animal. Lab. Anim. Sci., 23, 248-251.
Rygaard, J. (1973). Thymus & Self-Immunobiology of the Mouse Mutant Nude.
    F.A.D.L., Copenhagen.

New Animal Models in Pharmaceutical Research

W. A. Hiddleston

I.C.I Ltd., Pharms. Div., Alderley Park, Macclesfield, Cheshire, UK

ABSTRACT

In this paper, the potential use of the common marmoset, Callithrix jacchus, and the Gottingen minipig in the development and discovery of new pharmaceutical products is discussed. A brief description of the husbandry of both species is given as well as some of the purposes for which these species have been used. Whilst the marmoset has been found a satisfactory model of teratological and toxicological studies , the minipig has been found to be successful in pharmacological studies.

KEYWORDS

Callithrix jacchus; miniature swine; drug research.

INTRODUCTION

In the mid 1960's it became apparent that there was a need for an alternative non-rodent species to the dog or Rhesus monkey for the development and safety evaluation of new medicinal compounds. Ideally such a species would be a small non-human primate which would breed readily in captivity, be safe to handle and not present a health hazard to those who had to work with it.

Following reports that the common marmoset, Callithrix jacchus, had been succesffully bred and used in the laboratory it was decided to evaluate this species at ICI.

A colony was established in 1968 and between 1968 and 1972 this species was evaluated in toxicological, teratological and biological studies. At the same time various systems of breeding and housing were investigated and as a result of these investigations it was decided to invest in a breeding unit in 1972.

The common marmoset is a small non-human primate with a mature body weight of 300-400 gms. Breeding animals are housed as monogamous pairs. Breeding is not seasonal. Multiple births are the norm – less than 8% of offspring are singletons. The average gestation period is 140 days with a litter to litter interval of 158 days. On average, each pair will produce twins twice each year. The average mortality rate of unweaned animals is between 20–25% but this is inflated by the death of one member of each set of triplets. It is possible to rear these animals artificially but it is uneconomic, so no attempt is made to hand rear the animals. Occasionally, it is possible to cross foster these surplus animals. Sexual maturity is reached around 400 days. No difficulty was experienced in getting colony bred animals to breed and to rear their offspring.

Care and Husbandry

Adult marmosets are housed in breeding pairs in cages 50 x 50 x 75 cms. Each cage is provided with perches and a shelf or nest box. The perches are wooden and it will be found these animals chew these perches. This is a behaviour pattern which is seen in the wild when the marmoset gouges holes in the branches of trees which fills up with a sap which forms a major part of their diet in the wild.

Twins or triplets are born at intervals of 5 months. The male animal mainly carries the babies only giving them to the female to suckle. Conception usually takes place around the 16 day post partum. The young animals are weaned when they are 5–6 months old, either just before or shortly after the birth of the next animals. On weaning, the animals are allowed some time to stabilise in groups of 2 or 3 and then are released into gang cages where they remain until they become mature. On maturity these animals start to fight and unless separated, deaths occur. If it is proposed to use these animals for experimental purposes, they are caged as same sex pairs. Compatible pairs can be established at this time which will live happily together. Since marmosets are territorial by nature, it is difficult to introduce a mature animal into the territory of another of the same sex without much fighting. If it is decided to do this, it is best to introduce the pair simultaneously to a completely new cage and this may lead to the animals accepting each other.

Diet

The marmosets are fed a mixture of an expanded diet (analysis in Table 1). About 20 gms of dry diet is given to each pair daily. The diet is mostly softened by the addition of milk and cereal baby food, or it may be ground and mixed with orange. Fruit is also given, apples and oranges have proven to be best. It is necessary to feed the dry diet and fruit at separate times of day since the animals prefer the fruit and protein intake will be inadequate if they are given a free choice. The diet is supplemented by the administration of Vitamin D_3 once each fourteen days, 1000 i.u. per animal given orally. Ascorbic acid is added to the drinking water which is available at all times and 4 i.u. of Vitamin E is added to the food of each animal daily. No other supplements are routinely given.

The environment is maintained at a temperature of $75°F \mp 2$ and a humidity of 55% $\mp$ 5%. Initially with feral animals, the humidity was maintained at 65%. 15 air changes per hour are supplied with no re-circulation.

Spontaneous Disease

Bacterial diseases are more common than viral conditions. Enteric and pulmonary conditions are most commonly seen. In young, enterotoxaemia was identified and animals are now routinely vaccinated with an E. coli vaccine and this has led to a marked reduction in acute gastro intestinal problems. Spasmodic outbreaks of pneumonia have occurred and the most common organisms isolated are Alkaligenes, Bronchisepticus and Klebsiella. Middle ear disease is also seen from which Klebsiella can be isolated.

Marmosets are susceptible to the human Herpes simplex virus and this produces a fatal encephalitis in the marmoset. Measles and mumps have also been reported to cause disease and deaths in the marmosets. Tuberculosis has never been seen in any of the marmosets at ICI but has been reported once by Levy and Mircovic (1971).

One condition which has caused major losses in marmoset colonies throughout the world is the so called "Marmoset Wasting Syndrome". In my opinion, this label has been given to a number of different conditions for which there seems no apparent aetiology but many of which were either primary dietetic problems or secondary to dietary problems. In our own case, the incidence of this condition has dropped to insignificant levels following changes in our dietary routine.

Crude Oil	5.2%	Isoleucine	1.15%
Crude Protein	25.8%	Leucine	1.86%
Crude Fibre	3.2%	Phenylalamine	1.17%
Ash	6.5%	Valine	1.19%
N.F.E.	49.5%	Tyrosine	0.85%
Dig. Crude Oil	4.6%	Aspartic Acid	1.86%
Dig. Crude Protein	21.0%	Glutamic Acid	4.83%
Dig. Crude Fibre	1.6%	Proline	1.57%
Dig. Carbohydrate	42.4%	Serine	1.22%
T.D.N.	74.8%	Myristic Acid	0.3%
Gross Energy	3480 Cal/Kg.	Palmitic Acid	1.0%
Calcium	1.49%	Stearic Acid	0.3%
Phosphorous	1.02%	Oleic Acid	1.7%
Sodium	0.25%	Linoleic Acid	0.9%
Chlorine	0.37%	Linolenic Acid	0.2%
Magnesium	0.27%	Arachidonic Acid	0.3%
Potassium	0.96%	Vitamin A	31500 IU/kg.
Sulphur	0.30%	Vitamin D3	11500 IU/kg.
Iron	300 mg/kg.	Carotene	1.3 mg/kg.
Copper	12 mg/kg.	Vitamin B1	13.0 mg/kg.
Manganese	51 mg/kg.	Vitamin B2	9.8 mg/kg.
Cobalt	1082 mcg/kg.	Vitamin B6	14.7 mg/kg.
Zinc	26 mg/kg.	Vitamin B12	35.8 mcg/kg.
Iodine	1876 mcg/kg.	Vitamin C	2000.0 mg/kg.
Selenium	200 mcg/kg.	Vitamin E	61.5 mg/kg.
Arginine	1.58%	Vitamin K	2.3 mg/kg.
Lysine	1.40%	Folic Acid	6.5 mg/kg.
Methionine	0.46%	Nicotinic Acid	106.6 mg/kg.
Cystine	0.39%	Pantothenic Acid	70.9 mg/kg.
Tryptophan	0.30%	Choline	1.9 g/kg.
Glycine	2.43%	Biotin	0.3 mg/kg.
Histidine	0.56%	Inositol	1.7 g/kg.
Threonine	0.83%		

TABLE 1 Primate Diet – Calculated Analysis

Handling and Collection Techniques

Colony bred marmosets can usually be picked up without the necessity of
wearing protective gloves. The oral administration of compounds is easy,
the animals will drink many compounds voluntarily from a syringe or small
plastic catheter provided they are not bitter. Urine collection can take
place using rat metabowls. Cardiac measurements can be made by restraining
the marmoset and using needle electrodes. Heart rate and ECG's can be
measured in the conscious animal. ECG's give a clear pattern with easily
distinguishable P-QRS and T waves. Once the animals have been restrained
a few times they do not object to the restraint and soon settle well. A
special restrainer has been developed to allow conscious blood pressure to
be measured from the femoral artery. Various tail cuff methods were tried
but did not provide satisfactory readings. Urine samples can be collected
by using rat metabowls, glass metabowls giving better recovery of compound
than plastic or polycarbonate ones.

Experimental Usage of the Marmoset

Toxicological Studies

The marmoset was originally considered as an alternative to the dog for
toxicological studies. It had the advantage of having morphological, biochemical and haematological parameters similar to man.

It is a small primate requiring less space and less compound than either the
dog or Rhesus monkey. Tissues are more akin to the size of a rodent and may
require less histologists and pathologists time. It is possible to make
complete body sections to study drug distribution. The disadvantage of the
marmoset is that it is a primate which requires a carefully controlled
environment and a more labour intensive regime of husbandry than the common
laboratory species. The diet is much more expensive than other laboratory
species but since only small amounts are consumed the total cost of feeding
is low. The marmoset is also more susceptible to human viral infections as
compared to the rat or dog. The amount of blood or body fluids which can be
collected from the marmoset at any one time is small and micro methods have
had to be developed. This can present problems when drug metabolism studies
are required but by increasing the group size or having fewer sampling
points this can be overcome. Up to 5 samples can be collected from one
animal in a 24 hour period.

In ICI and some other companies, the marmoset has been used in toxicological
studies when the dog has been found to be unsuitable. There is at least
one pharmaceutical company where the marmoset is used as the species of
choice in preference to the dog or other larger primates in toxicological
studies.

Use of Marmosets in Teratology

In 1963 Benirschke and Visek recommended that the marmoset be considered as
a laboratory model for the evaluation of possible teratogens, a view that
was restated in a WHO report in 1967. The marmoset has a placenta which
has many similarities to the human placenta. Because of these similarities
Benirschke said that the marmoset should be second only to the chimpanzee
in its usefulness in determining the safety of drugs during pregnancy.
Published results of teratology studies support this (Poswillo 1972a; 1972b;
Phillips 1975; Siddall 1978).

Poswillo et al studied the effects of thalidomide and a number of other teratogens and concluded that the marmoset should command the attention of all concerned with developmental pathology. Foetal and early neonatal liver metabolism is similar to humans (Neubert 1979). Pregnancy may be determined by uterine palpation (Gengozian et al 1974; Phillips and Grist 1975; Siddall 1978) and may be timed accurately by means of serum hormonal assays (Hearn and Lunn 1975). Current work in progress has shown that a simple urinary hormone assay may be used to time pregnancy (in press).

Thalidomide induces a severe embryopathy following oral administration of doses as low as 9 mg/kg between days 30 and 50 of pregnancy, (Poswillo et al 1972; Siddall 1978). Embryological studies and timed dosing experiments with thalidomide have shown some delay in embryogenesis and limb development takes place between 40 and 50 days. The syndrome is similar to that seen in man with amelia and oto-mandibular defects. The effects of several other compounds on the marmoset foetus have been examined.

The Marmoset in Drug Metabolism Studies

The marmoset, due to its small size, presented problems in drug metabolism studies but micro techniques have been developed to enable the determination of the route and rate of elimination of compounds and also drug distribution throughout the body using whole body autoradiography. A surgical technique has been developed for the insertion of a bile duct cannula to allow collection of bile to monitor elimination of drug and its metabolites in the bile. Other fields in which the marmoset has been used are in the study of reproductive physiology and immunology (Hearn et al) and much work has been published on behavioural studies.

The marmoset has now been used in increasing numbers of laboratories for more than 10 years. It presents an opportunity to use a laboratory bred primate at a time when supplies of primates from the wild are disappearing for one reason or another and I feel certain that in future the marmoset will become widely accepted by the registration authorities and the biological users as one of the primates of choice. Whilst the marmoset was found to be a suitable species for toxicological and teratological studies and for certain other experimental uses, there were still many procedures which required a larger model particularly for surgical and pharmacological purposes.

It was for those purposes that the potential of the miniature pig appeared attractive. What was required was an animal in the 15-20 kg weight range which was docile, easy to breed in laboratory conditions and which preferably would be non-emotive. There is a potential to use certain non-domesticated species but thee are always objections from conservationists if it appears that a feral animal might become popular in the laboratory. The Gottingen strain of minipig appeared to satisfy these requirements and it was decided to evaluate this animal in ICI.

Care and Husbandry of the Miniature pig

Accommodation

The adult minipigs can conveniently be housed in the accommodation used for breeding dogs. A pen of 5ft x 4ft 6ins is adequate for a sow and litter. The temperature can be maintained around 65°F although additional heating in the form of an infra red lamp is provided at the time of farrowing. Weanling pigs can either be housed in floor pens or battery cages depending on the space available and the experimental requirements.

Diet

The animals are fed a modified pig diet developed by the University of Gottingen. The formulation is in Table 2. 350 gms of diet is given twice daily
to the adult breeding animals, young animals are fed according to appetite
and animals which are on experiment are fed 350 gms of maintenance diet once
daily to decrease the growth rate.

Breeding

The minipig reaches sexual maturity around 5 months of age – younger than the
domestic pig and it is our practice to mate them at this oestrus. The gestation period is the same as the domestic pig – 116 days. Parturition is
mainly uneventful. We have not had to carry out any surgical interference in
more than 250 pregnancies. The average number of animals born is 6.83 per
litter and weaned 5.73 per litter. Animals are weaned at 6 weeks of age and
the sows mated at the first oestrus post weaning. Fertility is good and it
is unusual for the animals not to conceive at this mating. At weaning, the
average weight of the piglets is 6.6. kg. The growth rates for these animals
is in Table 3. Adult breeding sows weigh 45-50 kg and the boars 65-70 kg.

	Maintenance	Breeding
	%	%
Barley	38	66.5
Dried grass	30	5
Bran	20	10
Soyabean meal	8	10
Fishmeal		5
Dicalcium phosphate	1.5	1.0
Limestone	1.0	1.0
Salt	0.5	0.5
Vitamin mixture	1.0	1.0

TABLE 2   Minipig Diet Formula

Problems of Husbandry and Disease

The Gottingen minipig is relatively resistant to infection and very few
problems have been experienced. It was found necessary to give all piglets
a prophylactic treatment with an iron dextran compound to prevent anaemia.
There is an incidence of post parturient mastitis which will result in loss
of piglets if untreated but as this responds well to antibiotics it does not
present a major problem. This colony has not been subject to outbreaks of
either enteric or pulmonary diseases. No endoparasites have been seen in
these animals.

Costs

The cost of producing one minipig to the weight at which it would be used for pharmacological studies is approximately 50% that of a dog.

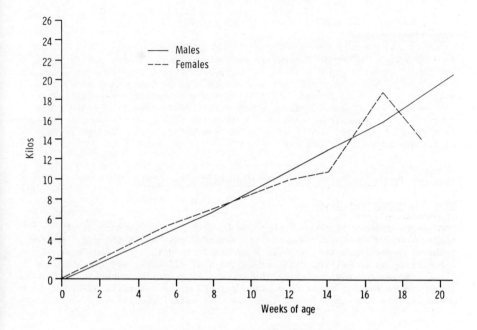

TABLE 3   Growth Curves of Minipigs

Techniques in which the minipig has been used

There is a resistance from most experimenters to change species especially
when species they are currently using are available and do not present any
major problems. To encourage a scientist to change from a dog, with which
he is accustomed to work, to a pig, was a major difficulty. However, once a
few scientists had used the minipig and found it to be a successful species,
this resistance diminished.

Anaesthesia

It was found that the minipig presented fewer anaesthetic problems than the
conventional pig.

Large Animal Immobilon (Etorphine) has proved very effective as a premedication prior to the administration of Fluothane/oxygen mixture as a general
anaesthetic. Simple procedures such as X-ray examination, endoscopy, cardiac
puncture, collection of blood samples and non invasive techniques which
require restraint, can be performed using Immobilon alone. Where general
anaesthetic is required, intubation can be performed in a relatively simple
manner. The animal is premedicated with Immobilon and laid on its back.
The throat is anaesthetised by spraying it with a local anaesthetic immed-

iately prior to the introduction of the endotracheal tube. Anaesthesia is
maintained using a Fluothane/oxygen mixture. Recovery from anaesthesia is
rapid, particularly if Revivon is given to counter the effects of the
Immobilon.

Drug Administration

It is a simple matter to administer drugs by intramuscular injection into
the thigh of the minipig. If it is desired to give a drug by oral administration it has been found that most drugs will be taken when added to a
small amount of normal food. If the substance is bitter, the addition of a
little sugar will usually overcome any reluctance to eat it. Tablets can
often be given sandwiched between 2 pellets of diet. Intravenous injection
is more difficult but the vessels in the ear can be used. Gavage is very
difficult in the conscious pig.

Surgical Preparations in Which The Minipig Has Been Used

Atrial and Venous Catheters

Due to the anatomy of the minipig, the carotid artery is more deeply
placed than in the dog. Cannulation is not so easy as in the dog. However,
catheters once implanted, work very successfully with a low incidence of
infection. An indwelling catheter is the most effective way of obtaining
blood samples and administering intravenous drugs in the conscious animal as
there are no readily accessible blood vessels. The recording of blood
pressure from the carotid catheters is very satisfactory.

Thoracic Surgery

In general, thoracic surgery is well tolerated by the minipig with good long
term survival. The implantation of left atrial and aortic catheters has been
successfully carried out. The implantation of aortic and oesophogeal grafts
have also been successfully carried out with good long term survival.

The implantation of artificial heart valves has met with poor success. Only
a small number have been attempted. Failure has been largely due to clotting on the valve. This may, however, be a feature of the valve used rather
than the pig. The pig survives a simple cardiac by-pass very well. However
it is difficult to cool the minipig due to the thick layers of subcutaneous
fat.

Tracheal pouches

Tracheal pouch preparations have been developed in the minipig for the
collection and evaluation of tracheal mucous and mucous secretion. These
pouches can be maintained provided they are carefully looked after for
periods of up to 10 months. It was found that the tracheal mucous of the
pig was frequently contaminated with bacteria and that daily flushing with
a dilute chlorhexidine solution was sufficient to prevent the pouch becoming
infected.

Infarction

Myocardial infarction has been produced in the minipig either by the introduction of a tiny copper coil into the coronary artery or by the infusion of
Sephadex beads. The resulting infacts are usually very clearly defined and
resemble human myocardial infarcts very closely. Unlike the dog, the pig
does not appear to develop a collateral circulation very easily so heart
failure can be induced by the myocardial infarcts which affect a large area
of cardiac muscle.

Thrombosis

A small number of tests using the Chan model for thrombosis production have
been performed. These have been fairly successful. It has been observed
that the clotting time of minipigs' blood varies over a wide range and also
that the animal appears to produce a hypercoagulable state. We are currently
gathering background information on the clinical chemistry and haematology
of the minipig.

Bile and Pancreatic Duct fistulae

The bile duct is situated very close to the pylorus and is quite large in
the pig when compared to that of the dog. Using a standard technique for
biliary cannulation with exteriorisation into a chenutal cannula, the
procedure works well and the pigs have shown no signs of developing jaundice.
The pancreatic fistula functions equally well but there was a tendency for
the cannula to be extended as with the gastric cannulae.

Gastric fistula and pouches

The pig stomach appears to have a tendency to extrude cannulae both Kemital
and Vitanium. This may be due to continued growth or it may be that the
stomach is more muscular and contracts more vigorously than other species.
The gastric mucosa tends to be rather loosely attached to the submucosal
layer and also tends to be folded. This leads to folds of mucosa closing
over the cannulae and eventually creates problems with drainage of acid.
Another problem with experiments involving the digestive tract is the
apparent slow gastro-intestinal motility. The stomach appears to be always
filled with partly digested food, so long periods of fasting are necessary
to allow the production of an empty resting stomach. However, long periods
of fasting appear to reduce the appetite stimulus in the pig and this may
cause problems in the animal refusing to eat when required.

Ulcer models

Attempts to produce peptic ulcers in the minipig have met with varying
degrees of success. Only limited work has been carried out in this area.
Endoscopic examinations can be carried out successfully in anaesthetised
pigs provided the animals have been deprived of solid food for a period of
24 hours prior to the examination.

The Gottingen strain of minipig has been evaluated as an alternative to the
dog in certain experimental programmes. Once the initial reluctance of the
investigator to use the pig has been overcome, it has proved to be equal to

the dog in many cases and preferable in some.

REFERENCES

Benirschke, K., 1963. Report to the commission on drug safety, in
  "Conference on Prenatal Effects of Drugs", pp.8–11 (Commission on Drug
  Safety, Chicago).
Gengozian, N., Smith, T.A. and Gosslee, E.G., 1974. External uterine pal-
  pation to identify stages of pregnancy in the marmoset, Saguinus fuscicollis
  ssp., J. med. Primatol. 3, pp. 236–243
Hearn, J.P. and Lunn, S.F., 1975. The reproductive biology of the marmoset
  monkey, in: "Breeding Simians for Developmental Biology", (Perkins and
  O'Donoghue, eds.) pp. 191–202, vol 6, Laboratory Animals Ltd., London.
Levy, B.M. and Mircovic, R.R., 1971. An epizootic of measles in a marmoset
  colony, Lab. Animal Care 21, pp. 33–39
Neubert, D., 1978. Metabolism of Xenobiotics in the Fetal and Neonatal
  Marmoset monkey (Callithrix jacchus), Role of Pharmacokinetics in Prenatal
  and Perinatal Toxicology, pp. 299–309.
Phillips, I.R., 1975. Macaque and Marmoset monkeys as Animal Models for the
  Study of Birth Defects, in: "Breeding Simians for Developmental Biology",
  (Perkins and O'Donoghue, eds.) pp. 293–302, vol. 6, Laboratory Animals
  Ltd., London.
Phillips, I.R. and Grist, S.M., 1975. The use of transabdominal palpation
  to determine the course of pregnancy in the marmoset Callithrix jacchus
  J. Reprod. Fert. 43, pp. 103–108.
Poswillo, DE., Hamilton. W.J. and Sopher, D., 1972a. The Marmoset as an
  animal model for Teratological Research, Nature (London) 239, pp 460–462.
Poswillo, D.E., Sopher, D. and Mitchell, S., 1972b. Experimental Induction
  of fetal malformations with "blighted" potato: a Preliminary Report
  Nature (London) 239, pp. 462–464.
Siddall, R.A., 1978. The use of marmosets Callithrix jacchus in teratological
  and toxicological research, Prim. Med., 10, pp. 215–224, Karger, Basel.
Visek, W.J., 1963 in: "Conference on Prenatal Effects of Drugs", pp. 42–45,
  (Commission on Drug Safety, Chicago).

Species Variation in Evaluation of
Safety of Drugs in the Developing Animal

W. J. Scott

Childen's Hospital Research Foundation, Elland & Bethesda Aves.,
Cincinnati, Ohio 45229, USA

ABSTRACT

Variation of teratologic response to chemicals administered during pregnancy
is a well known, widespread phenomenon. This brief review lists the three
sites responsible for determining teratologic outcome and gives examples of
how variation at these sites can lead to species variation in teratologic
response.

KEYWORDS

Species variation; mother; placenta; embryo.

INTRODUCTION

Safety evaluation of new drugs is done in lower mammals and thus the
phenomenon of species variation confounds the assessment of human safety
of new agents. With regard to teratology both ends of the spectrum, false
negatives and false positives lead to undesirable results. False negatives
could lead to clinical use of a potent human teratogen followed by
recurrence of a thalidomide-like epidemic of malformed children. False
positives on the other hand could lead to suppression of agents valuable
for therapy of human illness. Thus the choice of the species to conduct
safety evaluation studies is of great importance.

Before discussing the sites responsible for species variation in teratologic
response it is appropriate to discuss the scope of this phenomenon.
Attention is usually centered on agents which are teratogenic in one species
but said to be non-teratogenic in a second species. Perhaps the most often
cited example is thalidomide, which is a potent human teratogen but usually
is without effect on rat embryos.

Two other facets of species difference are equally important in routine
attempts to compare species response to a teratogen. These are: (1) the
dose/response relationship, especially the therapeutic/teratogenic ratio

319

and (2) the type of malformation produced across species lines. To continue
the analogy with thalidomide it is well known that the embryos of many
species of non-human primates are affected with similar if not identical
malformations following maternal thalidomide administration, and the dose
needed to induce such malformations is in the human therapeutic range
(Wilson, 1973). Thus we have some assurance that no species difference
exists in teratologic response to thalidomide between human and non-human
primates suggesting the utility of monkeys for screening of thalidomide
analogues and agents with similar chemical structure.

A degree or more removed from monkeys is the response of rabbit embryos to
thalidomide. First, the type of limb malformation is similar to those in
children since the preaxial portion of the limb is preferentially affected
(Vickers, 1967). Usually, however, the degree of reduction deformity is
less than that observed in human or monkey offspring. Secondly, the dose
needed to produce teratologic effects in rabbit fetuses is well above human
therapeutic levels, although the therapeutic/teratogenic ratio has not been
calculated for this species to my knowledge.

Further removed from the clinical situation is the response of some mouse
strains to thalidomide. Most mouse strains examined are resistant to
thalidomide teratogenesis but Giroud, Tuchmann-Duplessis and Mercier-Parot
(1962a, 1962b) demonstrated that moderately high doses of thalidomide were
teratogenic in some mouse strains. However, the malformations seen, cleft
palate, hare lip, craniorachischisis and cataracts are not usually
associated with primate fetuses exposed to thalidomide. With a single
agent then a whole spectrum of species variation is apparent. In comparison
to humans, numerous non-human primate species respond identically. Rabbits
respond with similar but less severe malformations and need higher drug
dosage. Some mouse strains are susceptible to thalidomide but the malformations are distinctly atypical of primate fetuses. Finally, most rat
stocks are completely resistant to thalidomide teratogenesis.

With the scope of species variation in teratologic response defined it is
appropriate to discuss the factors which contribute to dissimilar outcome.

There are three major sites which determine teratologic outcome in mammalian
pregnancies, the mother, the placenta and the embryo.

MOTHER

The interested reader is referred to Gillette (1977) for a comprehensive
discussion of the factors that affect drug concentration in maternal plasma.
Examples of how three of these factors, absorption, drug metabolism and
plasma binding, contribute to species variation in teratologic response will
be outlined.

It has been found that cyclopia can be produced in sheep and other ruminants
by ingestion of the weed Veratrum californicum. An alkaloid purified from
this week, cyclopamine, is capable of inducing typical malformations in
sheep (Keeler and Binns, 1968) but the plant or purified preparations given
to pregnant non-ruminants (rabbits, rats, pigs) was free of teratogenic
effects. Keeler (1970) deduced that the acid milieu of the non-ruminant
stomach might alter the structure of cyclopamine and went on to show that
cyclopian rabbit fetuses could be produced if sufficient alkali were
co-administered with the alkaloid.

The potential magnitude of ethanol as a human teratogen (Hanson, Streissguth and Smith, 1978) has prompted many attempts to produce an animal model of the human condition. Chernoff (1977) administered ethanol to pregnant mice and found an embryotoxic response including a specific pattern of malformations which he considers similar to the syndrome seen in humans. An important aspect of that study for this discussion was a marked strain difference, the CBA strain being more sensitive to alcohol teratogenesis than the C3H strain. Subsequently Chernoff (1980) showed that fetal abnormalities and maternal blood alcohol levels varied with maternal strain in the order CBA>C3H>C57. Convincing evidence that maternal metabolism was the basis of these strain differences was the level of maternal hepatic aldehyde dehydrogenase which varied inversely with maternal blood ethanol concentration.

Another possible means of species variation in teratologic response via maternal difference is the degree of plasma binding of a proximate teratogen. At roughly equivalent maternal doses of aspirin rats are teratogenically more sensitive than monkeys and this is correlated with a much higher level of salicylic acid in the rat embryo (Wilson and co-workers, 1977). Measurement of free and bound maternal plasma levels of this aspirin metabolite provided a rational explanation for the species difference in embryonic metabolite levels and presumably therefore for the difference in teratologic outcome.

These few examples serve to illustrate the contribution of maternal biotransformation and pharmacokinetics to species difference in teratologic response. Numerous other maternal parameters have been shown or could be predicted to likewise contribute to species variation. A recent publication (Gordon and co-workers, 1981) has in fact suggested that species variation in response to thalidomide could have a maternal metabolic basis.

PLACENTA

The second potential site of species difference in teratologic response is the interface between mother and embryo, the placenta. Documented examples of this organ being responsible for species differences are rare indeed due in large part to neglect of this structure by most investigators. The exception to this generalization is the work of Drs. Beck and Lloyd who have provided convincing evidence that some teratogens such as trypan blue act by interfering with the nutritive function of the yolk sac placenta (Beck, Lloyd and Griffiths, 1967). The importance of this work for the present discussion is that relatively few mammals utilize the yolk sac as an organ of embryonic nutrition. However, all of the species commonly used in the testing of new chemicals, rats, mice and rabbits, possess and utilize an inverted yolk sac placenta and thus the possibility for species variation is clear.

Stevens and Harbison (1974) examined the distribution of diphenylhydantoin in four species. They demonstrated that fetal levels of this agent were much higher in the mouse than rat in good agreement with the teratologic sensitivity of these two species. Furthermore they showed that maternal plasma levels were the same in these two species and suggested that placental transfer was the basis of the difference in drug concentration in the embryo.

EMBRYO

The secrets of normal embryogenesis and how it can be diverted to produce malformations have been slow to be uncovered. Thus the means by which species variation in teratologic response might occur at this level are for the most part not understood. One well studied example of variation in teratologic response, not between species, but between various strains of the same species, concerns the frequency of cleft palate production by glucocorticoids in mice (Kalter, 1954). Many factors have been suggested to underlie this phenomenon but one of the most recent concerns the level of glucocorticoid receptors within the maxillary mesenchyme. Salomon and Pratt (1979) reported a concordance between the amount of glucocorticoid specifically bound to fetal maxillary mesenchyme and the strain susceptibility to cortisone-induced cleft palate. Thus it seems that the greater the concentration of glucocorticoid receptors found in palate mesenchyme, the greater the susceptibility of that strain to cortisone-induced cleft palate. However, even this story is incomplete since there are a few exceptions to this generalization and more importantly the biological response to glucocorticoids responsible for non-closure of the palate is unresolved.

In our own laboratory we have suggested that species difference in teratologic response to carbonic anhydrase inhibitors is related to ontogeny of the target molecule, carbonic anhydrase. The prototype agent of this class, acetazolamide produces a very unique and characteristic limb malformation in most strains or stocks of rats and mice (Layton and Hallesy, 1965). On the other hand limb deformities are absent in monkey fetuses exposed to very high drug doses (Wilson, 1971). Carbonic anhydrase activity in these species revealed that monkey embryos had very low enzyme activity in comparison to rat embryos at the appropriate developmental stage (Scott and co-workers, in press).

In summary the examples of species difference in teratologic response presented here further justify the well worn phrase that no single species is routinely the best one for estimating potential effects of new chemical agents on human offspring. Clearly some information regarding the pharmacologic attributes of a new agent would help in choosing the proper species. Thus the study of species difference in teratologic response has a very practical purpose but information gathered from such work is also helpful in understanding mechanisms of teratogenic action.

REFERENCES

Beck, F., J. B. Lloyd, and A. Griffiths (1967). Lysosomal enzyme inhibition by trypan blue: A theory of teratogenesis. Science, 157, 1180-1182.
Chernoff, G. (1977). The fetal alcohol syndrome in mice: An animal model. Teratology, 15, 223-229.
Chernoff, G. F. (1980). The fetal alcohol syndrome in mice: Maternal variables. Teratology, 22, 71-75.
Gillette, J. R. (1977). Factors that affect drug concentrations in maternal plasma. In J. G. Wilson and F. C. Fraser (Eds.), Handbook of Teratology, Vol. 3, Plenum Press, New York. pp. 35-78.
Giroud, A., H. Tuchmann-Duplessis, and L. Mercier-Parot (1962a). Observations sur les répercussions tératogènes de la thalidomide chez la souris et le lapin. C. R. Soc. Biol., 156, 765-768.
Giroud, A., H. Tuchmann-Duplessis, and L. Mercier-Parot (1962b).

Thalidomide and congenital abnormalities. Lancet, 2, 298-299.

Gordon, G. B., S. P. Spielberg, D. A. Blake, and V. Balasubramanian (1981). Thalidomide teratogenesis: Evidence for a toxic arene oxide metabolite. Proc. Natl. Acad. Sci. USA, 78, 2545-2548.

Hanson, J., A. Streissguth, and D. Smith (1978). The effects of moderate alcohol consumption during pregnancy on fetal growth and morphogenesis. J. Pediatr., 92, 457-460.

Kalter, H. (1954). Inheritance of susceptibility to teratogenic action of cortisone in mice. Genetics, 39, 185-196.

Keeler, R. F. (1970) Teratogenic compounds of Veratrum californicum (Durand). Teratology, 3, 175-180.

Keeler, R. F., and W. Binns (1968). Teratogenic compounds of Veratrum californicum (Durand). Teratology, 1, 5-10.

Salomon, D. S., and R. M. Pratt (1979). Involvement of glucocorticoids in the development of the secondary palate. Differentiation, 13, 141-154.

Scott, W. J., K. S. Hirsch, J. M. DeSesso, and J. G. Wilson (in press). Comparative studies on acetazolamide teratogenesis in pregnant rats, rabbits and rhesus monkeys. Teratology.

Stevens, M. W., and R. D. Harbison (1974). Placental transfer of diphenylhydantoin: Effects of species, gestational age and route of administration. Teratology, 9, 317-326.

Vickers, T. H. (1967). Concerning the morphogenesis of thalidomide dysmelia in rabbits. Br. J. Exp. Pathol., 48, 579-591.

Wilson, J. G. (1971). Use of rhesus monkeys in teratological studies. Fed. Proc., 30, 104-109.

Wilson, J. G. (1973). An animal model of human disease: thalidomide embryopathy in primates. Comp. Pathol. Bull., 5, 3-4.

Wilson, J. G., E. J. Ritter, W. J. Scott, and R. Fradkin (1977). Comparative distribution and embryotoxicity of acetylsalicylic acid in pregnant monkeys and rats. Toxicol. Appl. Pharmacol., 41, 67-78.

Defined Laboratory Animals

T. Nomura and Y. Tajima

Central Institute for Experimental Animals, Kawasaki, Japan

ABSTRACT

In order to assure reproducible animal experiments, the experiments must be performed by appropriate methods using defined laboratory animals. The site and the course of the host response in animal experiments must be understood to make sure that a certain treatment always produces the same responses. When an animal is considered on the basis of its genes it is called a genotype and when the maternal effects are added, the animal is then known as a phenotype. It was formerly considered that the results of animal experiments were the direct response of the phenotype to the experimental procedure, but it has since become clear that the same results are not always obtained when the environment of the phenotype is varied and, therefore, a new type, the dramatype which is the result of the effects of the proximate environment on the phenotype is necessary. The dramatype must be uniform to achieve reproducible animal experiments and animals having such uniform dramatypes are defined laboratory animals. Control and testing are essential to achieve defined laboratory animals, and the performance or quality assurance test is a check of the inviariability of the status and quality of the animal. Current concepts and methods used in genetic and microbiological monitoring to assure this invariability are discussed.

KEYWORDS

Defined laboratory animal; experimental animal; laboratory animal; dramatype; performance test; genetic monitoring; microbiological monitoring; animal control; environmental control; proximate environment.

INTRODUCTION

In the course of development of new drugs, animal experiments are indispensable in evaluation of the efficacy and the safety of the drug which can be extrapolated to humans. Reproducibility of the results of such experiments is essential but the results are often difficult to reproduce because of the complexity of the factors involved, such as the genetic and microbiological background of the animals themselves, the environment in which the animals

are reared and the experimental environment and techniques used. To assure
reproducible animal experiments, the experiments must be performed by appropriate methods using defined laboratory animals.

In this paper, we would like to give an outline of defined laboratory animals
using the mouse as an example of the degree of quality to which laboratory
animals have progressed at present. Studies are now underway to apply the
concepts and methodology used with mice to other species and it is hoped that
this discussion will prove valuable for those involved in pharmacological
research.

CLASSIFICATION OF EXPERIMENTAL ANIMALS

First, we will discuss animals used for experiments, the so-called experimental
animals. Experimental animals are of various species and strains, and they
are reared in different environments. Their quality with respect to background and history is not always constant.

As shown in Table 1, experimental animals can be divided into three groups:
laboratory animals developed for research purposes and produced under controlled conditions; domestic animals produced without the controls required for
research purposes; and animals obtained in the wild state from nature.

TABLE 1 Classification of Experimental Animals

Group	Definition
Laboratory animals	Animals which are domesticated because of importance or need in research. They are bred and produced under controlled conditions for research purposes
Domestic animals	Animals which are domesticated for use in human society. They are bred and produced without the control required for research purposes
Animals obtained from nature	Animals which have been in nature. They are not produced or reproduced by humans

The reasons for dividing experimental animals into these three groups are as
follows. The results of animal experiments are affected by the origin and
rearing environment of the animal used. Therefore, it is important that this
origin and environment be clear and controllable. However, these factors
clearly differ among the three groups. Laboratory animals satisfy all of
these factors while those obtained from nature do not. Domestic animals are
intermediate between laboratory animals and those obtained from nature.
Therefore, it is essential that the group to which the animals belong be
known if the results of the experiments are to be evaluated precisely (Tajima,
1973). Defined laboratory animals are the most strictly controlled types of
all laboratory animals.

SITE OF THE RESPONSE TO THE EXPERIMENT
- DETERMINATION OF THE DRAMATYPE

The following is a discussion of the site and course of the host response in
animal experiments.

In animal experiments, the physiological and pathological responses of the
animal are observed. Therefore, it is necessary that the experimental conditions be controlled so that the responses to a certain treatment are
always the same.

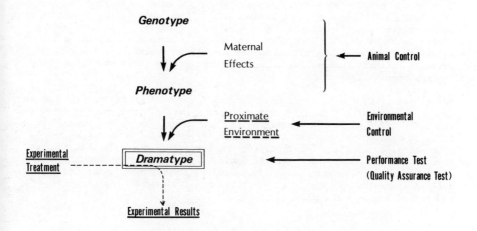

Fig. 1.   Determination of dramatype and controls and
testing to obtaining defined laboratory animals.

As shown in Fig. 1, animals begin life as fertilized eggs which receive many
different genes from both parents. When they are considered on the basis of
their genes, the animals are called genotypes. The fetus (genotype)is exposed
to various external factors in its maternal and development environment up to
the time of maturity, such as the environments within the oviducts and uterus
before and after implantation, and the environment during lactation. Thus,
the animal bodies are formed and on the basis of their characters, they are
then called phenotypes. In other words, the phenotype can be considered a
genotype with the addition of maternal effects. These effects differ in accordance with differences in the characters. For example, the morphological
and permanent physiological characteristics, such as differences in coat
color, skeleton and various enzymes, are not seriously affected by maternal
effects. Genetic malformations can also be considered part of this category.
On the other hand, induced malformations, such as cleft palates in newborn
mice from mothers which had been administered cortisone during pregnancy and
phocomelia of newborn macaca monkeys from mothers administered thalidomide
are characters (phenotype) strongly influenced by maternal effects.

Usually, the results of animal experiments are considered to be the direct
response of the phenotype to treatment. However, general experience shown
that the same responses, i.e. the same experimental results, are not always
obtained in animals of the same phenotype when these animals are moved to
different locations and are subjected to the same experimental treatment.

The reason for such differences appears to be the effects of the proximate environment on the animals. The physiological conditions of the animals are susceptible to change in accordance with different environmental conditions and it is only natural that different results will be obtained from the same experimental treatment when the animal's physiological functions are changed by differences in the environment. An example of this is the different LD50 values in toxicity tests and the different mortality rates for anaphylactic shock seen in the same phenotype of inbred mice at different temperatures (Nomura, 1967, 1968, 1969).

Therefore, the effects of the various environmental conditions under which animals are maintained and conditions during the animal experiments, i.e. the proximate environment, can not be neglected. When considering the effects of these proximate environmental factors on the phenotype, it is necessary to introduce a new concept "the dramatype" which is determined by the action of proximate environmental factors on the phenotype. Therefore, the results of animal experiments can actually be considered as the response of the dramatype to experimental treatment.

One important key in the evaluation of the results of animal experiments is the uniformity of the dramatype, i.e. uniform physiological status among the animals being used in the experiments at the time of the experiments. There-fore, it is absolutely essential to carefully control the genotype, the maternal effects on the genotype, the phenotype, and the proximate environ-ment of the phenotype which are the decisive factors for the dramatype. In other words, animals which have a uniform dramatype can be considered as defined laboratory animals. (This is the modification of the original concept of Russel and Burch, 1959).

CONTROL AND TESTING OF LABORATORY ANIMALS AND DEFINITION
OF DEFINED LABORATORY ANIMALS

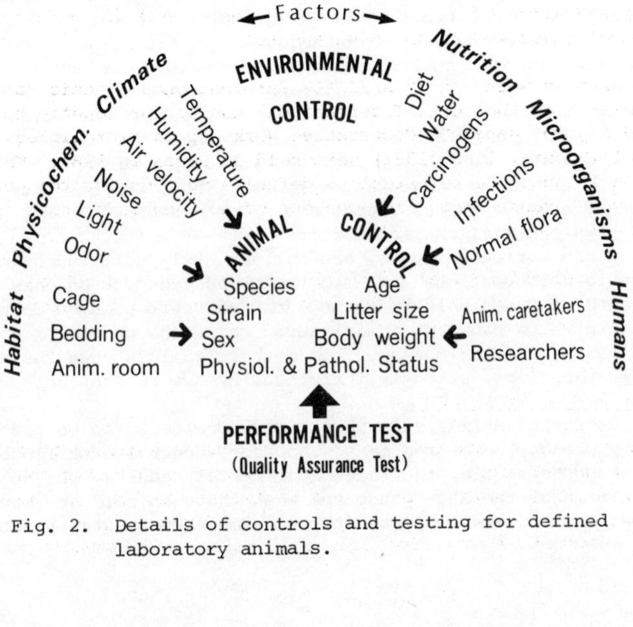

Fig. 2.   Details of controls and testing for defined
laboratory animals.

The different types of control and testing required to obtain uniform dramatypes are shown in Figs. 1 and 2. They consist of animal control, i.e. the
control of the animal itself, environmental control and the performance test
or quality assurance test. Animal control involves investigations covering
genetics, physiological, and pathological status (Genotype, maternal effects
and phenotype). Details of control factors are shown in Fig. 2.

Environmental control includes control of the environment in a narrow sense,
nutrition, and living things (microorganisms and humans). Details of these
factors are also shown in Fig. 2.

The performance test or quality assurance test is a check of the invariability
of the status and quality of the animal.

The defined laboratory animals must be those subjected to strict animal and
environmental control as mentioned above, but in addition, they must also be
those for which the dramatype has been monitored and confirmed by means of
performance tests or quality assurance tests.

The term "defined laboratory animals" was first mentioned at the ICLAS Symposium in 1969 (Hill, 1971), but at that time, the concept was only an ideal
since no definite methods for performance tests had been established. Thereafter, demands for the quality control of laboratory animals increased as
animal experiments became more precise and long-term, and it became evident
at this time that strict genetic and microbiological control of laboratory
animals was essential. It also became apparent that genetic and microbiological monitoring was necessary for the quality assurance of laboratory animals.

GENETICAL AND MICROBIOLOGICAL MONITORING AS A PERFORMANCE
TEST TO OBTAIN DEFINED LABORATORY ANIMALS

The International Council for Laboratory Animal Science (ICLAS) is promoting
a genetic and microbiological monitoring centre system program as one aspect
of the international standardization of laboratory animals, and this program
includes the preparation of an international genetic and microbiological
monitoring manual (Radzikowski and Nomura, 1981).

As one aspect of this work, an ICLAS/ICREW International Genetic Monitoring
Workshop (Committee of the ICLAS International Manual for Genetic Monitoring,
in press), and a joint Japan-US Cooperative Workshop on Microbiological
Quality Control (Nomura, 1980, 1981) were held in Japan in 1980. This monitoring system made it possible to establish definite methods for the performance
test or quality assurance test. The concept of defined laboratory animals
has become a reality.

This genetic and microbiological monitoring system involves periodic checks
of the genetic and microbiological quality of the animals to determine if
their quality remains invariable.

Outline of the Genetic Monitoring

The aim of genetic monitoring is to assure the genetic quality of laboratory
animals, mainly inbred mice, for the early detection of genetic contamination
and mutations, and thus improve the accuracy and reliability of the results
of animal experiments. Genetic markers which are located on loci of the
chromosomes are tested by morphological, biochemical and immunological methods.

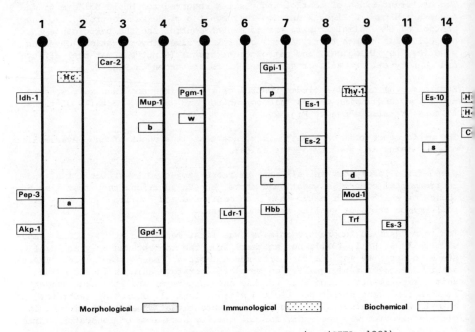

Fig. 3.　Genetic profile of mouse strains (CIEA, 1981).

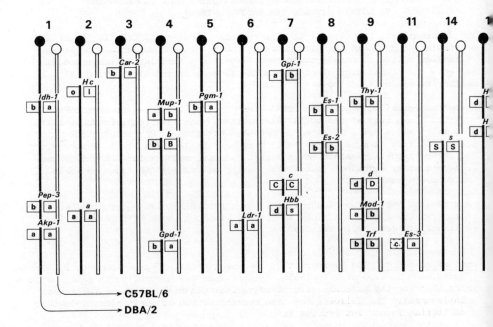

Fig. 4.　Genetic profile of C57BL/6 and DBA/2 (CIEA, 1981).

Chromosome No.	1	1	2	3	4	5	6	7	7	8	8	9	9	9	9	11	11	17	17
Locus	Idh-1	Pep-3	Akp-1	Hc	Car-2	Mup-1	Gpd-1	Pgm-1	Ldr-1	Gpi-1	Hbb	Es-1	Es-2	Thy-1	Mod-1	Trf	Es-3	H-2K	H-2D
A	a	b	b	o	b	a	b	a	a	a	d	b	b	b	a	b	c	k	d
AKR	b	b	b	o	a	a	b	a	a	a	d	b	b	a	b	b	c	k	k
BALB/c	a	a	b	l	b	a	b	a	a	a	d	b	b	b	a	b	a	d	d
CBA/J	b	b	a	l	b	a	b	a	a	b	d	b	b	b	b	a	c	k	k
C3H/He	a	b	b	l	b	a	b	b	a	b	d	b	b	b	a	b	c	k	k
C57BL/6	a	a	a	l	a	b	a	a	a	b	s	a	b	b	b	a	b	b	b
DBA/2	b	b	a	o	b	a	b	b	a	a	d	b	b	b	a	b	c	d	d
NZB/Jic	a	c	b	o	a	a	b	b	a	a	d	b	b	b	b	b	c	d	d

Fig. 5.   Genetic profile of main inbred strains
(CIEA, 1981).

The test results are compared with standard types and any abnormalities are determined. The following are the current concepts and methods used in genetic monitoring.

The seven morphological items, the four immunological items and the 16 biochemical items in genetic monitoring in our institute (CIEA) are shown in Fig. 3. As can be seen in the figure, these 27 items are distributed on 12 chromosomes.

As an example, a comparison of the genotypes of 2 strains (C57BL/6 and DBA/2) are shown in Fig. 4. In both strains, there are different genotypes at many loci.

Figure 5 shows the genotypes of each locus for main strains. Each of these strains has a different genetic profile and it is possible to identify each strain by examining its profile. It is also possible to detect very quickly any genetic contamination which occurs among the strains.

Outline of Microbiological Monitoring

The aim of microbiological monitoring is to make possible the correct analysis of experimental data by permitting the experimenter to know the microbiological background of laboratory animals. Microbiological monitoring is also a system for checking the accuracy of control of microorganisms in the experimental environment. The following are the current methods used in microbiological monitoring in our institute (CIEA).

Table 2 shows the selection standards of microbiological monitoring items.

T. Nomura and Y. Tajima

TABLE 2   Microbiological Monitoring Items for Mice and
          Rats (CIEA, 1981)

Category	Item	Methods* S	C	M
A	Salmonella spp.	0	0	
	Dermatophytes		0	
B	Sendai virus	0		
	Mouse hepatitis virus	0		
	Ectromelia virus**	0		
	Mycoplasma pulmonis	0	0	
	Pasteurella pneumotropica		0	
	Bordetella bronchiseptica***		0	
	Streptococcus pneumoniae***		0	
	Corynebacterium kutscheri	0	0	
	Tuzzer's organism	0		
	E. coli 0115a, cK(B)**		0	
	Giardia muris			0
	Spironucreus muris			0
C	Pseudomonas aeruginosa		0	
D	Syphacia spp.			0

* S:Serological   C:Cultivation   M:Microscopical
** Mice only *** Rats only.

Category A includes microorganisms pathogenic to both humans and rodents.
Category B includes potential pathogens for mice and rats. These pathogens
disturb animal experiments because they often kill the infected animals.
Category B also includes microorganisms which often cause inapparent infection
and alter the physiological status of animal responses to various experimental
treatments. Category C includes microorganisms which are usually harmless, but
under special experimental conditions such as irradiation experiments, can
become harmful. Category D includes parasites which are not pathogenic, but
are useful parameters for checking the microbiological control of rearing environments. Another selection standard for these items is that these organisms
be widely distributed throughout Japan. There are 14 items each for mice and
rats and they are checked by serology, cultivation and microscopy.

Genetic and microbiological monitoring is basically a form of quality control
which can be considered as equivalent to the performance or quality assurance
test.

CONCLUSION

To assure correct experiments, defined laboratory animals must be used. These
defined laboratory animals are those bred and produced under controlled conditions and maintained in a controlled environment, with clear genetic and
microbiological backgrounds obtained by regular monitoring. The use of such
defined laboratory animals is a prerequisite for obtaining reproducible
results in animal experiments.

REFERENCES

Committee of the ICLAS International Manual for Genetic Monitoring (Ed.) (in press). ICLAS Genetical Monitoring Manual. University of Tokyo Press, Tokyo.

Hill, B.F. (Ed.) (1971). Defining the Laboratory Animals. National Academy of Sciences, Washington, D.C.

Nomura, T., C. Yamauchi, and H. Takahashi (1967). Influence of environmental temperature on physiological functions of the laboratory mouse. In M.L. Conalty (Ed.), Husbandry of Laboratory Animals. Academic Press, London and New York. pp. 459-470.

Nomura, T., and C. Yamauchi (1968). Environments and physiological status of experimental animals. In O.Mühlbock, and T. Nomura (Eds.), Experimental Animals in Cancer Research. Maruzen Co., Ltd., Tokyo. pp. 17-35.

Nomura, T. (1969). Management of animals for use in teratological experiments. In H. Nishimura, and J.R. Miller (Eds.), Methods for Teratological Studies in Experimental Animals and Man. Igaku Shoin Ltd., Tokyo. pp. 3-15.

Nomura, T. (Ed.) (1980). Research on Preparation of Quality Standards of Laboratory Animals and Establishment of Checking Methods. Report of Grant-in-Aid for Special Project Research, The Ministry of Education, Science and Culture, Japan. Central Institute for Experimental Animals, Kawasaki.

Nomura, T. (Ed.) (1981). Promotion of an Exchange of Information between the United States and Japan concerning Quality Control of Laboratory Animals (1) Microbiological Quality Control. Report of Grant-in-Aid for Special Project Research, The Ministry of Education, Science and Culture, Japan. Central Institute for Experimental Animals, Kawasaki.

Radzikowski, Cz., and T. Nomura (1981). ICLAS Monitoring Centre System Programme. ICLAS Bull., No. 48, 6-8.

Russell, W.M.S., and R.L. Burch (1959). The Principle of Humane Experimental Technique. Methuen & Co. Ltd., London.

Tajima, Y. (1973). General concepts concerning new laboratory animals. Exp. Anims., 22, Suppl., 85-90.

Quality Control in Diets — the Attainable

J. K. Eva

Special Diets Services Limited, 1 Stepfield, Witham,
Essex, CM8 3AB, UK

ABSTRACT

Since the Good Laboratory Practice Regulations were first proposed (1976,
published Fed. Reg. 43.247.1979) there has been considerable interest in
diet quality with particular reference to contamination. Over the past 3
years, more than 200 batches of diets (6 different formulae) have been produced in a manner conforming with G.L.P. using modified methods of conventional diet manufacture. These diets have been tested for over 20 different
contaminants including heavy metals (5), other inorganic contaminants (3),
pesticide residues (6), mycotoxins (8) and microbiological activity (6).
The levels found are compared with published maxima (N.C.T.R. 1979 and E.P.A.
prop. reg. 44.91.1979) and the indications are that, for many contaminants,
these maxima are impossible to achieve. Problem contaminants include
Selenium, Cadmium, Lead, DDT and Fungal Spores.

KEYWORDS

Diets; quality; attainable quality; desirable quality; contamination;
variation; stability; cost.

INTRODUCTION

It is unfortunate that the "attainable" is not necessarily the same as the
"desirable", and it is equally unfortunate that idealism, whether of moral
or scientific origin, will make demands for quality which are impractical.
What makes it more difficult is that "quality" is such an all embracing term
which can rarely be defined simply, and yet, comprehensively. Quality in
diets relates to nutritional performance, to purity, to consistency in analysis, to appearance, to acceptability, to packaging, stability and many
other things besides. The main point to be made is that if diets are subject
to a quality specification covering a considerable number of parameters, and
if the tolerances applied are too severe, then the regularity of supply of
diet will be greatly at risk, and the price of diet will greatly increase.

This paper concerns commercially available diets, and the data presented relate to diets of British manufacture. As many of the raw materials used were
either produced or processed in the U.K., these data may not compare very
closely with similar data from diets of different origins.

In the U.K. the majority of diets for laboratory animals are manufactured to
fixed formulae, and no adjustments are made to these formulae to accommodate
variations in nutrient analyses of raw materials. Fixed formula diets usually
require fairly wide tolerance limits for nutrient contents, as raw materials
are subject to remarkably wide variations, even in the simplest parameters.

Basically, there are two factors affecting diet quality, and these are the
raw materials, and the machinery and methods used to convert these raw
materials into suitable diets.

DIET MANUFACTURE

The ideal mixing operation is one where all processes are isolated and
visible, where raw materials can be segregated and where all batch assemblies
are discrete. This ideal situation usually turns out to be one man with a
shovel who does all the work and a supervisor who watches him do it. Costs
are astronomical.

A more normal diet manufacturing unit is very complex and is designed for
large scale, semi-continuous production. There is still expert operation and
supervision, but as the processes are now hidden from view, it is necessary
to presume that all is operating properly and, in the final reckoning, quality
can only be determined by analysis. There are other disadvantages also.
There are areas which are inaccessible, where materials may get trapped and may
later cause contamination, so special cleaning procedures and a strict admin-
istrative protocol for production are necessary to ensure that inevitable
interbatch contamination is rendered insignificant. Contamination of one diet
with another, or with a simple raw material is usually of little importance,
and may well be incapable of identification, but there are contaminants which
are potentially dangerous. Historically, diets for laboratory animals have
been made by manufacturers of feeds for farm animals, and such feeds contain
many non-nutritive additives, most of which are medicinal in purpose.
Contamination of a laboratory diet with a medicinal product could have
disastrous results, not perhaps to the animals being fed, but certainly to
the validity of the test results. The only sensible way of eliminating the
possibility of such contamination is to prohibit medicinal products from the
production site. There are two sites in the U.K., dedicated to quality diet
production, where medicinal products are banned and where such contamination
is impossible.

Manufacturing methods and machinery can be responsible for other, cruder,
forms of contamination. Apart from foreign materials which may, inadvertently
pass into the machinery with a raw material, the machinery may fracture, nuts
and bolts may come loose, bits may fall off, so protective devices have to be
installed to screen off such contamination and these include screens, cleared
by rotating brushes or by vibration, to remove large lumps, or to remove dust
and broken pieces from pelleted diets, and magnets to remove ferrous metals -
and fortunately, most metallic contamination is magnetic.

In our experiences, pieces of metal have been found in a diet meal assembly,
and unfortunately, these particular pieces of metal were themselves part of
a screen installed to remove such contamination. If the screen itself breaks,
pieces of it may well end up in the diet. Examples of the metallic debris
collected by the magnets include particles of iron, which are inevitable when
iron machinery is used, nuts and bolts which seem to appear by some form of
instantaneous creation and a wide miscellany of nails, welding rod, marker
pens and knives which have somehow found their way into a diet mix. Finally,
material screened from the pelleted diet includes lumps of damp material
created from the hot damp dust produced with the freshly made pellets. There
is also fine dry dust created by abrasion of the pellets as they pass through
the machinery and there are odd foreign pellets proving the point that there
are inaccessible parts of the machinery where material can get trapped, later
to be released. Considerable attention to maintenance, administration and
cleaning is therefore necessary to ensure optimum quality with optimum
production.

DIET INGREDIENTS

Raw materials are also sources of contamination which may vary from bits of
metal and pieces of wood to weed seeds and other unwanted matter and finally
to micro-contaminants of many types.

Basically raw materials are of two different types:-

Micro-nutrients are usually synthetic, chemically pure materials, vitamins,
amino acids and inorganic salts. As their inclusion rates in diets are low,
they are usually premixed before inclusion. Premixes can be tested before
use and their inclusion can be accurately controlled, but premixing can
create problems in respect of stability and, consequently, their manufacture
requires considerable care. Premixing does however permit a guaranteed
inclusion and the efficient dispersion of many micro-nutrients and the
analyses of these are very much easier and more accurate in the premix than
in the diet where their dilution is much greater and there is more chance of
interference.

Macro-nutrients, comprising cereals, cereal byproducts and proteins, provide
two basic problems - their bulk and their variability. Quality specifications
are not easy to define and their bulk interferes with monitoring. For
instance, in the U.K., barley is defined as containing not more than 4% of
materials other than barley grain. In a 20 tonne bulk load, 4% is 800 kg
and vibration in transit may cause separation so that, when the bulk load is
tipped, the first part off may be almost pure barley while the last part may
be chaff, straw and husk with very little barley grain.

Variations in certain parameters for various raw materials are illustrated
in Table 1. Compared with the found averages, variations of $\pm$ 30% for
moisture and fat and $\pm$ 15% for protein are not uncommon and clearly
illustrate the difficulties of diet formulation and the need for sensible
tolerance limits for fixed formula diets.

TABLE 1   Nutrient Variations in Raw Materials - 1979

Raw Material	No. of Samples	Test	Range %	Mean %	Spec %	Mean as % of Spec
Wheat	70	Moisture	9.8-15.9	13.0	16.0 max	81.3
		Protein	8.3-12.8	10.4	11.0	94.5
Maize	45	Moisture	11.1-15.6	13.2	16.0 max	82.5
		Fat	1.4- 3.8	3.1	3.5	88.6
		Protein	8.0-10.5	8.7	9.0	96.7
Barley	25	Moisture	10.5-17.0	13.8	16.0 max	96.3
		Fat	1.0- 2.3	1.5	1.5	100.0
		Protein	8.1-12.6	9.7	10.0	97.0
Oats	10	Moisture	8.7-12.9	11.3	16.0 max	70.6
		Fat	4.5- 7.0	5.5	4.5	122.2
		Protein	8.5-10.8	9.5	11.0	86.4
Wheatfeed	45	Moisture	9.7-15.1	13.5	16.0 max	84.4
		Fat	1.6-4.7	3.3	3.5	94.3
		Protein	11.0-15.2	14.6	15.0	97.3
Ext. Soya Bean Meal	30	Moisture	11.8-14.2	13.2	15.0 max	88.0
		Protein	40.0-44.0	41.4	43.0	96.3
Meat and Bone Meal	30	Moisture	3.2-10.2	7.2	10.0 max	72.0
		Fat	6.4-13.7	8.8	9.0	97.8
		Protein	44.6-55.9*	48.9	48.0	101.9
Meat Meal	30	Moisture	2.7- 7.8	5.4	7.0 max	77.1
		Fat	25.7-38.9	31.7	30.0	105.7
		Protein	48.9-60.8	53.2	54.0	98.5
White Fish Meal	25	Moisture	4.2-10.6	7.1	10.0 max	71.0
		Fat	4.1- 7.7	6.1	7.0	87.1
		Protein	61.7-67.2	63.9	65.0	98.3
Herring (type) Meal	10	Moisture	7.1-11.5	8.6	10.0 max	86.0
		Fat	7.9- 9.1	8.7	9.0	96.7
		Protein	64.4-68.2	66.6	70.0	95.1
Dried Yeast Unext.	10	Moisture	2.0- 8.5	6.7	10.0 max	67.0
		Protein	32.3-47.8	43.6	45.0	96.9

*In the U.K. "Meat and Bone Meal" contains less than 54% Protein.

Raw material micro-contaminants show even greater variability and these are illustrated in Table 2. Factors of greater than 100x the minima found are not uncommon and, for instance, the maximum Malathion level found in Wheat is nearly 2000x the minimum detectable level. Fortunately, most contaminant findings are low but these results clearly illustrate the danger in adjusting formulae to accommodate nutrient variations - a contaminant could be increased out of all proportion with only a minor change in the formula.

TABLE 2   Found Contamination in Raw Materials - U.K. 1979

Contaminant		Cereals	Cereal Byproduct	Vegetable Proteins	Animal Proteins	Fish Meals	Grass Meals
$NaNO_2$	ppm	ND-4	ND-3	ND-3	ND-100	ND-7	ND-10
$NaNO_3$	"	ND-23	ND-29	ND-9	ND-200	2-33	ND-4000
Pb	"	ND-1.00	ND-1.00	ND-4.00	2.0-30.0	1.0-10.0	ND-10.0
As	"	ND	ND	ND	ND-5.0	2.0-12.0	ND-5.0
Cd	"	ND	ND-0.2	ND-0.3	ND-4.0	ND-1.2	ND-1.0
Hg	"	ND-0.08	ND-0.06	0.01-0.03	ND-0.02	0.10-0.25	ND-0.05
Se	"	0.03-0.16	0.04-0.90	0.09-0.26	0.04-0.10	1.00-1.30	ND-0.05
Dieldrin	ppb	ND	ND-8	ND-6		ND-23	
DDT's	"	ND-94	ND-70	ND-50		ND-80	
Lindane	"	ND-13	3-48	1-10		2-10	
Heptachlor	"	ND-30	ND-10	ND-4		ND-5	
P.C.B's	"	ND	ND	ND		ND	
Malathion	ppm	ND-36.0	ND-1.0	ND-0.01		ND	
Aflatoxins	ppb	ND-8.0	ND	ND-60		ND	ND
T.V.O.	/g	10^3-10^7	10^3-10^6	10^5-10^7	10^4-10^6	10^3-10^5	10^4-10^7
Meso.Spores	"	10^2-10^5	10^2-10^4	10^4-10^6	10^3-10^5	10^2-10^4	10^4-10^6
Coliforms	"	Rare	Rare	Rare	Frequent	Frequent	Frequent
E.Coli 1	"	"	"	"	"	"	"
Salmonellae	"	ND	ND	ND	Rare	Rare	Rare
Fung.Spores	"	10^2-10^4	10^2-10^4	10^3-10^4	ND-10^4	ND-10^4	10^2-10^3
Antibiotics	"	ND	ND	ND	ND	ND	ND

notes:-   Rare - found in not more than 10% of samples tested.
          Frequent - found in more than 20% of samples tested.
          E.Coli 1 - confirmed in about 10% of samples in which
                     Coliforms were found.

The majority of micro-contaminants found in diets directly reflect the
levels of those contaminants in the raw materials. In considering attainable
quality in diets it is necessary to have some idea of desirable quality and
Table 3 illustrates various published values - there is considerable
divergence of opinion.

TABLE 3   Published Levels of Contaminants - Desirable Maxima

Contaminant		N.C.T.R. 641-4-2090c 1975	E.P.A. 44.91.40 CFR770-772 1979	N.C.T.R. 1979	GV-SOLAS 1978	No Effect Level ?
F	ppm	35.0				
Se	"	0.05-0.50	0.10-0.60	0.05-0.65		0.025-0.50
Cd	"	0.5	0.16	0.25	0.5	1.0
Hg	"	1.0	0.1	0.2		1.0
As	"	1.0	1.0	1.0		5.0
Pb	"	1.2	1.5	1.5		5.0
P.C.B's	"	1.0	0.05	0.05		0.5
DDT's	"	0.15	0.1	0.1		1.0
Dieldrin	"	0.1	0.02	0.02		0.1
Lindane	"	0.1	0.02	0.2		0.5
Heptachlor	"	0.1	0.02	0.02		0.1
Malathion	"	0.5	2.5	5.0		5.0
$NaNO_2$	"					10.0
$NaNO_3$	"					?
Nitrosamine	ppb		10.0	10.0		
Aflatoxins	"	5.0	5.0	5.0		10.0
Oestrogenic Act.	"	5.0	1.0			
B.H.A.	ppm			50.0		
Ethoxyquin	"			50.0		
Tot.Viable Orgs.	/g	100,000		100,000	100,000	
Mesophilic Spores	"	30,000		30,000		
Coliforms	"			5		
E.Coli Type 1	"					
Salmonellae	"	Absent		Absent	Absent	Absent
Fungal Spores	"		Absent	100		
Antibiotic Act.	"					Absent

CONTAMINATION IN DIETS

Contaminant levels found in over 250 batches of diets manufactured on plants
dedicated to quality diet manufacture since 1978 are illustrated in Table 4.

TABLE 4   Found Contamination in Diets

Contaminant			Mean	Range
Pb	(+Meat & Bone Meal)	ppm	2.9	0.5 - 6.5
"	(- " " " ")	"	1.3	0.5 - 4.0
Cd	(+ " " " ")	"	0.65	0.2 - 1.1
"	(- " " " ")	"	0.35	0.05 - 0.9
NaNO$_3$	(+Grass Meal)	"	440.0	1.0 -900.0
"	(- " ")	"	15.8	1.0 - 70.0
NaNO$_2$		"	1.8	1.0 - 7.0
F	(+Meat & Bone + Phosphate)	"	43.4	11.0 - 70.0
"	(+Phosphate only)	"	18.3	10.0 - 35.0
"	(Low Phosphate only)	"	5.1	1.0 - 11.0
Hg		"	0.02	0.01 - 0.12
As		"	0.3	0.20 - 1.10
Se		"	0.19	0.02 - 0.66
Lindane		1978 "	0.017	0.001- 0.170
(overall Mean 0.013 ppm)		1979 "	0.023	0.001- 0.300
		1980 "	0.006	0.001- 0.035
		1981 "	0.004	0.001- 0.011
Heptachlor		1978 "	0.001	0.001- 0.011
(overall Mean 0.004 ppm)		1979 "	0.008	0.001- 0.065
		1980 "	0.003	0.001- 0.010
		1981 "	0.001	0.001- 0.002
Dieldrin		1978 "	0.003	0.001- 0.120
(overall Mean 0.003 ppm)		1979 "	0.006	0.001- 0.035
		1980 "	0.002	0.001- 0.014
		1981 "	0.001	0.001- 0.002
DDT's		1978 "	0.033	0.001- 0.250
(overall Mean 0.023 ppm)		1979 "	0.039	0.001- 0.165
		1980 "	0.011	0.001- 0.070
		1981 "	0.008	0.001- 0.018
Malathion		1978 "	0.190	0.02 - 1.00
(overall Mean 0.148 ppm)		1979 "	0.330	0.02 - 4.80
		1980 "	0.030	0.02 - 0.09
		1981 "	0.025	0.02 - 0.06
Total Viable Organisms		/g	7300	1000 - 75000
Mesophilic Spores		"	3400	100 -100000
Fungal Spores		"	83	ND - 1100

Cadmium and Lead are quite specifically related to formulation, significantly higher levels being found in diets containing Meat and Bone Meal. Lead levels are 3x higher and Cadmium levels are 2x higher than those levels found in diets not containing this ingredient. With respect to certain published permitted maxima, there is no way in which diets containing Meat and Bone Meals could be made in the U.K. to comply regularly with a Lead limit of 1.5 ppm, and no diet at all would regularly comply with a Cadmium limit of 0.25 ppm.

Certain other contaminants also show specific raw material relationships - Nitrate levels are very high in diets containing Grass Meal and Fluoride is related both to Meat and Bone Meal and to Mineral Phosphates. For the majority of these contaminants there are no real problems in achieving levels similar to, or rather less than, published maxima.

Selenium presents a problem. In the diets considered here, Selenium is a
contaminant, but Selenium is also an essential micro-nutrient and minimal
levels of 0.025 - 0.10 ppm have been proposed. With a detection limit of
0.02 ppm, there have been about 30 occasions when the found level was less
than 0.1 ppm and 10 occasions when less than 0.025. If Selenium supplement-
ation was prescribed in order to achieve levels of not less than 0.1 ppm,
there would be a very real risk of exceeding the maximum permitted level.

For pesticide residues, the published maxima vary considerably and, for
instance, Heptachlor has exceeded 0.02 ppm about 5 times. Lindane has
exceeded this level 26 times and Dieldrin 4 times. DDT has exceeded 0.1 ppm
10 times and Malathion has exceeded 0.5 ppm 16 times. P.C.B's have never
been detected. The detection limit for all chlorinated pesticides is 0.001
ppm and for Malathion 0.02 ppm.

MICROBIOLOGICAL CONTROL AND DIET STABILITY

It is in the area of Microbiology that diet processing conditions have a very
considerable effect. Most pelleting processes use steam and this, together
with the extra heat generated by friction and pressure at the die face, kills
off many of the micro-organisms present in the raw materials. An unprocessed
mixed meal may contain millions of organisms per gram and correct processing
will reduce the level to tens of thousands at the most. At the same time
viable E.Coli and Salmonellae will be destroyed. Compared with the various
proposed maxima there are no difficulties in producing diets with low microbial
populations. Fungal spores are rather more difficult as they are fairly heat
resistant and there is every likelihood that, however efficient the process,
the fungal spore count will exceed the proposed maximum of 100/g.

The use of steam, efficient though it may be in producing pellets of good
physical quality which are also clean, has one disadvantage in that the
pellets, when produced, are damp with moisture contents ranging from 16-25%.
Damp pellets will very quickly go mouldy. Normal pelleting practices as
applied to farm feeds are not so concerned with microbiological cleanliness
and neither are they concerned with a long usable life, so normal practice
simply cools pellets in a stream of ambient air during which time the moisture content may fall to 13-16%. Such pellets will show considerable microbiological activity, they will go mouldy and rancid, and most vitamins will
very quickly be destroyed. The diets considered here have been dried with
heated air at a minimum 90°C, apart from further reducing the microbial
population, the moisture content is also reduced to not more than 12.5%, and
given satisfactory storage conditions, clean dried diets remain stable and
usable for prolonged periods of time. Trends in storage for moisture,
microbiological activity, rancidity development and loss of Vitamin A are
illustrated in Figs. 1 - 4.

It must be explained that these results are for storage in the U.K., where
neither the temperature nor the humidity achieve such extremes as are
experienced in Japan.

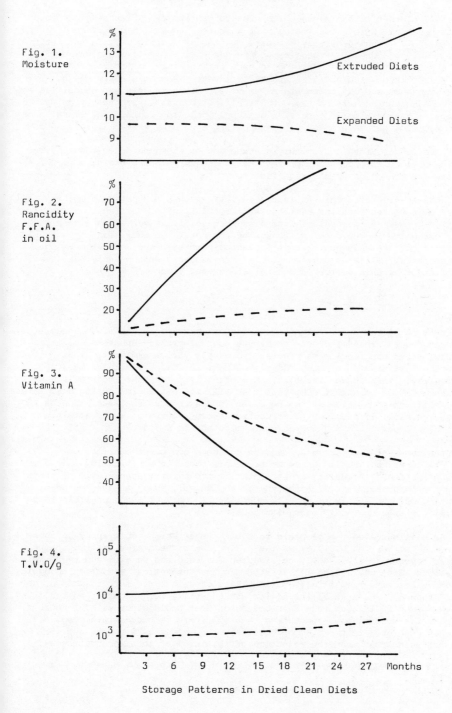

Fig. 1.
Moisture

Extruded Diets

Expanded Diets

Fig. 2.
Rancidity
F.F.A.
in oil

Fig. 3.
Vitamin A

Fig. 4.
T.V.O/g

Storage Patterns in Dried Clean Diets

There are other contaminants which must be mentioned. Aflatoxins have been
detected 4 times in diets in the past 4 years - once at 6 ppb, once at 3 and
twice at 1.5 - the generally accepted maximum is 5 ppb. Certain raw materials
are likely sources of Aflatoxins and in the U.K. there is legislation limiting
Aflatoxin contents in feeds, and indeed, prohibiting the importation of certain materials which contain detectable levels. The main materials at risk
are Groundnut and Cotton and to a lesser extent, Soya Bean and Maize. In the
U.K. Groundnut and Cotton are not normal ingredients in laboratory animal
diets. Other Mycotoxins are also assayed, including Ochratoxin, Zearalenone
and Patulin, but have never yet been detected at a detection limit of 5 ppb.

Antibiotic Activity is routinely checked and has been detected once only,
this was in a diet containing Grass Meal, and no animal protein, a factor
which may or not be of any significance.

Nitrosamines, Oestrogenic Activity and Antioxidants are not assayed, and it
must be admitted that the real reason for this lack of testing is cost. The
cost of assaying the contaminants discussed so far is very high - over £300
per batch and inclusion of Nitrosamines and Oestrogen would more than double
this cost. Antioxidants are not included in these diets and although the
concentrated fat soluble vitamins will contain some antioxidant, the level
in diets from this source is unlikely to exceed 1 ppm.

           COST

Cost is of course a very significant factor in achieving attainable quality.
Compared with diets manufactured before Good Laboratory Practice was introduced, diets now require manufacture to a very strict protocol, plant hygiene
needs maintaining at a higher level, microbiological cleanliness has, of
necessity, improved and stability in storage is of greater importance. All
these will add to normal diet costs, as will the extra time during which diets
are awaiting completion of the necessary and extensive analyses. On the
negative side, limitations to production because certain raw materials and
types of product are prohibited, will also add to costs.

In the commercial world, provided the customer can pay the price, a
manufacturer can usually be found to supply goods to any practicable quality
specification. If quality constraints are too severe, supply will be affected,
and for laboratory animals, indeed for any animal, human beings included, a
continuous food supply is of paramount importance. It seems sensible that
quality standards should recognise this fact.

Table 5 illustrates the probable rejection rates which could apply to these
diets if either the N.C.T.R. or the E.P.A. maxima became mandatory. Reject
rates approaching 100% could be expected for Lead and Cadmium and 5-30% for
Pesticide Residues. Also illustrated are the theoretical maxima which would,
from experience, result in rejection rates of either not more than 1% or not
more than 5%. Even at 5% the maxima are generally much higher than published
levels, and 5% is much more than a manufacturer could carry without increasing
costs. It must also be remembered that 5% refers to batches produced, not
tonnes of diet. In the U.K. batches vary from about 5-25 tonnes and a 5%
reject rate could mean the rejection of about 10% of total production by
weight.

TABLE 5   Probable % Rejection Rate depending upon Limit Applied

Contaminant		N.C.T.R. Limit	N.C.T.R. Reject Rate	E.P.A. Limit	E.P.A. Reject Rate	Max. limit for 1% Reject	Max. limit for 5% Reject
Se(min)	ppm	0.05	7	0.1	15	ND(0.02)	0.025
" (max)	"	0.65	nil	0.6	nil	0.4	0.3
Cd(+Meat & Bone)	"	0.25	97	0.16	100	1.0	0.9
" (- " " ")	"	0.25	72	0.16	95	0.8	0.65
Pb(+ " " ")		1.5	79	1.5	79	6.0	5.5
" (- " " ")	"	1.5	22	1.5	22	3.5	2.5
As	"	1.0	nil	1.0	nil	1.0*	0.6
Hg	"	0.2	nil	0.1	2	0.08	0.06
F (Low Min.P)	"					15.0	15.0
" (High Min.P)	"					35.0	30.0
" (+Meat & Bone)	"					80.0	65.0
NaNO$_2$						6.0	5.0
NaNO$_3$ (+Grass)	"					800.0	400.0
" (- ")	"					50.0	30.0
Nitrosamine	ppb	10.0		10.0			
Aflatoxins	"	5.0	1	5.0	1	3.0	ND(1.0)
Oestrogenic Act.	"			1.0			
B.H.A.	ppm	50.0					
Ethoxyquin	"	50.0					
P.C.B's	"	0.05	nil	0.05	nil	ND(0.001)	ND(0.001)
DDT's	"	0.1	10	0.1	10	0.2	0.1
Dieldrin	"	0.02	5	0.02	5	0.05	0.02
Lindane	"	0.1	5	0.02	30	0.2	0.1
Heptachlor	"	0.02	5	0.02	5	0.05	0.02
Malathion	"	5.0	nil	2.5	5	4.0	0.7
Tot.Viable Orgs.	/g	1×10^5	nil			8×10^4	2.5×10^4
Mesophilic Spores	"	3×10^4	5			4×10^4	1.5×10^4
Coliforms	"	5	1			10	Absent
E.Coli Type 1	"					Absent	Absent
Salmonellae	"	Absent	nil			Absent	Absent
Fungal Spores	"	100	20	Absent	70	1000	400
Antibiotic Act.	"					Absent	Absent

If this is pleading in defence of the diet manufacturer it is because many of the quality constraints relating to diets resulting from Good Laboratory Practice appear to have been set without regard to the difficulties related to achieving quality of the desired standard. *As an example, and no doubt something similar applies in many countries, U.K. legislation prescribes contaminant maxima in raw materials and feeds and for instance, Fish Meal is permitted to contain a maximum of 10 ppm of Arsenic. If a diet formula prescribes 10% of Fish Meal, and many diets do prescribe this amount, there is a good chance that a maximum level of 1.0 ppm would be exceeded and although, in the U.K., we have not yet experienced levels higher than 1.0 ppm, it does not mean to say that we never will. There is similar legislation for Fluorine (150 ppm in most raw materials), Aflatoxin B$_1$ (at 50 ppb) and Mercury (0.5 ppm). There could well be occasions when the only materials available contain these maxima, and depending on formulation, the maxima could be exceeded in the diet.

J. K. Eva

This paper is essentially about contamination, and there are many other contaminants which have not been mentioned. Good Laboratory Practice requires
that diets must not contain contaminants at interfering levels - the interpretation of this requirement needs the services of a fortune teller or a
prophet, as in many animal tests the interferences may not be known. In the
U.K. the principle of testing all batches of diets for all the contaminants
mentioned has, so far, proved satisfactory. If any other contaminant is
found to require assay, then this would be a matter for arrangement between
diet user and diet supplier.

NUTRIENT VARIATIONS IN FIXED FORMULA DIETS

Little has been said about nutrients, other than that tolerances should recognise methods of formulation and the excessive natural variations of raw materials. Table 6 illustrates results over 3½ years on 125 batches of a single,
fixed formula rodent diet. Also indicated are the $\pm$ 10% tolerances allowed
in the E.P.A. proposals and the tolerances permitted in U.K. legislation.

TABLE 6 Nutrient Variations in Fixed Formula Diets

		Calc. Level	Found Mean	Range	Tolerance Limits E.P.A.	Tolerance Limits U.K.
Moisture	%		11.3	9.6 - 12.5	10.0	
Fat	"	3.3 DM	3.5	2.8 - 4.5	3.15- 3.85	2.7 - 5.1
Protein	"	22.2 "	22.1	20.2 - 23.8	20.0 - 24.4	20.0 - 26.0
Fibre	"	5.5 "	4.0	2.2 - 6.6	3.6 - 4.4	2.0 - 5.5
Ash	"	7.7 "	6.9	5.5 - 8.8	6.2 - 7.6	5.0 - 8.5
Carbohydrate	"	61.2 "	63.5	60.5 - 67.0	57.0 - 70.0	
Calcium	"	0.96	1.03	0.75- 1.45	0.93- 1.13	0.85- 1.30
Phosphorus	"	0.80	0.83	0.55- 1.10	0.75- 0.91	0.61- 5.00
Sodium	"	0.35	0.32	0.20- 0.70	0.29- 0.35	0.20- 0.60
Chloride	"	0.47	0.63	0.35- 1.10	0.57- 0.69	0.40- 0.80
Potassium	"	0.77	0.97	0.40- 1.60	0.87- 1.07	
Magnesium	"	0.24	0.20	0.08- 0.36	0.18- 0.22	0.10- 0.50
Iron	mg/kg	119	207	100-325	186-228	100-300
Copper	"	17	19	8- 32	17- 21	9- 29
Manganese	"	68	73	40-110	66- 80	43-105
Zinc	"	26	49	25- 75	44- 54	23- 76
Vitamin A	iu/kg	9.1	11.4	7.0 - 17.0	10.3 - 12.5	7.5 - 14.3
Vitamin E	mg/kg	84.0	95.4	40.0 -180.0	86.0 -105.0	65.0 -123.0

notes:- DM = Dry Matter.   Tolerance Limits calculated from Found Means.

CONCLUSION

Obviously I cannot comment on American ideas of tolerance limits, I can only
say that British legislation is based essentially on experience - or should I
say, on those levels which are attainable in practice. From a pharmacological
point of view, I am not qualified to define the quality constraints satisfactory for pharmacological purposes. What I have tried to do is to indicate the
standards which are regularly attainable in the U.K., which provide no threat
to the continuity of diet supply and which do not add too greatly to the
present high cost of research.

Problems and Improvements in the
Development of Good Laboratory Practice

P. D. Lepore

U. S. Food and Drug Administration, Rockville, Maryland, USA

ABSTRACT

The U.S. Food and Drug Administration published Good Laboratory
Practice Regulations (Title 21, Code of Federal Regulations, Part
58) for Nonclinical Laboratory Studies (GLPs) intended to assure the
quality and integrity of safety data collected on drugs, food
additives and medical devices. The GLPs which became effective on
June 20, 1979 apply to all laboratories involved in safety
assessment. The GLPs do not describe the "science" of safety
assessment nor do they mandate specific study plans or standard
operating procedures; rather, they stipulate those laboratory
practices and procedures essential to the proper collection and
documentation of safety data. Accordingly, they contain sections on
all features of toxicology laboratory operation - organization and
personnel, facilities, equipment, testing facilities operation, test
and control articles, protocol for a nonclinical laboratory study,
and records and reports. U.S. laboratories have made excellent
progress in adopting GLPs. In FY 1980 only 3 of 130 laboratories
inspected were seriously out of compliance. Generally, GLPs have
had a beneficial impact on toxicology testing. The quality of final
reports received by FDA has improved and the data provide a sound
basis for agency decision-making. Further, as results of FDA's
inspections show, both U.S. and foreign laboratories recognize that
GLPs provide sound guidance on the conduct of toxicology testing.

KEYWORDS

Toxicology; safety assessment; drugs; food additives; medical
devices; regulations for laboratories

INTRODUCTION

For the past several years, the U.S. Food and Drug Administration
(FDA) has operated a Toxicology Laboratory Monitoring Program which
is intended to ensure the quality and integrity of the safety data
submitted to FDA in support of the approval of regulated products.
This objective is achieved by regulations (Good Laboratory

Regulations, GLPs) (Anonoymous, 1978) setting forth the minimum
standards for quality toxicology testing and by laboratory
inspections made to determine whether the standards are being
achieved. The objective encompasses all products regulated by FDA
that require the submission of an application for use, including
human and animal drugs, feed and food additives, human biological
products and medical devices, color additives, and electronic
products that emit radiation. The complete range of toxicology
tests from in vitro mutagenicity tests to in vivo chronic toxicity
and carcinogenicity studies are covered. The objective includes
sponsor, contractor, university and government laboratories that
actually perform the toxicity test or that contribute data
supportive to a safety study.

Impetus for the institution of FDA's Toxicology Laboratory
Monitoring Program originated from a series of laboratory
inspections that were made by FDA during 1975. The inspections
examined toxicology data collected in testing facilities of both
major pharmaceutical firms and private contract laboratories. These
inspections revealed a variety of testing deficiencies that
undermined the quality of the study results. The major deficiencies
that were cited can be summarized as follows:

1. Experiments were poorly conceived, carelessly executed, or
inaccurately evaluated or reported.

2. Technical personnel were unaware of the importance of adherence
to protocols, accurate observations, proper administration of test
article, and accurate recordkeeping.

3. Management did not ensure critical review of data or proper
supervision of personnel.

4. Studies were impaired by protocol designs that did not allow the
evaluation of all available data.

5. Assurance could not be given that personnel involved in the
studies had suitable scientific qualifications and adequate
training.

6. There was evidence of improper laboratory procedures, animal
care, and data management.

7. Drug sponsors did not adequately monitor the studies performed
in whole or in part by contract testing laboratories.

8. Likewise, sponsors failed to verify the accuracy and
completeness of the final reports.

The seriousness of these findings coupled with the fundamental
importance of proper safety evaluation of regulated products
prompted several congressional hearings. As a consequence, in 1976
FDA was given new resources to implement a program to ensure that
the listed deficiencies did not recur.

PROGRAM MILESTONES

The Toxicology Laboratory Monitoring Program officially began when

FDA published proposed regulations on good laboratory practice
(Anonymous, 1976). Since that time, a number of significant
activities have occurred: Laboratory inspections were started
(December 1976); public hearings on the proposal were conducted
(February, 1977); the results of the first 40 laboratory inspections
were evaluated (October, 1977); an economic-impact assessment of the
proposed regulations was prepared (February, 1978); final
regulations were published (December, 1978); conferences on the
interpretation of the final regulations were held (May, 1978); final
regulations became effective (June, 1979); and a conference report
was published (August, 1979).

SCIENCE AND PROCESS

Understanding the GLPs requires making a distinction between the
"science" of toxicology and the "process" of toxicology testing.
The proper evaluation of product safety results from a mixture of
good science and adequate process. Science determines the study
objectives, the adequacy of the protocol in satisfying the
objectives, and the conclusions to be drawn from an established set
of data. The science of toxicology is in a state of flux, and
newer, more efficient test protocols are constantly being developed.
On the other hand, process determines suitable study conditions as
well as those laboratory features, practices and procedures that are
essential to valid data collection and study documentation.

Therefore, the GLPs do not address the "science" of toxicology; this
task is left to the expert toxicologists in industry, academia and
government. Rather the GLPs do address the "process" of toxicology
testing, since the testing deficiencies described earlier represent
failure in study process.

GLP CONCEPTS

Although the GLPs contain a number of specific provisions, five
general concepts encompass all operational aspects of the
regulations. These concepts can be labeled tools, rules,
characterization, documentation, and quality assurance.
Accordingly, a well-managed laboratory must provide the proper tools
for quality testing. The tools include personnel trained and given
sufficient time to do a good job and facilities and equipment that
can achieve their intended function and that are used in accord with
known instructions. Similarly, a laboratory must provide adequate
rules for study conduct. These include protocols and standard
operating procedures that are clear, well-written, and
understandable. Next, attention must be given to the procedures for
characterization of the test article. The identity of the test
article should be confirmed and the amount of test article
administered to the test system should be as specified in the
protocol. Also, good laboratories have sound procedures for study
documentation. Data are collected, recorded, stored, and reported
so that a third party can determine that the results presented in
the final report are fully documented in the study records.
Finally, and most importantly, laboratories should have a system of
quality assurance to verify that the entire experimental process
occurs as planned.

THE PRINCIPAL GLP PROVISIONS

The GLPs contain provisions that deal with laboratory personnel, facilities and equipment. Each laboratory should have a sufficient number of trained personnel to allow a study to be conducted as directed by the protocol. Documentation of personnel training should appear in the study records as summaries of training and experience and as discrete position descriptions. Employees having illness that can affect study results should be excluded from participation in the study. Facilities should be of suitable size and construction, and adequate space provided for separation of activities and functions that are capable of interferring with proper study conduct. The GLPs do not require dedicated space for each activity but space should be utilized in a manner that prevents mix-ups. Equipment should be designed and located to function in accord with the protocol and the standard operating procedures. The equipment should be maintained, cleaned, and calibrated to ensure proper use, and such operations should be described in the standard operating procedures.

The GLPs also contain provisions that address standard operating procedures and protocols. FDA is convinced that clearly written standard operating procedures are essential components of the data collection process. Although standard operating procedures should be written for most laboratory operations, the GLPs describe some twelve areas for which standard operating procedures are mandatory. These include animal care, laboratory tests, necropsy, histopathology and other methods of test system observation. Specific standard operating procedures should be readily available in the immediate work area and provision should be made for periodic updating. Changes in standard operating procedures are to be authorized in writing and deviations in actual practice from existing standard operating procedures are to be documented in the study records. The GLPs also require the preparation of a clearly written, complete protocol that is understood by study personnel. Each study should have a specific protocol that addresses items such as objectives, methods, experimental design, records and several other study characteristics. The laboratory should have a formal procedure by which the study director can amend the protocol.

The characterization and control of test articles are important study areas discussed in the GLPs. Test articles should be characterized before the study starts but test article stability can, if necessary, be determined concurrent with the conduct of the study. The characterization should be sufficient to permit the preparation of subsequent batches of test article similar enough to the initial batch to ensure valid testing. Test article containers should be properly labelled and reserve samples taken and stored for possible reanalysis. Use and distribution throughout the laboratory should be controlled and documented to afford an accurate accounting of actual use. Mixtures of test article with carriers, diluents, and animal feed should be tested at least once for homogeneity and periodically for concentration. Reserve samples of mixtures of test articles are not required.

The major processes associated with study conduct include data collection, recording, analysis, reporting and storage. Data should

be collected and recorded in accord with the protocol and the
standard operating procedures. Specimens derived from the test
system should be labeled with appropriate identifying information.
Once a measurement has been made, the data should be recorded
promptly, accurately, and legibly in ink. Data entries are to be
dated on the day of entry and signed by the person entering the
data. Reasons should be given for changes in data entries. The
person making the change should initial and date the changed entry.
Data evaluation should also be done in accord with the protocol and
standard operating procedures, and the final report should fully
describe the experimental findings and conclusions. The final
report should be signed by the study director and should contain the
signed and dated reports of other scientists contributing to the
study. It is not necessary to include all raw data in the final
report, but the storage location of the raw data should be given.
Changes in the final report are to be made in the form of dated
amendments, prepared by the study director, that clearly identify
the change and provide satisfactory reasons for it. At the
conclusion of the study, all records are to be kept in suitable
archives accessible only to authorized individuals.

Many of the GLP principles that have already been discussed
represent nothing more than common sense applied to toxicology
testing. Those principles represent actual practice in most
laboratories. The novel aspect of the GLPs is the application of a
quality assurance function that is distinct and organizationally
independent from the study conduct function. The Quality Assurance
Unit monitors each study to assure that facilities, equipment,
methods, practices, records and controls are as specified in the
GLPs. Specifically, the quality assurance unit should maintain a
master schedule sheet that describes all ongoing studies and their
current status. The purpose of the sheet is to identify those study
phases that are to be inspected by the quality assurance unit. The
results of the inspections are to be communicated periodically to
management and to the study director. Finally, the quality
assurance unit is to review the final report of each study to verify
that the report accurately reflects the data collected. The purpose
of the quality assurance unit is not to criticize the science of the
study but rather to verify the process that was used.

FDA'S LABORATORY INSPECTION PROGRAM

FDA estimates that some 550 laboratories throughout the world
conduct toxicity testing that falls under the GLPs. Of these, 400
are located within the United States. The agency attempts to
inspect each domestic laboratory at least once every two years and
each foreign laboratory at least once every five years. The kinds
of inspections made include a surveillance inspection of ongoing
practices and procedures and a data audit inspection which involves
checking a final report for conformity with the study data. About
half of the inspections are made by a team composed of an FDA field
investigator and a headquarters scientist. After the inspection a
report is prepared and forwarded to headquarters for review and
evaluation. The results of FDA inspections that were made in fiscal
year 1980 show that U.S. laboratories have made excellent progress
in adopting the GLPs. Of the 130 inspection reports that were

reviewed, 102 laboratories were classified as being essentially in compliance with the GLPs, 25 laboratories exhibited only minor variances, and 3 were found to be seriously out of compliance. For the out-of-compliance laboratories, significant problems were found in standard operating procedures, amending of data sheets, and protocol completeness and revision. These problems are quite minor compared to those found by FDA in 1975.

SUMMARY

The GLPs were intended to improve the quality and integrity of safety data collected on regulated products. FDA's experience shows that the GLPs have exerted a beneficial impact on toxicology testing. The quality of final study reports received by FDA continually improve and the resulting data provide a sound basis for agency decision making. The results of FDA inspections show that both U.S. and foreign laboratories have recognized that GLPs provide sound guidance on the conduct of toxicology testing.

REFERENCES

1. Anonymous (1976). Nonclinical Laboratory Studies, Proposed Regulations for Good Laboratory Practice. Federal Register, 41, 51206-51229.

2. Anonymous (1978). Nonclinical Laboratory Studies, Good Laboratory Practice Regulations. Federal Register, 43, 59986-60025.

Index